What Are My Chances?

What Are My Chances?

Ben Eiseman, M.D.

THE SAUNDERS PRESS

W. B. Saunders Company

Philadelphia • London • Toronto

THE SAUNDERS PRESS/SAUNDERS PAPERBACKS
W. B. Saunders Company
West Washington Square
Philadelphia, Pennsylvania 19105

IN THE UNITED STATES
DISTRIBUTED TO THE TRADE BY
HOLT, RINEHART AND WINSTON
383 Madison Avenue
New York, New York 10017

IN CANADA
DISTRIBUTED BY
HOLT, RINEHART AND WINSTON, Limited
55 Horner Avenue
Toronto, Ontario
M8Z 4X6 Canada

Library of Congress Cataloging in Publication Data

Eiseman, Ben
What are my chances?

1. Prognosis
2. Life expectancy
3. Medicine—Decision-making
4. Surgery—Decision-making

I. Title, [DNLM: 1. Prognosis—Popular works, WB142 E36w]
RC80.E37   616.07′5   79-67118

W.B. Saunders Company ISBN 0-7216-3344-7
Holt, Rinehart and Winston ISBN 0-03-056739-4

Print Number 9 8 7 6 5 4 3 2

First Edition

Designed and produced by Stanley S. Drate/Folio Graphics Co., Inc.

Contents

What Are My Chances?

I
Opening Chapters

1. Disease, Responsibility, and Risk in a No-Risk Society

For thousands of years, man lived in constant awareness of the intimacy of death. If he had children, he anticipated that one of four would die during childhood. Epidemics of little-understood diseases swept away many adults. Survivors could anticipate crippling disabilities from diseases such as poliomyelitis or tuberculosis, or disfigurement from infections such as smallpox.

In this century, life expectancy has almost doubled. In 1900, a newborn child had an average life span of about forty years. Now it is over seventy and climbing. In short, we are the first generation with a reasonable chance to live until we wear out rather than having our lives cut short by acute illness.

This startling change has attracted the attention of such diverse groups as social planners, nursing home proprietors, insurance actuaries, and of course, politicians. But one important aspect of this change has been largely overlooked. It is the effect such health security has had on man's attitude toward both his physician and disease. Whereas in 1900 man could only vainly hope for a long life, he now not only hopes for but demands it. When anything interferes with his good health, he feels cheated and wants to fix the blame on the person at fault.

The causes of this amazing change of attitude are several. For one, it reflects our remarkably short memory. The dangers of diseases which were so real thirty to forty years ago are now no more a threat than are the Black Plague or miasma.

Also, it reveals modern man's almost childish confidence in the power of science. In America, in particular, we feel that if sufficient personal resources and money are devoted to a problem, it can automatically be solved. If a president says we will land on the moon within a decade, the footprints are planted there in the dust as predicted. If a president asks for our dimes to conquer poliomyelitis, it is soon accomplished by the simple act of eating a block of sugar to which a few drops of liquid have been added. No disease can withstand knowledge, energy, and money—so goes the false but generally accepted premise.

Throughout the century we have stampeded toward a riskless society. Government, functioning as the corporate embodiment of society, has responded to the wishes of its constituents. Thus it set out to protect the poor from starvation and providing security for those not able to fend for themselves—the very young, the very old, the insane, the mentally and physically handicapped. Once the list begins, its growth becomes difficult to stop: the educationally handicapped, minorities, those with end-stage renal disease, whales, porpoises. They all deserve and have received protection. And where government has not provided total protection, private insurance companies have been created to supplement the effort.

Such protection and the resulting near-riskless existence has been the source of much debate by both political liberals and conservatives. Regardless of the merits of minimizing risk, much of our world now lives in a society dedicated to that principle. The effect of man's attitude toward the risk of disease is predictable, for disease has always been one of the first risks against which man has wanted protection. Good health is now considered a basic right guaranteed by God (or, at least, government). Like clean water and electricity, health and health care is a public utility, and those who dispense it can line up behind our colleagues who administer other public services. Those once called physicians now are often called "health-care dispensers."

The medical profession itself must bear responsibility for another influence in the change in attitude of patients toward illness. We have over-sold our product and created an image of ourselves far more effective than reality. With the subtle goadings of the news media, who make good copy of "doctor stories," physicians have assumed an aura of omnipotence. At the slightest scientific provocation, a physician can be found who will predict startling breakthroughs lurking just beyond the horizon. These phantoms always seem to remain hull down with only a wisp of smoke promising their actual existence.

Such publicity is obviously highly flattering to the physicians, but as happens with any inaccuracy after the truth is known, it takes its toll. The public, eager for good news even if it isn't the truth, has developed a false image of the powers of physicians in controlling disease. Thus when a member of one's family is stricken by disease, shock and letdown follow. As a result the "consumers" (as government health-care planners now call patients) become frustrated with their assigned health-care providers (i.e., the doctors).

The relationship now resembles that of the owner of an old and battered automobile who takes his car to a garage mechanic. The mechanic is expected to identify the problem immediately, correct the trouble, and have the machine operating as good as new by Tuesday morning (early). Once an agreement has been reached as to a usual and reasonable fee for the job, responsibility for the problem is shifted entirely from the car's owner to the mechanic. Anything that complicates perfect performance thereafter is considered to be due to poor service.

An entire segment of the legal profession is earning a living from the development of a similar attitude between patient and physician.

Most physicians foolishly have gone along with this unrealistic image. We have been reluctant to admit our fallibility. We have also failed to emphasize to patients their own responsibility for their disease.

Parents of teenagers soon learn the consequences of assuming their children's responsibility to work out problems. If the parents unwisely take on the child's burden, the child is, of course, only too willing to unload it. The wise parent provides sympathy and support but makes it clear that adults solve their own problems. Likewise, just because people are sick does not mean they automatically should be deprived of the opportunity to make decisions.

Many physicians feel it is their professional duty to make all decisions for their patients. They emphasize that the subtleties of clinical medicine are so complex that it is unfair to ask a patient to share the responsibility. In some parts of the world this is the customarily accepted doctor-patient relationship. But in America, the patient usually wants some part in plotting the course of his treatment. He wants to be kept informed and to share authority in determining his fate.

The exact proportions in which the physician and patient decide to share responsibility inevitably vary with every patient's doctor and every disease. But regardless of the proportion, both persons should begin with the same perception of the problem. This means that both should understand the implications of prognosis, or prediction of what may happen next, which is best expressed by numerical probabilities. It is to provide such data for a number of common situations that this book is designed.

It would be presumptuous to suppose that availability of prognostic data will automatically change the sense of risk and responsibility for disease by patients reared in essentially a no-risk society. But with the data easily available, there can at least be no excuse for patients remaining ignorant of their odds. They can find out for themselves what their chances are.

2. Probabilities, Or How to Use This Book

An intelligent person who is told by a physician that he has an illness wants to know what the diagnosis implies. What will it mean to his future? Will he get well, and if so, how soon and with what disability? What, in short, are his chances? Although few people think of it in these terms, they want to be informed about probabilities. Probabilities of symptoms progressing or going away spontaneously; likelihood of requiring an operation and the chances of cure; complication—or not surviving. Although all such questions are seldom fully expressed, they usually go through a patient's mind. Following the shock of being told one has a serious disease, and trying to cope with the stress of being in the doctor's office or in the hospital, a patient frequently forgets (or is reluctant because of fear) to ask the very questions which have such an important bearing on the many plans he may then have to make.

This book is intended to give the patient and his family answers to some of these questions in a simple, readable form that can be studied at home after a diagnosis has been made by a physician. The more a patient understands about the anticipated future course (prognosis) of his illness, the better equipped he will be to make the many decisions in his private life that may be necessary.

Use it, if you will, as the handicapper's manual of disease. It quotes past performance of illness in the same way as a racetrack program shows the records of the horse and jockey, helping a person to decide how to bet.

Many ordinarily meticulous people are remarkably casual when it comes to decisions concerning their health. Those who would never risk a business deal on chance accept foolish guidance from uninformed strangers at cocktail parties when it comes to medical matters. Men glory in analyzing statistics concerning automobiles, race horses, and municipal bonds; women do the same before buying washing machines. Yet both often shun the equivalent hard data that affect good health and illness.

The reason for this anachronistic behavior by usually rational people is not difficult to understand. Faced with serious illness, we are all cowards. We hear what we want to hear and filter out what conflicts with our hopes. Given a little time, we can find some well-meaning but equally uninformed "authority" to reinforce our bias.

Another explanation is the suddenness with which an illness presents itself. People before the age of about sixty have a vague sense of immortality. Illness and its consequences are for someone else, and the ravages of old age are a long way off. Consider, for example, how few people have even made a will. When illness strikes, a person is often emotionally unprepared and cannot quickly adapt to the logical process of decision-making that characterizes ones usual thought patterns.

Because this book primarily involves numbers that help predict the usual course of a disease, it is important to indicate their source. Each is a compilation of data published in reputable medical and surgical journals. In *Prognosis of Surgical Disease* (W. B. Saunders Company, 1980), a book written for physicians by the present author, the actual references are annotated.

Development of reliable data of this kind is relatively recent and represents an important part of the advancement of medicine into the dignity of an applied science. In the early days, a physician predicted the outcome of illness almost solely on the basis of his own experience. Adding to this the teachings of an older physician, the data base might be doubled. But recollections of one's own experience are notoriously inaccurate, be it of one's athletic prowess in high school or the course of illness of a patient under one's care. We tend to remember triumphs and forget failures.

Although medical literature is designed to help physicians profit from the experience of their predecessors, it was largely anecdotal until a few years ago. Prestigious physicians thundered in print, "This is what I believe and therefore this is how I do it," without providing adequate evidence to confirm their prejudices. Case reports were predictably brilliant successes. Failures, like military defeats, found few historians.

But during the past fifty years, scientific medicine has demanded sound evidence before undertaking treatment. This has assumed particular importance with the discovery of new drugs and operations having great potential for doing either good or harm. The computer is, of course, ideally suited for recording and analyzing such data, which now forms the basis for accurately predicting the prognosis of many diseases.

The reader of this book is assumed to be familiar with the concept of probability, a term increasingly common in Western life. Daily we learn on television the probability of rain or snow, expressed as a percent. People understand that when a probability of rain is 75%, or even 95%, rain is not an absolute guarantee. Sports, and particularly baseball, has become the great popularizer of statistics. Sports fans think in percentages as they scan the won-and-lost column or the frequency that a quarterback completed a pass or was sacked. When it comes to a much more serious game—health—most people are comfortable with transferring these thought patterns to the probability of cure, recovery, mortalities, or expected length of survival.

A caveat, or word of warning, should be made concerning the interpretation of medical "fact" and statistics, including the ones in this book. People are not inbred mice; they differ. The average height of American males might be stated as being five feet 10 inches. But every child cannot anticipate growing to exactly that size. Some will be five feet, and a few seven feet tall. Similarly, if a person with a given type of tumor finds in this book that the quoted probability for him to live five years is only 20%, he should realize that he may very well outlive the prediction by many years. By analogy, he may be the seven footer, not merely five feet, ten inches.

There will be those who will protest that they do not want to become involved with the gloomy possibilities of their illness or the probability of complications in an anticipated operation. They will say they leave all this to their physician, in whom they have complete confidence. This is fair enough and an accepted way for a person to shift responsibility from his own shoulders to another's. But physicians have to base their opinions on analyses of probabilities, and an increasing number of patients are becoming interested in sharing in the decision-making process that is so vital to their own future. The necessity of informed consent before an operation is the prime example of this trend.

But apart from the legal aspects of the problem, most patients want to know something of the anticipated course of their disease. If nothing else, they want to know the probability of cure and the likelihood of whether a prescribed medication or operation will cure or benefit the condition.

In diagram form, these thought processes might look like the diagram that follows, which is what we know as a decision tree:

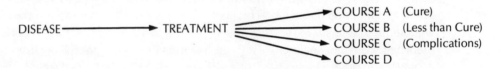

Having thought through the possibilities, the intelligent patient then wants to know the probabilities. In decision-tree form, this is:

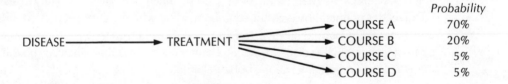

When the physician and patient have provided the leaves on the bare branches of the decision tree by understanding both the expected quality and duration of life with each option, they will be in a good position to choose the course that will give them the best chance of benefit with the least risk. As in poker, if they know the odds (probabilities) they will have a far better chance of winning than a beginner who relies on intuition and luck. The poker expert, for example, knows the following probabilities if he draws three cards to a pair:

	Probability
No improvement	60%
Getting 2 pair	20%
Getting 3 of a kind	12.5%
Getting 4 of a kind	2.7%

Graphically this would look like:

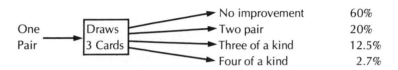

No improvement	60%
Two pair	20%
Three of a kind	12.5%
Four of a kind	2.7%

These probabilities form the basis of decision, but the decision itself must be determined by what sort of risk the player wants to take. The expert knows that only a fool relies on drawing one card to an inside straight (probability of benefit, 9%, or one chance in eleven). The sad fact is that many who would never take such a silly risk in a poker game, when all that can be lost is money, will blithely accept those stakes in a much more serious game involving life.

It must be emphasized that this is not a textbook of medicine from which a patient might, without the help of a physician, "doctor" himself and make clinical decisions about treatment or predict with accuracy how long he is going to live. When our automobile sputters we ask the opinion of a good mechanic, and after preliminary sparring and an uneducated look under the hood, we usually take his advice about having the oil filter changed or buying a new set of spark plugs. So, too, should the fifty-five-year-old, long-time smoker, when he begins to spit up blood, visit a knowledgeable physician before he decides he has lung cancer and is doomed. He needs his physician to interpret his symptoms and signs and make appropriate diagnostic tests. He may have nothing more than a simple cold, in which the probability of spontaneous cure within days is 100%.

Such a warning would seem unnecessary, but knowing the tendency of people for self-diagnosis, even this disclaimer may not stop the enthusiast from using this book as a do-it-yourself medical textbook—which it certainly is not.

3. An Explanation of Terms

Although every effort has been made to avoid using highly technical terms, certain words in this book may be unfamiliar to some readers. To avoid confusion, a few definitions follow.

PROGNOSIS: Prognosis means the anticipated future progression of a disease. It is the answer to the important question, "What are my chances?" The prognosis of a given disease is reached by determining the usual course of a similar disease in many other people. At best, it records in numerical form the characteristic or predictive course.

COHORT: Cohort, as used in this book, refers to a group of people matched as closely as possible by age, sex, race, etc., to a person, except that the members of the cohort do *not* have the disease under consideration. In some cases, such as in the discussion concerning smoking, the cohort is matched as a "control," e.g., a non-smoking person or group. The cohort is the standard by which a patient's prognosis is compared.

SURVIVAL: Survival means that the patient is alive. It is more accurate to speak of a survival rate than it is to speak of a cure. Because a patient with a tumor is alive (surviving) a year after an operation does not mean he or she is cured, since the tumor may recur two, five, or even ten years later.

Because most tumors recur within two–four years, physicians usually refer to the probability of survival at five years (the five-year survival rate) as the means of comparing methods of treating most diseases. For example, the five-year survival rate for a given tumor, left untreated, might be only 10%, whereas if operated upon and removed, the survival rate might be 70%—a 60% improvement.

MORTALITY RATE: Mortality rate, or death rate, means the probability of dying of a disease or operation. When used in reference to an operation, it usually refers to the chances of dying anytime during the period of hospitalization in which the operation is performed. The likelihood of dying during the operation itself is usually very low (less than 1% for most elective operations). A mortality rate of 15% for a very serious operation would mean that of a hundred patients undergoing the procedure, fifteen would not leave the hospital alive. Of these, perhaps one might die in the operating room, five of a heart attack during the days or weeks following the operation, two of a stroke, three of kidney failure, and four of the progress of the disease.

In considering mortality in older people, it is well to remember that the mortality rate of merely being eighty years of age, even without an acute illness, is about 1% per month.

COMPLICATIONS: The single word "complications" is used to describe a variety of events that might mar an otherwise smooth clinical course. Complications that are frequent, unique, or particularly serious are specifically described.

RADIATION: The benefit of x-radiation in the treatment of many tumors is well known to most readers. But X rays can be delivered to tumors in a variety of ways—using different sources for the X rays, varying the dosage, and changing the time schedule in which treatments are given. Even though these details of X ray therapy may alter tumor response, no attempt is made in this book to describe the intricacies of treatment. Commonly accepted means of X ray treatment are considered typical.

CHEMOTHERAPY: Chemotherapy means the treatment of a disease with a drug. In this book, the word refers only to the drug treatment of tumors. There are many types of anti-cancer drugs that can be used alone or in combinations and although change in drug regime alters tumor response, the differences are usually slight. As with radio-therapy, only the usual or characteristic response after treatment with commonly used drugs is cited.

SYMBOLS: Several shorthand symbols have been used in the text:
$<$ = less than
$>$ = more than
$\pm$ = plus/minus, used before a number to indicate that the number quoted is an approximation

This book is not light reading, but serious illness should not be taken lightly. Some readers will take exception to the pessimistic nature of some of the statistics and accompanying text. The numbers, however, accurately reflect the unpleasant prognosis of many serious diseases. They also indicate that major operations and other forms of treatment are themselves often perilous.

Apology may be more in order for an occasional tone in the text that some readers might find depressing. The prognosis of a grave illness can be described as providing a 20% chance that the patient will be alive in five years. On the other hand, it could be said that there is an 80% chance the patient will be dead. A glass of water can be described as half empty or half full.

An Explanation of Terms

Since many of the readers of this book will themselves be patients seeking reference for their own disease, the text tends to emphasize the positive. In fact, numbers speak for themselves, and patients will interpret them according to their own philosophies. In my own experience, most patients and their families are better served by facing facts. Fantasies, future hopes, and fabrications, under whatever sobriquet, become doubly cruel when the unpleasant truth inevitably becomes evident. I might add, however, that many respected colleagues disagree with the philosophy of this approach.

This book, filled with data predicting the probabilities of cures and complications of disease, will be launched into an increasingly litigious society. There may be surprise at the high incidence of failure and complication associated with many accepted forms of treatment. In the current state of the art, however, the patient with a serious illness must accept the fact that any treatment involves risk.

II
Your Chances

1. Life Expectancy

Age	Male	Female	Age	Male	Female	Age	Male	Female
0	68.7	76.5	28	43.6	50.4	56	19.5	25.0
1	68.9	76.6	29	42.6	49.5	57	18.8	24.2
2	68.0	75.6	30	41.7	48.5	58	18.1	23.4
3	67.0	74.7	31	40.8	47.5	59	17.4	22.6
4	66.1	73.7	32	39.9	46.6	60	16.8	21.8
5	65.1	72.8	33	39.0	45.6	61	16.1	21.0
6	64.2	71.8	34	38.1	44.7	62	15.5	20.2
7	63.2	70.8	35	37.1	43.7	63	14.9	19.5
8	62.2	69.8	36	36.2	42.8	64	14.3	18.7
9	61.2	58.9	37	35.3	41.8	65	13.7	18.0
10	60.3	67.9	38	34.4	40.9	66	13.1	17.3
11	59.3	56.9	39	33.5	40.0	67	12.5	16.5
12	58.3	55.9	40	32.6	39.0	68	12.0	15.8
13	57.3	64.9	41	31.7	38.1	69	11.4	15.1
14	56.3	53.9	42	30.8	37.2	70	10.9	14.4
15	55.4	63.0	43	30.0	36.3	71	10.4	13.7
16	54.4	62.0	44	29.1	35.4	72	9.9	13.1
17	53.5	61.0	45	28.3	34.5	73	9.5	12.5
18	52.6	60.1	46	27.4	33.6	74	9.0	11.9
19	51.7	59.1	47	26.6	32.7	75	8.6	11.3
20	50.8	58.1	48	25.7	31.8	76	8.2	10.7
21	49.9	57.2	49	24.9	30.9	77	7.8	10.2
22	49.0	56.2	50	24.1	30.1	78	7.5	9.7
23	48.1	55.2	51	23.3	29.2	79	7.1	9.2
24	47.2	54.3	52	22.5	28.3	80	6.8	8.7
25	46.3	53.3	53	21.8	27.5	81	6.5	8.3
26	45.4	52.3	54	21.0	26.6	82	6.2	7.9
27	44.5	51.4	55	20.3	25.8	83	6.0	7.4
						84	5.7	7.1
						85	5.4	6.7

2. Risks in Everyday Living

AUTOMOBILE (Yearly risk)

One in 20 (5%) chance of accident

One in 83 (1.3%) chance of accident in which someone is injured

One in 3,570 chance of accident in which someone is killed

One death per 296,000 vehicle miles

URBAN BUS AND TAXIS

One death per 769,000 miles

TRAIN

One death per 2,000,000,000 passenger miles

DOMESTIC U.S. COMMERCIAL AIRLINES

One death per 2,400,000,000 passenger miles

PRIVATE FLYING

One death per 9,000 flying hours, or about 1,350,000 miles

One non-fatal injury per 20,000 flying hours, or about 3,000,000 miles

(Data from National Transportation Safety Board)

CHANCE OF DEATH IN HAZARDOUS SPORTS

(Approximated by dividing *estimated* number of participants in the sports by the reported deaths from that sport)

Sport	Chances of Death per Year Per Participant
Airplane racing (closed course)	45
Bicycle racing	10,600
Boxing	7,000
Football:	
Sandlot	1,000,000
High school	100,000
College	20,000
Professional	1,500
Gliding (soaring)	2,500
(One per 25,000 hours of gliding)	
Hang gliding	428
Hot-air ballooning	250
Mountaineering	2,000
Parachuting	714
Scuba Diving	18,000

(Data from Accident Facts-National Safety Council 1978)

PROBABILITY OF INJURY*PER SEASON IN VARIOUS SPORTS

Sport	Probability (%) of Injury Each Season
Wrestling	29.6
Football (fall)	24.0
Ice hockey	21.3
Basketball	16.7
Volleyball	16.7
Tennis	12.5
Soccer	12.2
Football (spring)	10.5
Cross country	9.7
Gymnastics	9.4
Lacrosse	9.1
Indoor track and field	8.9
Outdoor track and field	8.3
Baseball	6.8
Swimming and diving	2.2

(Data from National Injury/Illness Reporting System, 1978)

*Injury defined as that which keeps the athlete out of participation one week or any dental injury.

3. Smoking

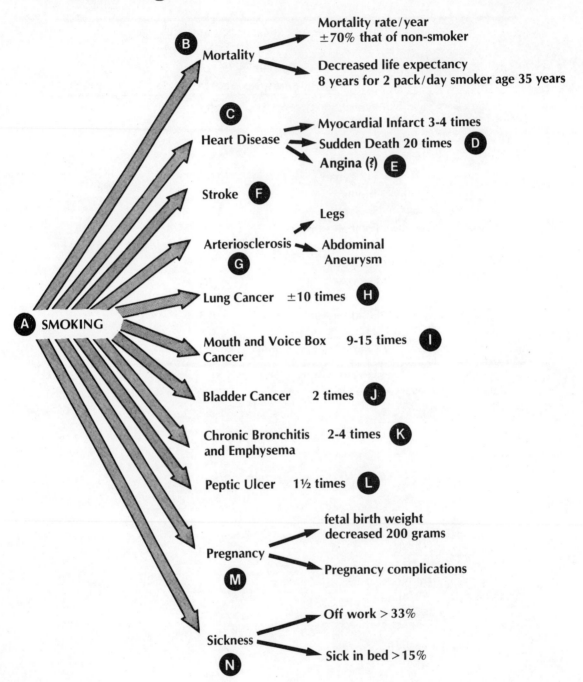

SMOKING

Mortality (B)
- Mortality rate/year ±70% that of non-smoker
- Decreased life expectancy 8 years for 2 pack/day smoker age 35 years

Heart Disease (C)
- Myocardial Infarct 3-4 times
- Sudden Death 20 times (D)
- Angina (?) (E)

Stroke (F)

Arteriosclerosis (G)
- Legs
- Abdominal Aneurysm

Lung Cancer ±10 times (H)

Mouth and Voice Box Cancer 9-15 times (I)

Bladder Cancer 2 times (J)

Chronic Bronchitis and Emphysema 2-4 times (K)

Peptic Ulcer 1½ times (L)

Pregnancy (M)
- fetal birth weight decreased 200 grams
- Pregnancy complications

Sickness (N)
- Off work > 33%
- Sick in bed > 15%

A Smoking affects life expectancy, amount of sickness, and chances of developing many diseases. For example, 280 people in the U.S. die every day from lung cancer, which is usually related to smoking. This is equivalent to deaths caused by the daily crash of a large passenger plane carrying smokers only. The risk is dose-related; the more cigarettes smoked each day, and the longer one smokes, the greater the risk. The discontinuation of smoking does not remove the accumulated past risk, but definitely reduces it. Men are slightly more at risk than women, but that difference is small. Cigar and pipe smoking offers slightly less risk. Smoking always involves "inhaling" to some degree. Low-tar cigarettes and filters decrease the risk, but do not eliminate it.

B Each year that a person continues to smoke, his chances of dying are 70% greater than those of a non-smoker of the same age (called by statisticians a cohort). For example, if at a given age in any one year ten non-smokers would be expected to die, seventeen smokers would also be expected to die. This is called the mortality ratio of smokers (death rate of smokers/death rate of non-smokers).

The relationship to the number of cigarettes is as follows:

EFFECT OF SMOKING ON MORTALITY RATE

| | AGE | | |
Cigarettes per day	30–34 years	35–44 years	45–54 years
None	100	100	100
10		144	144
10–20	127	179	164
21–39	176	223*	210
Over 40	233	272	213

(The higher the mortality rate the greater is the probability of dying in that year)

*For example, a thirty-five-year-old, twenty-five-cigarette-per-day smoker has almost two and one-fourth times greater chance of dying (223) in a given year than his non-smoking cohort. (If 100 cohorts will die, 223 smokers can be expected to die.)

Smoking decreases life expectancy as follows:

YEARS OF LIFE EXPECTANCY LOST BY SMOKING

Cigarettes per day	AGE		
	30 years	*40 years*	*50 years*
None	0	0	0
1–9	4.6	4.3	3.8
10–19	5.5	5.2	4.6
20–39	6.1*	5.5	5.1
Over 40	8.1	7.6	6.3

---

*This means that a thirty-five-year-old, twenty-five-cigarette-per-day smoker is cutting off an expected 6.1 years from his life expectancy.

Death in smokers is due most frequently to 1) heart disease, 2) lung cancer, and 3) chronic lung disease (emphysema).

C Smoking increases the chances of developing narrowing of the arteries (arteriosclerosis) in the heart (coronary arteries). Smokers have about three to four times the risk of dying of heart disease than do non-smokers. In those smoking thirty-five or more cigarettes per day, the risk is about ten times greater. Those who survive a heart attack and continue to smoke have double the risk of another attack.

D Sudden death is the first sign of heart disease in 20% of patients with coronary artery disease. This risk of sudden death is twenty times more frequent in smokers. Smokers of over twenty cigarettes per day have a three and one-third times greater chance of having a heart attack than do non-smokers.

E There is no certain evidence that smoking increases the chances of developing angina (pain over the heart with exercise). But patients who already have angina almost always notice that they develop pain more quickly if they continue smoking. Their tolerance to exercise is decreased.

F Although smoking does not seem to increase the risk of stroke, women who take oral contraceptives and smoke are twenty-two times more likely to have bleeding around the brain (subarachnoid hemorrhage) than are their matched cohorts taking the "pill" who do not smoke. Smoking seems to increase this risk from oral contraceptives.

G About 90% of those whose arteries to the legs are so narrowed that they have pain on walking are smokers. When operation for arteriosclerosis of the legs is necessary those who continue to smoke are 3 times more likely to clot off the arterial graft than are non-smokers. Many vascular surgeons will not operate on a patient who will not promise to quit smoking after the operation. The chance of developing an aneurysm of the aorta is five times greater in one-pack-a-day smokers and eight times greater in two-pack-a-day smokers than is the risk in non-smokers.

H There is overwhelming evidence that lung cancer is associated with smoking. Only 8–10% of lung cancers are curable. Twice as many people die of lung cancer every day than die in automobile accidents. Cigarette smokers are about ten times more likely to develop lung cancer than are non-smokers. This risk is increased to twenty times in two-pack-per-day smokers. The longer one smokes, the greater the risk. Starting to smoke during the teens increases the length of exposure (since few persons ever totally stop smoking) and therefore increases the likelihood of developing and dying at an early age of such a lung cancer. Women are possibly slightly less at risk, but not by much. Lung cancer kills more women than does cancer of the uterus.

I Cancer of the larynx is fifteen times more frequent in men smokers and nine times more common in women smokers than in their cohort non-smokers. The combination of smoking and alcohol is particularly likely to be associated with this type of cancer and cancer within the mouth.

J Smoking about doubles the risk of developing bladder cancer, probably because some of the chemicals in tobacco are passed out in the urine.

K Smoking destroys lung tissue. This can be proven with accurate measurement of lung function (and by athletes who smoke and get out of breath more quickly). It increases the risk of chronic bronchitis and emphysema by two and one-half times in one-pack-per-day smokers and four times in two-pack-per-day smokers. Emphysema is a disease that blocks the expulsion of air from the lung during expiration. It causes shortness of breath and infection in the lung, and is the third most common cause of death in smokers.

L A smoker has a half again (1.5) greater chance of developing a duodenal or gastric ulcer than does a non-smoking cohort.

M Infants born to women who smoke during pregnancy are an average of 200 grams smaller than those born to women who do not smoke. There is also an increased chance of complication during the pregnancy and delivery. This risk is almost abolished if the woman totally stops smoking during pregnancy, even if she smoked previously.

N Smokers get sick more often than non-smokers. Compared to non-smokers of the same sex loss of time from the job is 33% greater in men smokers and 43% greater in women smokers. Smokers average about 15% more bed-confining illness than do non-smokers.

4. Obesity

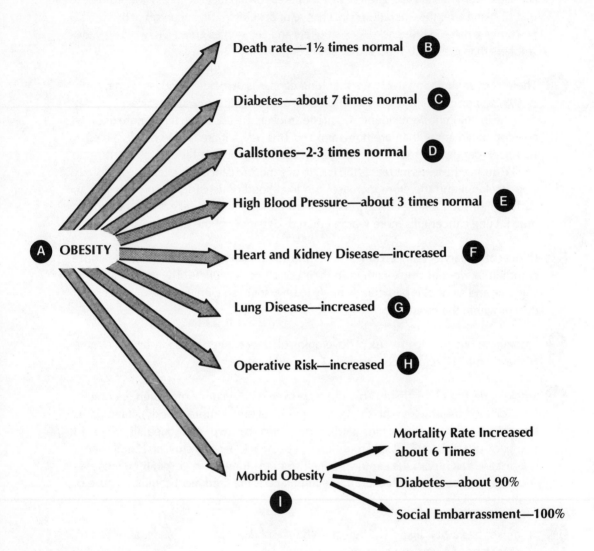

A OBESITY

Death rate—1½ times normal B

Diabetes—about 7 times normal C

Gallstones—2-3 times normal D

High Blood Pressure—about 3 times normal E

Heart and Kidney Disease—increased F

Lung Disease—increased G

Operative Risk—increased H

Morbid Obesity I

Mortality Rate Increased about 6 Times

Diabetes—about 90%

Social Embarrassment—100%

A People who are excessively fat are said to be obese. Obesity is usually measured as the percent of the patient's weight above the ideal weight. For example, if a person weighed 182 pounds (82.5 kilograms), but should weight 165 pounds (75 kilograms), he would be 17 pounds (7.5 kilograms), or 10% overweight. Obesity is a serious threat to good health, decreasing life expectancy and increasing the chance of developing many serious diseases.

B Life expectancy for those who are more than 15% overweight is reduced in direct proportion to the degree of obesity.

INCREASED MORTALITY AS RELATED TO OBESITY*

% Overweight	Increased Chance of Dying During any Given Year
15–20%	10%
25–35%	30%
Greater than 35%	50%
100%	600%

*The increased likelihood of an obese person dying compared to a person of normal weight dying during a given year. Thus a person who is 25% overweight has a 30% greater chance of dying during any year than a cohort of normal weight.

The effect of obesity (100 pounds overweight) on life expectancy is approximately as follows:

Years of Age	Percent Decrease in Life Expectancy	
	Men	Women
20–29	80	34
30–39	69	52
40–49	52	50
50–64	31	38
All ages		
20–64	50	47

This shows that obesity in the young is a more serious threat to life than in the elderly.

A fifty-year-old man whose suitable weight is 179 pounds (77 kilograms) can expect to live 24 more years. If he is 100 pounds (45 kilograms) overweight his expectancy is decreased by 31% to only 17 more years. For those overweight more than 30%, the increased probability of dying of complications of obesity is:

	INCREASED RISK OF AN OBESE PERSON DYING OF COMPLICATIONS OF OBESITY	
	Men	*Women*
Diabetes	3.83	3.72
Gallbladder disease	2.08	2.83*
Cardiovascular (heart disease)	1.49	1.77

*For example, an obese woman has between two and three times the likelihood (actually 2.83) of dying of gallstones than if she were of normal weight.

C The risk of diabetes is increased about seven times in the obese. The greater the obesity, the higher the risk. Losing weight decreases insulin requirements.

D The obese have an accumulative risk of developing gallstones far out of proportion to their non-obese cohorts. Overall, the risk is about twice normal. Correlated with age, the probability is:

Years of Age	*Risk of Gallstones*
55	2½ times normal
45–54	3 times normal
35–44	3 times normal

E About 30% of obese people (those whose body weight is 25% above normal) have high blood pressure.

G Increased weight interferes with normal breathing in many ways. Abdominal fat compresses the lungs, thereby increasing the work of breathing and for some reason, the very obese have changes in their brain that decrease the rate at which they breathe.

H Obesity adds many serious risks to a patient who must undergo anesthesia and an operation, the greatest being an increased likelihood of pneumonia or collapse of the lung. Such patients also have an increased risk of developing wound infections and blood clots in the veins of the legs (thromophlebitis, Chapter VI).

I People who are twice what their normal or ideal weight should be are said to be "morbidly obese." Their excess body fat is literally life-threatening. The risks in the morbidly obese are approximately:

Life expectancy decreased by	±10 years
Hypertension increased risk	10%
Diabetes increased	90%
Social embarrassment is universal	

Emotional factors usually contribute to obesity of this degree.

5. *Alcoholism*

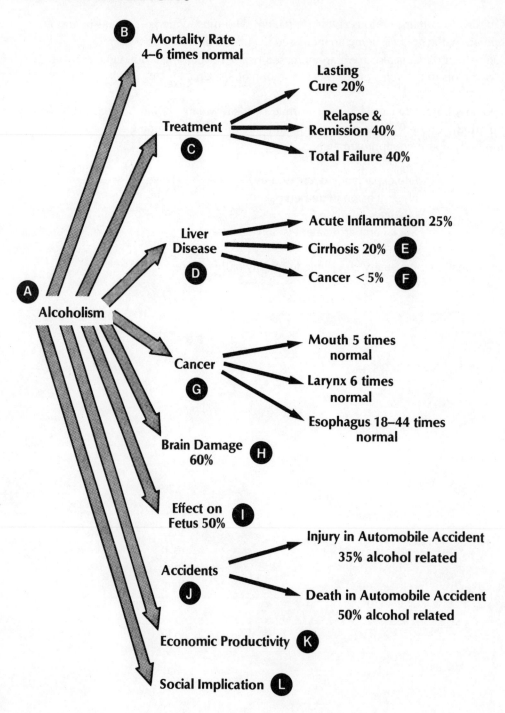

B Mortality Rate
4–6 times normal

Treatment C
- Lasting Cure 20%
- Relapse & Remission 40%
- Total Failure 40%

Liver Disease D
- Acute Inflammation 25%
- Cirrhosis 20% E
- Cancer < 5% F

A Alcoholism

Cancer G
- Mouth 5 times normal
- Larynx 6 times normal
- Esophagus 18–44 times normal

Brain Damage 60% H

Effect on Fetus 50% I

Accidents J
- Injury in Automobile Accident 35% alcohol related
- Death in Automobile Accident 50% alcohol related

Economic Productivity K

Social Implication L

A Although sociologists and moralists may argue about when a social drinker becomes an alcoholic, from the medical and physiologic point of view it occurs when a person drinks 50–80 grams of alcohol *every day*. Fifty grams per day is the more commonly accepted figure. This is the equivalent of three whiskeys or mixed drinks, five beers, or one-third of a pint of 80-proof whiskey. These figures are based on 1½ ounces (45 milliliters) of whiskey per drink of 80-proof (40%) alcohol. This equals about 15 grams of alcohol per drink. Drinks mixed at home are often stronger. The usual bottle or can of beer is 12 ounces (360 milliliters) and is about 4% alcohol. This contains about 12 grams of alcohol. There are about nine million such alcoholics in the United States. About 35% of the adults who drink are either actual or potential problem drinkers.

B An alcoholic has about four times the probability of dying in any one year than does a non-drinker of the same age, sex, and similar social and economic condition. This risk is dose-related: two times for social drinkers, four times for spree drinkers, and about six times for the established chronic alcoholic.

Frequent causes of death of the alcoholic are accidents, homocide, suicide, liver disease in the young and middle-aged, and alcohol-related cancers in older drinkers.

C Despite treatment, the chances for total and permanent cure of an alcoholic are only about 20%. Another 40% will periodically stop, but will have relapse when they drink again. A final 40% will never respond to treatment and continue drinking.

D Alcohol damages the liver. About 25% of chronic alcoholics will suffer at least one attack of severe inflammation of the liver (acute alcoholic hepatitis), which usually requires hospitalization and results in at least temporary yellow color to the skin (jaundice). For this type of hospitalized alcoholic, the mortality rate for the acute episode is about 10%.

E For reasons that are not clear, only about 20% of chronic alcoholics develop the liver condition called cirrhosis. Why the other 80% who drink just as much do not develop cirrhosis is not known. It is not fully explained by diet, vitamins, or the type of alcoholic beverage used. Cirrhosis may result in liver failure, ascites (fluid in the abdomen), and bleeding from the lower end of the esophagus. It is the fourth most common cause of death in adult males in the United States.

F The probability that even a confirmed alcoholic will develop liver cancer is less than 5%, but 70% of those with liver cancer are alcoholics with cirrhosis, confirming a definite relationship between alcoholism and this highly lethal (99%) tumor.

(G) Alcoholics are particularly liable to develop cancers of the mouth, upper airway, and upper intestinal tract. The increased probability of certain cancers in alcoholics compared to non-alcoholics is dose-related to the amount of alcohol consumed:

- Mouth and tongue: about five times
- Larynx (voice box): about six times
- Lung: two times
- Esophagus: eighteen times as frequent. If an alcoholic also smokes, the risk of esophageal cancer is increased to forty-four times that of a non-smoking, non-drinking cohort.

(H) Chronic alcoholics suffer brain damage even before they have evidence of liver disease. About 60% have intellectual impairment, and about half will show actual atrophy (withering) of brain tissue that can be recorded by special X-ray studies (CAT Scan).

(I) Children born to chronic alcoholic women who continue to drink 4–5 drinks per day during the first six months of pregnancy have about a 50% chance of suffering from a condition known as the *fetal alcohol syndrome*. This probability is dose related and may run as high as 90% with even heavier drinkers. Such children have mental retardation, birth defects, abnormal (jittery) behavior after birth, and do not grow normally.

(J) Alcoholics are accident-prone, creating a danger when you consider that one of every fifty automobile drivers is under the influence of alcohol at any given time. This does not necessarily mean that he is either drunk or an alcoholic, but judgment, vision, and response time are affected. One-third of all non-fatal and one-half of all fatal accidents are alcohol related.
   The probability of alcohol involvement in other accidents is:

- Fatal Burns: about 30%
- Drowning: about 20%
- Fatal falls: about 45%
- Homocide victim: 50%
- Industrial accident: about 30%
- Suicide: about 15%

(K) Although most alcoholics are economically independent, probably they lose productivity earlier than non-drinkers and, as a group, earn $2,000 a year less than non-alcoholics of the same background.

L The social risk of alcoholism is difficult to compute. The chance of a broken home, marital unhappiness and finally divorce is apparently increased. Quoted figures vary from "no change" to "ten times the frequency of divorce than non-alcoholics."
Association of various crimes with alcohol are:

- Assault: 60% of offenders
- Homocide: 30–80% offender
         50% victim
- Rape offender: 10–70%
- Robbery offender: 10–70%

(Source: "Alcohol and Health-3rd. Special Report to U.S. Congress," Department of Health, Education and Welfare, 1978)

6. Sexual Intercourse

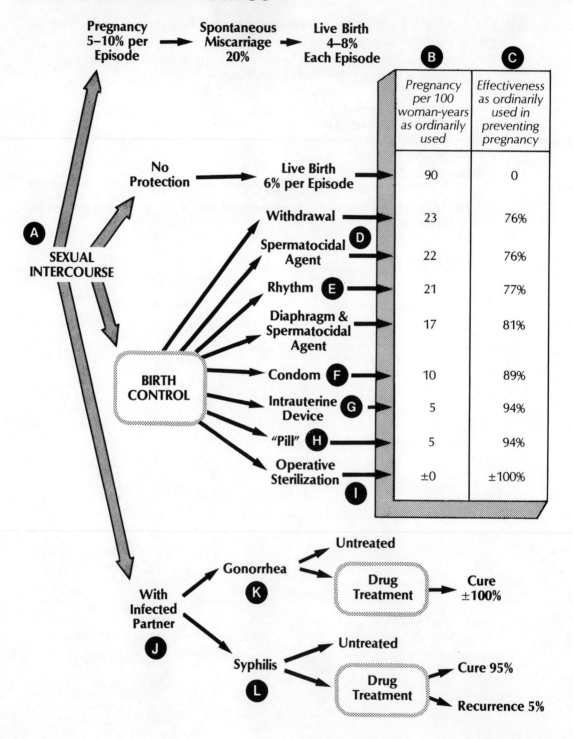

Pregnancy 5–10% per Episode	→	Spontaneous Miscarriage 20%	→	Live Birth 4–8% Each Episode

	B Pregnancy per 100 woman-years as ordinarily used	**C** Effectiveness as ordinarily used in preventing pregnancy
A SEXUAL INTERCOURSE → No Protection → Live Birth 6% per Episode	90	0
Withdrawal	23	76%
Spermatocidal Agent **D**	22	76%
Rhythm **E**	21	77%
Diaphragm & Spermatocidal Agent	17	81%
Condom **F**	10	89%
Intrauterine Device **G**	5	94%
"Pill" **H**	5	94%
Operative Sterilization **I**	±0	±100%

BIRTH CONTROL

With Infected Partner **J**

Gonorrhea **K** → Untreated
Gonorrhea **K** → Drug Treatment → Cure ±100%

Syphilis **L** → Untreated
Syphilis **L** → Drug Treatment → Cure 95%
Drug Treatment → Recurrence 5%

A The probability that a couple will become pregnant depends upon their relative fertility. About 15% of couples are infertile. In about one-half of cases, the problem is with the male; in the other half, it is with the female or with the couple together. Infertility is correctable in about one-half of the cases. Maximum fertility is at twenty-four years of age.

The likelihood of pregnancy is between 5–10% with each episode of unprotected intercourse. One in five pregnancies (20%) will end in a spontaneous abortion (miscarriage). There is, therefore, about a 4–8% likelihood that any one episode of unprotected intercourse will result in a live birth. One can reasonably assume that a pregnancy will result from every sixteen episodes (6%) of unprotected intercourse.

B Likelihood of pregnancy is commonly measured by the chance of pregnancy per year in a married couple. The ordinary young couple averages about 150 to 200 acts of intercourse per year after the first year of married life. The likelihood of pregnancy is 0.85–0.9 per year, so among one hundred women, one can expect 85–90 pregnancies per year. This term "one hundred woman-years" is the 100% baseline for measuring the effectiveness of birth-control devices.

Young couples having more frequent intercourse (more than four times per week) have a 95% probability of producing a pregnancy in six months if no safeguards are taken. There is only a 16% chance of pregnancy in wives of men over thirty-five years of age in a similar period if intercourse is less frequent than twice a week.

C Effectiveness of birth-control techniques depends upon the meticulousness with which the technique is employed. A comparison of the effectiveness of birth-control measures as employed by intelligent, careful couples and the average U.S. experience follows. It shows how errors in using birth-control techniques often account for unwanted pregnancies.

D A special foam or jelly designed to kill the male sperm (spermatocide) placed in the vagina before intercourse is only about 76% effective in preventing pregnancy as practiced by the ordinary couple.

E The ovary of a woman produces an egg ready for fertilization about every twenty-eight days. Normally this occurs midway between the woman's menstrual periods. Intercourse at that time (ten to eighteen days after menstruation period) has the greatest likelihood of resulting in a pregnancy. Intercourse just before or immediately after the period (days one to ten or days eighteen to twenty-eight) has the least chance of resulting in a pregnancy.

EFFECTIVENESS OF BIRTH-CONTROL TECHNIQUES
PREGNANCIES WITH CAREFUL USE OF TECHNIQUES COMPARED WITH AVERAGE U.S. EXPERIENCE IN COUPLES WHO DID NOT WANT MORE CHILDREN

TECHNIQUE	CAREFUL USE OF TECHNIQUE		AVERAGE U.S. EXPERIENCE	
	Pregnancies per 100 woman-years	*Effective-ness*	*Pregnancies per 100 woman-years*	*Effective-ness*
No protection	90	—	90	—
Douche	?	?	40	56%
Lactation (Breastfeeding)	25	72%	40	56%
Coitus Interruptus	9	90%	20–25	72–78%
Rhythm	13	86%	21	76%
Spermatocidal Foam	3	97%	22	76%
Diaphragm plus Spermatocide	3	97%	17	81%
Condom	3	97%	10	89%
Intrauterine Device	2	98%	5	94%
Condom plus Spermatocide	1	99%	5	94%
"Pill"	0.34	99%	4–10	89–96%
Sterilization	±0	±100%	±0	±100%

Source: R. A. Hatcher, *Contraceptive Technology: 1976–77* (J. Wiley & Sons, 1976).

"Rhythm" is the term used in describing the method of avoiding intercourse between days ten and eighteen after menstruation in order to prevent a pregnancy. Because the time of ovulation cannot be precisely predicted, rhythm as ordinarily practiced is only about 76% effective in avoiding pregnancies (twenty-one for every one hundred woman-years).

 A condom is a thin, tight-fitting cover to the penis, which keeps the male sperm from entering the vagina. It is about 89% effective in preventing pregnancy, reducing the likelihood of pregnancy to about ten per one hundred woman-years. Carefully used, it is about 96% effective in avoiding venereal disease if intercourse is with an infected partner.

G Intrauterine devices placed within the uterine cavity (womb) by the physician well before intercourse are about 98% effective under the most ideal conditions and about 94% effective with average couples.

H "The Pill" contains a sex hormone that stops the ovary from producing an egg ready for fertilization. If taken continuously every day by a woman, it is more than 99% effective in reducing the likelihood of pregnancy. Effectiveness is decreased to 89–96% if the woman is not careful about taking the pill. There are rare serious side effects of the pill, but it is extremely effective if the woman is careful in its use.

I Only under unusual circumstances will operative sterilization fail to prevent pregnancy.

J Gonorrhea and syphilis are the two most common diseases resulting from sexual intercourse (venereal disease). There is a 35% likelihood of contracting either or both of the diseases with each episode of intercourse with an infected partner. With repeated episodes, the likelihood rises to about 75%.

K Gonorrhea usually becomes evident 2–4 days after intercourse; in males, by a discharge of pus from the penis, and in women, by a discharge from the vagina. Untreated, the likelihood of complications include:

In men
- Narrowing (stricture) of the urinary passage: 1%
- Arthritis: 1%
- Inflammation in scrotum (epidymitis): 5–10%

In women
- Inflammation of the uterus, tubes, and ovaries (referred to as *pelvic inflammatory disease)*: 20%
- Sterility: 25% (10% with one episode; 75% with greater than three infections)

Prompt treatment of gonorrhea with antibiotics is approximately 95% curative in both men and women, and leaves no long-term complicating effects. There is no immunity to gonorrhea; it can afflict a person just as likely on re-exposure as it did the first time. Recurrence of a discharge after early treatment and no re-exposure is, about 40% of the time, apt to be due to an organism other than gonorrhea.

Sexual Intercourse

 Although syphilis is far less frequent than it once was, the disease is still common. The chances of getting syphilis from intercourse with an infected partner is about 50%. The first sign is usually an ulcer on the genitals, but if this passes unnoticed there may be no symptoms for many months. During this time, however, the patient is infectious and spreads the disease to a partner in intercourse. A blood test can determine whether a person has syphilis.

The effects of untreated syphilis are disastrous, including mental disease or involvement of almost any organ in the body. A child born of a syphilitic mother contracts the disease.

Treated promptly and thoroughly there is almost 100% chance of cure. Recurrence is possible in about 5% of cases, but these too are curable.

III
Head & Neck

1. Head Injury

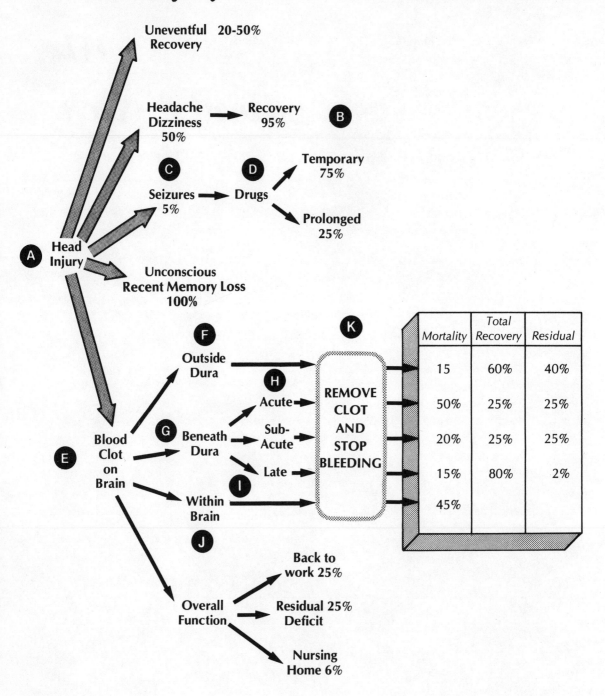

Uneventful Recovery 20-50%

Headache Dizziness 50% → Recovery 95%   **B**

C Seizures 5% → **D** Drugs → Temporary 75%
Drugs → Prolonged 25%

A Head Injury

Unconscious Recent Memory Loss 100%

E Blood Clot on Brain

F Outside Dura

G Beneath Dura

H Acute
Sub-Acute
I Late

Within Brain

K REMOVE CLOT AND STOP BLEEDING

Mortality	Total Recovery	Residual
15	60%	40%
50%	25%	25%
20%	25%	25%
15%	80%	2%
45%		

J Overall Function → Back to work 25%
Overall Function → Residual 25% Deficit
Overall Function → Nursing Home 6%

A A severe blow to the head usually produces a short period of unconsciousness. This is called concussion. Duration of the knockout roughly reflects the severity of the injury. The nerve cells in the brain simply fail to work for a short time after the blow and then return to normal activity. Occasionally there may be some memory loss (amnesia) for the events immediately preceding the injury. It is as though the most recent data received just before the accident had not had time to be stored in the computer.

B Headache, dizziness, confusion, and occasionally vomiting may occur immediately following injury. Most will disappear within 1–3 days. The severity of the injury does not always dictate the likelihood of such symptoms. Children often have severe symptoms immediately following injury, but few permanent problems thereafter. Just because a child after injury is unconscious, vomits after he wakes up, and is confused, does *not* mean he will have permanent brain damage.

Injuries that occur on a job or where there are legal implications associating the accident with likelihood of compensation are more likely to be associated with complications and complaints!

C Seizures are episodes of uncontrollable movements of some part of the body, such as the arms or legs. (Recurrent seizures are called epilepsy.) During the seizure, the patient may vomit and be confused and sleepy for a short time thereafter.

The likelihood of seizures occurring after head injury is related to the severity of the injury and the length of the period of unconsciousness. Following closed head injuries such as a blow to the head, only 5% of patients will be expected to have seizures. With injuries such as gunshot wounds that penetrate the skull, the probability of later seizures is 33%.

Adults who have loss of memory within less than twenty-four hours after the accident usually never have subsequent seizures. Although the first seizure may start at any time after the accident, if none has occurred during the first six months after injury, the likelihood of ever having epilepsy is less than 2%.

D Various drugs decrease the likelihood of seizures. In about 75% of patients, such medication can be stopped within a year after the injury. In the others, the drug may have to be taken for many years. Although frightening to the bystander, epileptic fits, or seizures, are generally not dangerous to the patient unless he is flying an airplane or driving a car or is in some way in a position to hurt himself by falling. Only about 20% of all seizures are due to previous head injury.

E The brain is packaged inside the skull, which is a firm, unyielding, protective box. If accident breaks a blood vessel within the skull, the resulting blood clot (hematoma) can squeeze the soft underlying brain against the rigid skull, interfering with brain activity. Such clots can form within the brain substance (intracranial hematoma), underneath the brain covering called the dura or outside the dura (extradural or epidural hematoma) just beneath the skull. Of all patients hospitalized for head injury, about 7% will have a blood clot in one of these sites. About twice as many of the hematomas will be beneath the dura as outside it.

F Bleeding outside the dura immediately under the skull (extradural or epidural hematoma) usually makes itself known within a few hours after injury, and if not treated by emergency operation may quickly be fatal by pressing on the brain and stopping its function. Chances of survival are about 85%, depending mainly on how promptly the bleeding is recognized, the skull opened, the pressure taken off the brain, and the bleeding stopped. About fifty percent of those who survive the injury and operation will be perfectly normal; 25% will have occasional seizures, and approximately 25% will have some sort of permanent disability resulting from the accident.

G Expectancy when bleeding occurs beneath the dura (subdural hematoma) depends in a large part on how soon after the injury the pressure on the brain begins to produce symptoms. Those causing symptoms within three days are called acute subdural hematoma and are the most dangerous. Those occurring between three days and three weeks are considered subacute, and those that do not declare themselves until after three weeks are called chronic subdural hematomas.

H The outlook for an acute subdural hematoma is not as good as for one that does not cause symptoms until later. Chances of survival from such an injury are about 50%. Of the survivors, one-half will return to some type of work, and only 5% will have to live dependently in a nursing home.

I At the other end of the spectrum, are those with chronic subdural hematoma who may require operation weeks after the injury. Survival after operation is approximately 85%, all but 20% of whom can anticipate total recovery. The younger the patient the better the chance for a good result.

J A severe blow to the head may cause bleeding into the brain, just as an injury to the thigh causes a black and blue spot in the muscles of the leg. Such intracerebral (inside the brain) clots cannot be removed without disturbing surrounding tissue. Almost half (45%) of patients with severe injuries that produce an intracerebral bleed will not survive.

K These brain operations consist of removing a segment of the bony skull, taking out the offending clot, and stopping the bleeding. They are usually performed under general anesthesia. Recovery may be slow and reoperation is necessary in about 1% of patients to remove more clots.

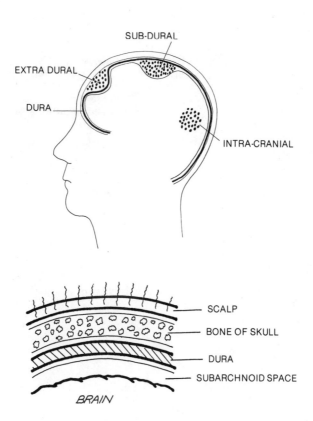

2. *Meningioma*

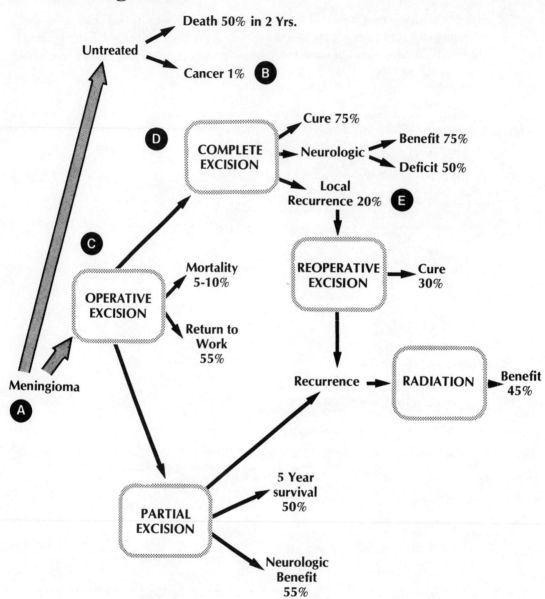

Death 50% in 2 Yrs.

Untreated

Cancer 1% **B**

Cure 75%

D

COMPLETE EXCISION

Neurologic

Benefit 75%

Deficit 50%

Local Recurrence 20% **E**

C

OPERATIVE EXCISION

Mortality 5-10%

Return to Work 55%

REOPERATIVE EXCISION

Cure 30%

Meningioma

A

Recurrence

RADIATION

Benefit 45%

PARTIAL EXCISION

5 Year survival 50%

Neurologic Benefit 55%

A The membranes covering the brain are called the meninges. Tumors of this thin sheet are called meningiomas. Although these tumors are benign, they continue to grow, press on the brain, cause signs of brain disturbance, and will ultimately kill if not removed.

Frequently, there is a one-to-two year delay from first symptom to diagnosis.

B Only a very few (if any) turn into a malignant cancer and spread. But meningiomas often recur locally.

C Operative removal involves taking off some of the bone of the skull and removing the tumor. The chance of death, of cure, and of leaving the patient with a nerve deficit depends mainly on the site of the tumor and its size. Certain parts of the brain are more accessible than others, and meningiomas overlying these areas can be widely and safely excised with a good chance of cure. Other areas are difficult for the surgeon to reach, and tumors in these areas often cannot be totally removed. There is a 5–10% chance that the patient with a meningioma will not survive the operation and subsequent hospitalization. The risk mainly depends on the location of the tumor. Three-quarters of those who survive will have signs of brain abnormality resulting from the tumor. One in five can anticipate some permanent nerve loss as the result of the operation. Of the 90–95% of patients who leave the hospital, 55% are able to return to work.

D Ability to completely excise the tumor depends primarily on its size and location at the time of operation.

E Recurrence is usually at the site of the original tumor and characteristically shows up five-to-six years after original excision.

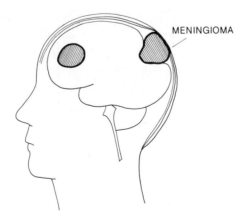

MENINGIOMA

TUMOR WITHIN BRAIN

3. Spinal Cord Injury

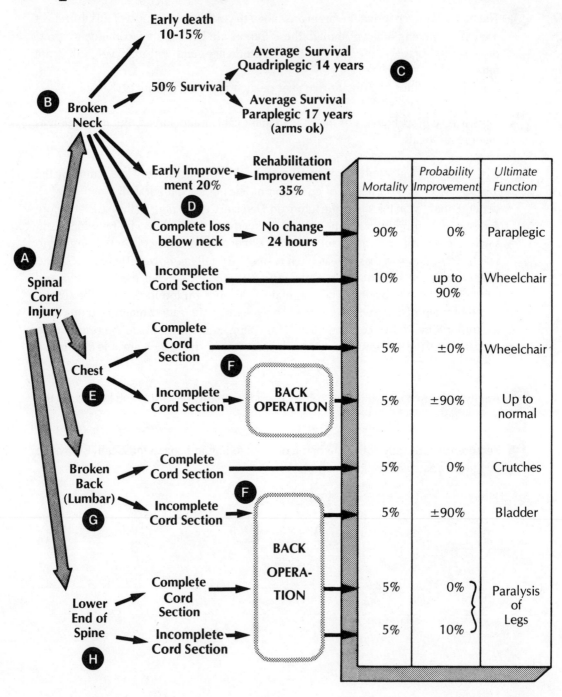

Early death
10-15%

Average Survival
Quadriplegic 14 years   **C**

B Broken   50% Survival
Neck   Average Survival
Paraplegic 17 years
(arms ok)

Early Improve- Rehabilitation
ment 20%   Improvement
                35%
                D

Complete loss   No change
below neck   24 hours

A   Incomplete
Cord Section
Spinal
Cord
Injury

| | Probability | Ultimate |
Mortality	Improvement	Function
90%	0%	Paraplegic
10%	up to 90%	Wheelchair
5%	±0%	Wheelchair
5%	±90%	Up to normal
5%	0%	Crutches
5%	±90%	Bladder
5%	0%	Paralysis of Legs
5%	10%	

Complete
Cord
Section
F
Chest   BACK
E Incomplete OPERATION
Cord Section

Complete
Cord Section
F
Broken
Back
(Lumbar) Incomplete
Cord Section
G

BACK
OPERA-
TION

Lower   Complete
End of   Cord
Spine   Section

Incomplete
Cord Section
H

42

A Nerve fibers packed together like electric wires in a telephone cable pass from the brain down a canal in the backbone (vertebral column). The nerves carry messages to and from the brain. When the vertebrae are broken, there is an obvious possibility that the spinal cord running through the center of the vertebral column may also be injured. Once such a nerve is cut, it will not regrow. Any improvement in function is due to compensatory action by muscles whose nerve supply has not been damaged.

B Cord damage in the neck has less chance for recovery than damage lower down the back. Early death is usually due to severance of the nerves controlling breathing.

C A quadriplegic has no function of arms, legs, or other areas served by nerves that go out of the spinal cord below the neck. Although average survival is fourteen years, the lack of sensation below the neck causes lifelong problems, with ulcers of the skin, urinary-tract infections, and problems with the bowels or lungs. Up to 50% of well-motivated quadriplegics using a special wheelchair can lead useful lives and hold productive jobs. Paraplegics, in contrast, have function of their arms but no other nerve activity below that level. On the average they live longer (about seventeen years) than quadriplegics, but have many of the same subsequent problems.

D The most significant indication for the chances of recovery in a person following spinal cord injury is whether some of the nerves passing through the area of injury are still intact upon first examination. If the injury is complete twenty-four hours after inception (no nerve function below the site of injury), then the patient and his family must face the fact that there will be no significant return of function thereafter. On the other hand, if some of the nerves are still working, there is a good chance that there will be some return of function in damaged but not destroyed nerves within the following four weeks. After a month, no further return of nerve function can be expected.

E Injuries severe enough to break that portion of the backbone containing the spinal cord often cause damage to organs within the chest and abdomen, which, of course, have an expected mortality and complications not associated with spinal cord damage.

F Back operations performed after spinal cord injury merely provide room for swelling in the injured cord, thus avoiding additional nerve damage. The operation cannot repair spinal cord nerves already severed in the spinal cord.

G Most broken backs involve the spinal column below the chest (the so-called lumbar area). Such injuries may cut the nerves to the legs. If there is no return of function within twenty-four hours, there is essentially no chance that there will be any thereafter.

H Although the spinal cord itself stops high in the lumbar area, nerves to the legs, bowels, and bladder continue on within the bony spinal canal, down almost to the end of the spine. Injuries in this area may cause paralysis of the legs or difficulty with controlling the bowels or urine.

4. Ruptured Intervertebral Disc

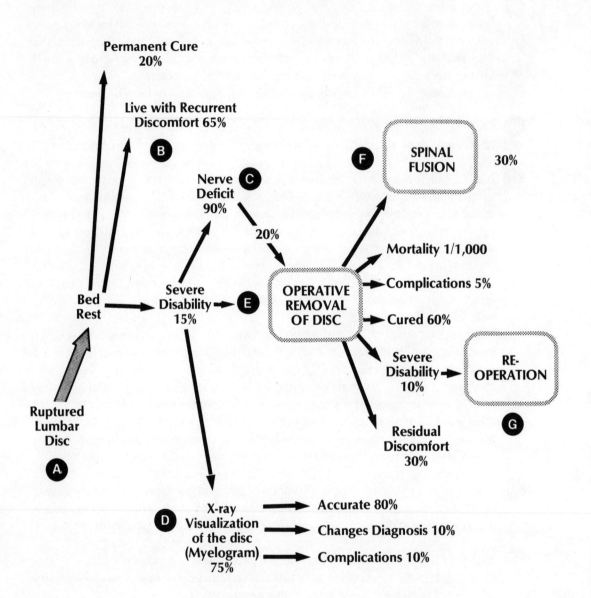

Permanent Cure
20%

Live with Recurrent
Discomfort 65%

B

Nerve
Deficit **C**
90%

20%

F SPINAL
FUSION   30%

Bed
Rest

Severe
Disability **E**
15%

OPERATIVE
REMOVAL
OF DISC

Mortality 1/1,000

Complications 5%

Cured 60%

Severe
Disability → RE-
10%   OPERATION

G

Residual
Discomfort
30%

Ruptured
Lumbar
Disc

A

X-ray
D Visualization
of the disc
(Myelogram)
75%

Accurate 80%

Changes Diagnosis 10%

Complications 10%

A The intervertebral disc normally fits like a thick cushion between adjacent vertebra in the spinal column. The disc is designed to take up the shocks between the bones. Its interior is a firm but compressible material, surrounded and contained by a circular capsule. When the disc ruptures, material from its interior pushes out through the capsule and presses on the nearby nerves from the spinal cord. Pressure on the nerves by the protruded disc substance causes pain or loss of nerve activity. Ninety-five percent of such ruptured, or herniated, discs occur in the small of the back at the lower end of the spine. There are many other causes of back pain that masquerade as a ruptured disc.

B Bed rest is the basis of non-operative treatment of a ruptured disc and, in time, usually gives relief from pain. Traction merely guarantees immobilization and allows inflammation around the area to subside. One to two weeks of bed rest may be required and provides long-lasting cure in 20% of patients.

Two-thirds of patients with a ruptured disc are willing to put up with the recurring episodes of pain and discomfort and do not require operation. Between attacks, which can come on suddenly with apparently little provocation, there may be no symptoms.

C If, in addition to pain, pressure on the nerves by the herniated disc produces muscle weakness or loss of sensation in the legs, then the chances of cure without operation are decreased. Twenty percent will totally recover without operation, but an equal number (20%) will require early operation for relief of pain. About 60% will recover from the immediate attack and chance another attack and further nerve injury.

D Even if the diagnosis of a ruptured disc is almost certain, the surgeon, before deciding to operate, will usually want to obtain evidence of the abnormality by X-ray examination. This study is performed by instilling a dye solution into the area around the spinal cord, which shows up on the X-ray film and indicates where the disc protrudes abnormally into the spinal canal.

This procedure (myelogram) is 80% accurate in localizing the site of rupture and actually changes the suspected diagnosis in 10% of patients. But as with any procedure, it has chances of temporary complications such as pain, retention of urine, or even, very rarely (about 0.1%), seizures or muscle weakness.

E Operation (laminectomy) is done under general anesthesia through the back. Some bone is removed from the vertebrae to expose the disc material where it presses on the nerves. The disc space between the vertebrae is then scraped out so that no further disc material will be pushed against the spinal cord.

Ruptured Intervertebral Disc

Sometimes, more than one disc must be explored. Mortality is about 0.01%, and the chance of a serious complication in the early days after operation is about 1%. This includes increase of pain or muscle weakness after operation or, very rarely, damage to the large arteries or veins that lie just in front of the disc.

F Sometimes the surgeon chooses to join or fuse the two bony vertebrae on each side of the ruptured disc in the hope of producing a stronger back. The relative gain and loss of adding fusion to simple disc removal is:

	No Fusion	Fusion
Bed rest	2–3 days	7–10 days
Hospitalization	7 days	14 days
Limited activity	10 weeks	28 weeks
Fusion failure		10%
Recurrent symptoms	35%	35%

G After removal of a disc, about 10% of patients will have so much continuing pain that they need a second operation. The causes are likely to be:

- Another herniated disc: 22%
- Recurrent pressure from disc material at the same site: 31%
- Adhesions around the operative site: 12%
- A piece of bone pressing on the nerves: 5%
- Instability of spine: 30%

Recurrence of symptoms after operation is particularly likely to occur in patients where compensation and/or a lawsuit are involved.

Chances for cure from a second operation for disc is the same as for the first procedure. For third or subsequent operations, however, the likelihood of cure falls rapidly, since only 10% of patients are likely to have a good result.

5. Schizophrenia

A Schizophrenia is the term used for a group of serious mental disorders that, in general, eventually results in personality deterioration. There are about one million schizophrenics in the U.S. The disease is typified by acute episodes usually lasting several weeks or months and interspersed by periods of remission, during which the personality returns toward, but seldom to normalcy. Ultimately, there is almost always some progressive personality deterioration. The diagnosis of schizophrenia must be made only by a trained physician, for it has serious implications.

B Eighty percent of first episodes usually occur between the ages of fifteen and twenty-five. The younger the age at onset, the worse the prognosis. Factors associated with a better prognosis include acute onset associated with a stressful or threatening situation, the presence of depression, previous good social adjustment, and onset in middle life or later. Onset after age forty-five is very rare.

About 60–80% of patients will have to be hospitalized with the first attack.

C Before the modern era of drug therapy and better understanding of the disease, the outlook for a schizophrenic was bad. Only about 15% recovered from the first attack, and 60% ended up with prolonged hospitalization. Only about 2% were cured. Essentially, all had progressive deterioration of the personality.

D Modern treatment usually includes one of the several effective drugs, psychotherapy by a physician, and, very importantly, support by the patient's family and associates. Psychotherapy can be given either individually or in groups. The combination of these three kinds of treatment has dramatically changed the outlook for a schizophrenic patient and the probability of keeping him within the community, rather than in the hospital. There is about a 5–15% chance of serious complications and a 80% chance of minor or transient complications involved in the use of antipsychotic drugs in treatment, depending on length of time and total dose.

The likelihood of response in the first attack is:

- Beneficial response: 80–90% (usually within three to six weeks)
- Ultimate discontinuance of drug support: 50%
- Required hospitalization within two years: 50%
- Ultimate prolonged hospitalization: 25%
- Ability to live outside the hospital and have a productive social life: 15–40%

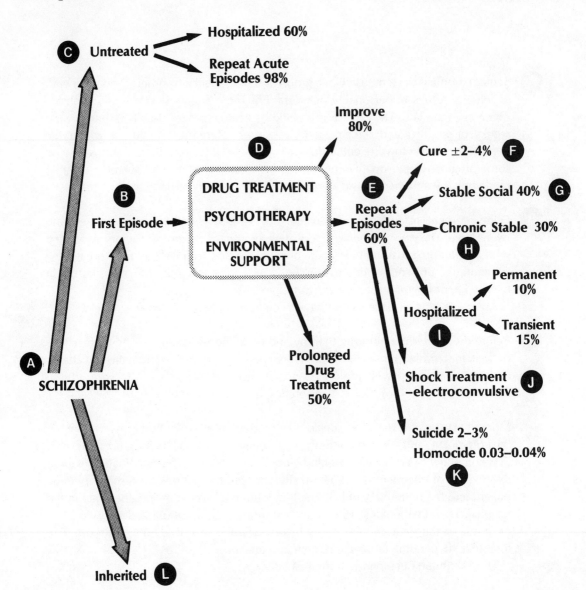

E Remission of symptoms after the first attack may last a few months or many years. Ten to fifteen percent of patients will relapse within a year. When a relapse occurs, as it does in about 50–80% of the cases, depending on whether treatment has continued, it is often (60% of the time) precipitated by some acute or chronic emotional stress. Such a relapse may consist of an increase of symptoms, without a frank, complete breakdown or decompensation. But with each relapse there is often additional deterioration of the personality. Such deterioration occurs more rapidly after the second and subsequent relapses.

F Complete remission or "cure" occurs in about 2–4% of patients.

G About 40% of schizophrenics will stabilize and lead—what to the outsider seems to be—a normal life outside of the hospital. They will, however, require drug support, at least intermittently, to control symptoms, particularly when threatened by stressful life situations. They are socially and economically independent, although somewhat impaired in level of function, and only during relapses do they have frank personality disorders.

H Another 30% will be incapacitated, but with drug, psychotherapy, and family support, will be able to live outside the hospital most of the time. They are considered to be in a stable chronic condition.

I Only about 25% will require appreciable hospitalization. Of these, about 15% will only need intermittent hospital care. The other 10% will have to be kept permanently in the hospital for their own and society's best interests.

J Electroconvulsive (shock) treatment is now used in only about 15% of schizophrenics, when other treatment fails. It is effective in bringing about a remission in about 50% of cases. Personality deterioration results from more than forty treatments.

K About 2–3% of schizophrenics will commit suicide, although attempts are much more frequent. A schizophrenic is no more likely to commit homocide than anyone else. If he does, it is liable to be during a period of acute upset.

L The likelihood of inheritance of schizophrenia is:

- With one schizophrenic parent: 10–12%
- With both parents schizophrenic: 35–44%
- With a schizophrenic uncle, aunt, or grandparent: 2–3%
- Regardless of family history: about 1%

These odds may be important in decisions regarding having children, sterilization, or even marriage.

6. Manic Depression

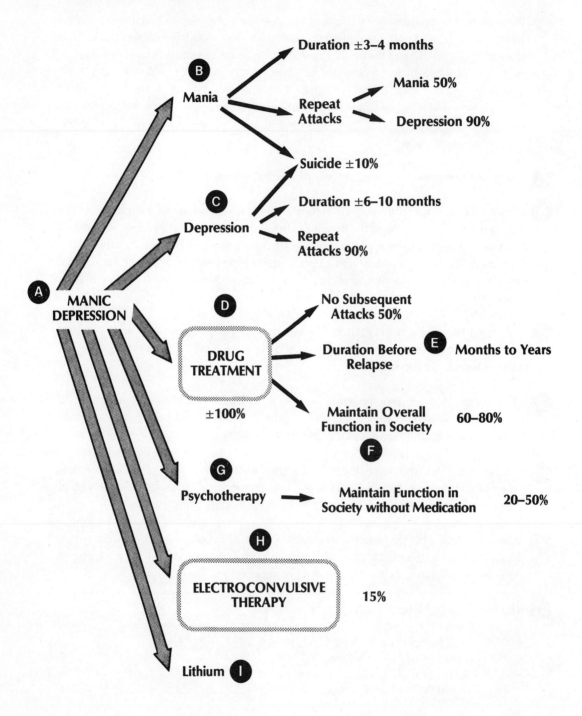

B Mania
- Duration ±3–4 months
- Repeat Attacks
  - Mania 50%
  - Depression 90%
- Suicide ±10%

C Depression
- Suicide ±10%
- Duration ±6–10 months
- Repeat Attacks 90%

A MANIC DEPRESSION

D DRUG TREATMENT
±100%
- No Subsequent Attacks 50%
- Duration Before Relapse — **E** Months to Years
- Maintain Overall Function in Society 60–80% **F**

G Psychotherapy → Maintain Function in Society without Medication 20–50%

H ELECTROCONVULSIVE THERAPY 15%

Lithium **I**

A Everyone has mood swings. In a few people, these changes become so extreme that they interfere with normal living. When depressed, nothing seems to go right. Unchecked pessimism seems to overwhelm the person. At the opposite extreme is the manic, whose uncontrollable enthusiasm overthrows all inhibitions, which may get out of hand in wildly erratic behavior. Wide and frequent deviations from normal are called manic depression. About 60–70% of patients will intermittently be purely depressed, while 30–40% will ultimately demonstrate both aspects of the disease. Repeated manic episodes without depression is rare. The manic-depressive person is likely to maintain his personality between episodes.

B The first *pure manic* break characteristically lasts three to four months, but there may be wide variations. A second attack can be expected in about 75% of cases and a third in about 65%. There may be months to years between attacks. About 80–90% require hospitalization. Thirty to fifty percent have the first attack before age twenty-five. About 20% of those in a severe attack will attempt suicide, of which about half will be successful.

C Depression will be the first manifestation in about 90% of manic-depressives. Twenty to thirty percent will be between the ages of fourteen to twenty-five years. Duration of the first *pure depressive* attack averages about six to nine months, with wide variations. Recovery without treatment is usually gradual over several months' time. About 50% will require hospitalization for periods of about three to ten weeks. Pure depressives often have months or years between attacks. A single depressive attack without any subsequent episodes is probably a different disease from manic-depressive illness.

D Three groups of drugs (antipsychotics, antidepressants, and lithium) have significantly altered the natural course of manic depression. An acute manic episode will respond to drug treatment within two weeks 80–90% of the time. Acute depressive episodes will respond 60–70% of the time with medication, whereas repeated depressive episodes can be controlled successfully about 50% of the time with medication. Twenty-five percent of patients with manic-depressive illness can safely be removed from drug treatment after they sustain a period of a year or two without subsequent episodes. With drug treatment, hospitalization for the first attack of either mania or depression is usually less than two months and may be as short as two weeks. Approximately 10% of patients with recurrent episodes may become disabled enough from their illness to be unable to return to a fully productive social existence.

E Characteristically, a relapse of a manic episode or a depressive episode will occur in approximately 50% of patients in spite of drug treatment. In the presence of drug treatment, these recurrences tend to be less severe than the first attacks. The likelihood of suicide increases with subsequent attacks of both depression and mania. In perhaps 25% of the cases, subsequent attacks of mania and depression are less responsive to drug treatment and lead to more chronic personality deterioration.

F Ultimate ability to live socially productive lives is possible in between 60–80% of the patients.

G Psychotherapy and environmental support remain significant components to the treatment of acute episodes, and psychotherapy, associated with drug treatment between episodes, can be very useful for helping the patient find ways of coping with normal life stresses without becoming ill.

H Electroconvulsive therapy (ETC) is very useful in the treatment of the acutely depressed patient. It usually requires six to nine treatments in the hospital spread over a two to three week period. Its most dramatic effect is during an acute attack of depression, preferably a first attack, where it will shorten the depressive episode in 70–80% of the cases. This treatment almost always provides some temporary memory impairment. In over 90% of the cases, this memory impairment is cleared within six weeks after the treatments are over. As is true for the use of ECT in the treatment of schizophrenia, the use of more than forty or fifty electroconvulsive treatments has been reported to lead to some deterioration of personality. Electroconvulsive therapy is most often used in situations where the suicidal danger is judged to be so high that waiting for the medication to take effect is too dangerous or where the use of antidepressant drugs has not proved to be productive. Nevertheless, for some patients, perhaps 10–20% of those with serious depressive episodes, it remains the single most effective treatment.

I Lithium helps prevent subsequent severe attacks in about one-half of these patients. It is effective for one to two years in about 70% of manics and about 40% of those in the depressive state. It is least effective in those with pure depression. There are disturbing side effects in about 20% of those taking the drug.

7. Suicide Threat

A A suicide threat must be taken seriously. Suicide is the third leading cause of death in children and teenagers, and about 12% of those who threaten it will ultimately make the attempt. About half of those who actually kill themselves have spoken to someone of suicide within one to twelve months prior. If others do not respond positively and provide some evidence of support, the risk of suicide is increased. Approximately 80% of people who kill themselves have visited a physician with vague symptoms (e.g., aches and pains or insomnia) within six months of their deaths. Fifty-five percent of those dying by ingestion of an overdose of a sedative obtained a lethal amount of the drug in one prescription from their physician. Patients may not volunteer thoughts of suicide but will usually admit to them if asked directly. Factors increasing the risks of a serious or successful suicide attempt include:

- A plan, and the means to carry out the attempt
- A feeling of hopelessness
- Depression, especially when accompanied by signs such as serious appetite or weight changes or sleeplessness
- Recent separation from a loved one
- Past history of a suicide attempt, especially if there have been two or more previous attempts
- Family history of suicide
- Social isolation
- Persistent complaints of insomnia
- Presence of psychosis
- A written suicide note
- Male, over age forty
- Poor health

B Suicide before age ten is exceedingly rare. Sixty-six percent of all suicide attempts among teenagers are associated with disturbed relations with parents or boyfriends or girlfriends. Fourteen percent are associated with school problems, and a like number with sexual conflicts. Ten percent are associated with pregnancy.

About 3–4% of children with psychiatric disorders will try to commit suicide. Most attempts are performed as a spur-of-the-moment, quick impulse, half of which occur within three minutes of an emotional crisis. Boys are three times as likely to attempt suicide as are girls.

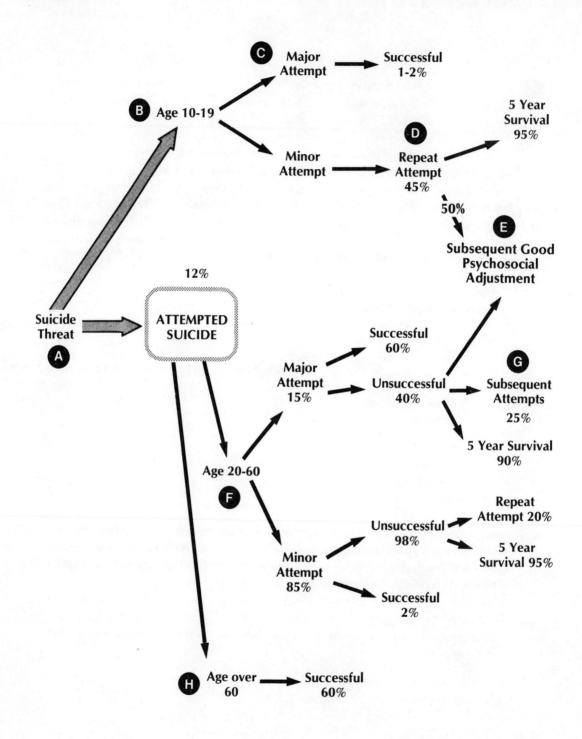

C Major attempts at suicide are characterized by a serious intent to die. They combine a high probability of death, such as shooting, hanging, or drowning, with a low probability of rescue, for example, being carried out in a remote place without a telephone. Twenty-five percent of serious attempts are by ingestion. Survival after a serious attempt at suicide is usually due to happenstance, such as the unexpected interruption by someone. Major attempts occur three times more frequently among men than they do among women. Minor attempts (low lethality of method with high probability of rescue) are three times more likely to be used by women. Without conscious intent, however, the patient may misjudge the circumstances and die accidentally.

D Once a teenager has attempted suicide, there is about a 50% chance that he will try again. Repeated attempts are more common in children and adolescents with poor social interactions. Repetitive attempts are less likely if family, friends, and physicians respond positively and are supportive.

E Half of the teenagers who make a serious suicide attempt will subsequently make good social adjustments. About 60-70% of adults will do so.

F In adults, the average age for a major suicide attempt is fifty-one years and for a minor attempt, thirty-four years. The older the patient, the more likely the attempt is to be premeditated, major, and successful. Almost 70% of major attempts in this age group are successful. Of those who live, 25% will try again, in which case the ultimate mortality from suicide is about one in four.

G As in all age groups, the more the attempts—regardless of whether major or minor—the greater the probability that one will be successful.
Family, friends, and physicians can go only so far in preventing successful future suicide attempts. No one can be watched twenty-four hours a day forever, and if a patient is bent upon suicide, there is often little even a psychiatrist can ultimately do to stop him. The family members must resign themselves to this fact. In particular, a patient must not be allowed to gain emotional power over his family or a physician by threatening suicide. Such threats are signs of a serious emotional disease and must be treated as such.

Suicide Threat

 Those over sixty who try suicide usually have cooly contemplated the act and are reacting depressively to a tragedy, such as loss of a spouse, or the occurrence of an incurable disease. Success in this age group is about 60%.

8. Hyperthyroidism

A The thyroid gland secretes a powerful substance (thyroid hormone) that circulates in the blood and, like a central thermostat, helps control the rate at which many organs function. When the thyroid puts out too much of this hormone (hyperthyroidism), many other organs work at an abnormally fast rate, and the patient becomes thyro-toxic. The amount of thyroid hormone secreted can be decreased by specific drugs, by radioactive iodine that concentrates in the thyroid, or by surgically removing part of the gland.

B Once a patient becomes thryo-toxic, the symptoms in 75% of cases usually progress and even cause death from heart failure in 10% of those affected. In 25% of patients, the disease, for unknown reasons, will spontaneously wax and wane, getting better for a time but then almost always getting worse.

C Certain drugs (Thiocarbazides, Propylthiouracil, and Tapazol) depress thyroid secretion and form the basis of drug treatment. They may produce prolonged "cure" or remission in 25–50% of patients. The various complications of taking the drug (itching, joint pain, jaundice, etc.) are related to the dose of the drug required.

D Another group of drugs (such as Propanolol) control some of the more serious symptoms of hyperthyroidism due to overactivity of the heart, but do not decrease overactivity of the gland.

E The thyroid selectively traps and concentrates iodine. By giving radioactive iodine, a high dose of radiation can be delivered directly to the thyroid, which decreases its production of thyroid hormone. A single dose can be expected to induce a "cure" (remission) in 85% of patients. This will last for ten years in 50% of patients. But in the other half, the radioactivity will overshoot and cause abnormally *decreased* function in 15% of patients within one year. Thereafter, an additional decreased function (myxedema) will occur in 2–3% of patients per year.

F In 15% of patients, the first dose of radioactive iodine is not sufficient to bring thyroid function quite to normal. At least one (and often several) more doses must be given. Such multiple doses of radioactive iodine will bring about normal thyroid activity in about 5% of patients, but increases the likelihood of abnormally decreased thyroid activity (myxedema).

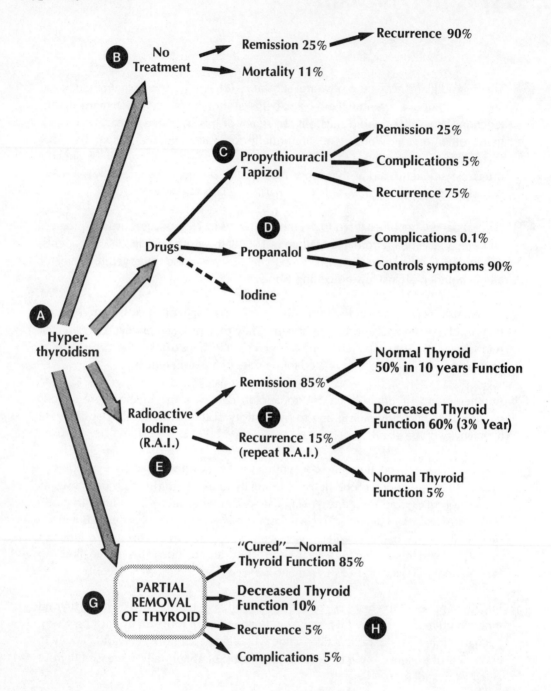

G Operative removal of part of the thyroid gland (thyroidectomy) is usually performed under general anesthesia, requires three-to-seven days of hospitalization, and has a mortality essentially no different than that of anesthesia (less than 0.1%). The various possible complications are described in "Thyroidectomy," page 64.

The nerves of the vocal cords lie very close to the thyroid gland and there is always a slight (less than 0.4%) chance they can be injured. So, too, can the parathyroid glands.

H The surgeon must estimate the amount of thyroid tissues he should remove to cure the overactive gland. If he takes out too little, he will not cure the overactivity; if too much, myxedema will result. In about 85% of patients, the surgeon estimates correctly and the patient has normal thyroid function. But even in the best hands, occasionally (about 5% of the time) too much gland is left, and some signs of hyperthyroidism remain. This may require some radioactive iodine for correction. Conversely, in about 10% of cases, too much gland is removed, and the patient has a decreased thyroid function (myxedema). This is corrected by taking thyroid hormone by mouth.

9. Thyroid Nodule

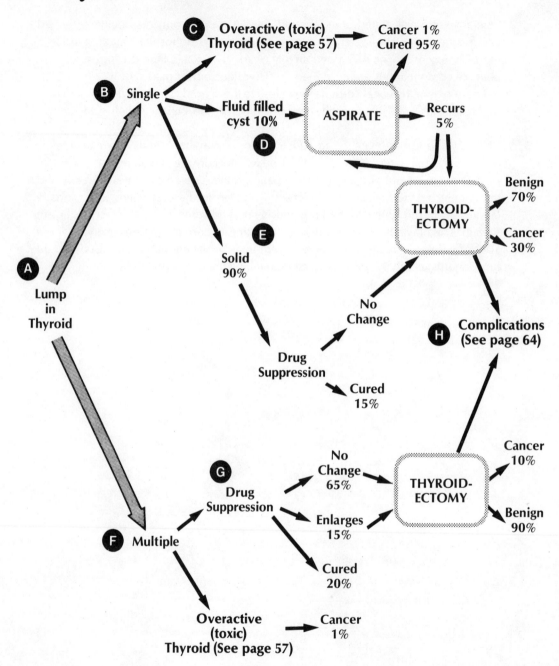

C Overactive (toxic) Thyroid (See page 57) → Cancer 1% Cured 95%

B Single

D Fluid filled cyst 10% → ASPIRATE → Recurs 5%

THYROID-ECTOMY → Benign 70% → Cancer 30%

A Lump in Thyroid

E Solid 90%

Drug Suppression → No Change / Cured 15%

H Complications (See page 64)

G Drug Suppression → No Change 65% / Enlarges 15% / Cured 20%

THYROID-ECTOMY → Cancer 10% → Benign 90%

F Multiple

Overactive (toxic) Thyroid (See page 57) → Cancer 1%

A The thyroid gland lies in the middle of the neck and normally is so small and inconspicuous it can hardly be felt. The appearance of a lump (nodule) in the gland is as abnormal as a lump in the breast and raises the same question: "Is it cancer?" The chances (15-20%) are about the same for a thyroid lump being cancerous as they are for a lump in the breast being cancerous.

B A single nodule is more likely to be cancer than is a gland filled with nodules.

C Rarely (only 1% of the time) will a solitary nodule that causes overactivity of the thyroid (see Hyperthyroidism," page 57) be the site of cancer. Thyroid overactivity caused by such a nodule is cured by removing the lump of overactive tissue.

D Ten percent of single nodules are simply fluid-filled cysts. They often can be detected either by their feel or by special studies using ultrasound. Such cysts can be punctured with a needle and the fluid drawn off and examined under the microscope. This will cure 95% of them. When the other 5% recur, needle drainage can again be performed. If after the second aspiration the mass recurs, it should be removed.

E Most lumps (90%) in the thyroid are solid and not fluid-filled. Thyroid hormone derivations taken by mouth over a three to six month period will make 15% of such solid nodules disappear. In the remainder (85%), the nodule, along with surrounding normal thyroid tissue, should be removed by an operation. Eighty percent of solitary lumps will be benign; 15-20% cancerous.

F More than one nodule (multiple nodules) in the thyroid may result from iodine deficiency in the diet, is six to nine times more frequent in women, and increases in occurence with age. About half of those who seem to have only a solitary nodule have in fact several nodules, which become apparent when the gland is removed. About 10% of suspicious lumps in a multinodular gland turn out to be cancer.

G Suppression with thyroid hormones makes about 20% of such lumps disappear just as it does with a solitary nodule. In the other 80% of patients where the lump remains, removal should be done to determine whether the lump is cancerous. Only 10% turn out to be cancer.

H Details of thyroidectomy are described on page 64. Mortality and serious complications following removal of a thyroid nodule should be under 1%. Hospitalization is usually three to five days. So little gland is removed with the nodule, that underactivity of thyroid function (myxedema) is extremely rare (less than 5%) when the operation is performed merely to remove a nodule.

10. *Thyroid Cancer*

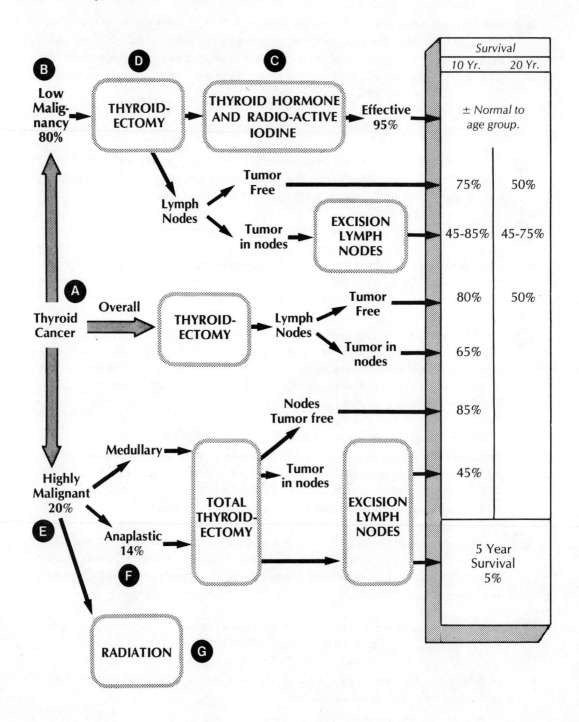

A There are many types of thyroid cancers. Some are so slow growing that they act almost as though they were benign, but left untreated they will ultimately spread widely. Other cell types grow very quickly from the start. Cancer of the thyroid often first appears in people under the age of forty.

B Eighty percent of thyroid cancers grow slowly. Of these, 60% are of one cell type (papillary), and most of the rest (20%) of another (follicular). The latter grows more quickly and is more likely to spread to lymph nodes in the neck outside the gland.

C Slow-growing tumors have many characteristics of normal thyroid cells, and they usually respond to drugs that depress the growth of normal thyroid cells, such as thyroid hormone and radioactive iodine. The combination of thyroid hormone and radioactive iodine decreases the size of these tumors and may improve cure rate.

D Many different types of operations are used to treat slow-growing thyroid cancers. They differ in the amount of thyroid gland and adjacent lymph nodes in the neck that are removed. In about half of the cases, there are several sites of tumor within the gland, complicating the decision as to how much of it should be removed.

When the tumor has spread to the nearby lymph nodes in the neck, they, too, must be removed in order to have a chance for cure. (See "Thyroidectomy," page 64, and "Radical Neck Dissection," page 70, for the implications of excision of lymph nodes in the neck.

E Twenty percent of all thyroid cancers grow and spread quickly. Of these, about one-third are so-called "medullary" tumors, which often occur in several members of a family and are associated with other tumors in other endocrine glands, such as the adrenals.

F The fastest-growing thyroid cancer (anaplastic) is highly malignant. Its growth seldom slows down either after removal by operation, radiation, or drug therapy. Only about 5% of patients with this relatively uncommon tumor survive five years.

G Radiation will not cure thyroid cancers, but helps contain tumor cells within involved lymph nodes and delays further spread. Unfortunately, highly malignant thyroid tumors seldom respond to X-ray therapy.

11. Thyroidectomy

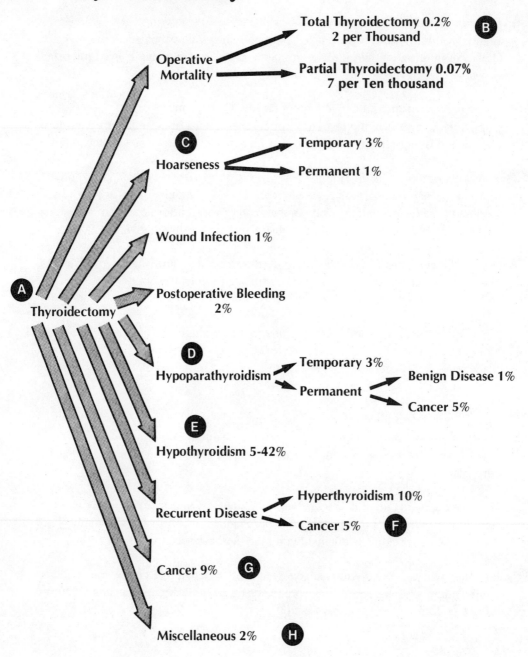

A Thyroidectomy

Operative Mortality
- Total Thyroidectomy 0.2% 2 per Thousand **B**
- Partial Thyroidectomy 0.07% 7 per Ten thousand

C Hoarseness
- Temporary 3%
- Permanent 1%

Wound Infection 1%

Postoperative Bleeding 2%

D Hypoparathyroidism
- Temporary 3%
- Permanent
  - Benign Disease 1%
  - Cancer 5%

E Hypothyroidism 5-42%

Recurrent Disease
- Hyperthyroidism 10%
- Cancer 5% **F**

Cancer 9% **G**

Miscellaneous 2% **H**

A The thyroid gland is usually removed either for cancer or because it is producing too much thyroid hormone with resulting hyperthyroidism. The probability of cure and complications following thyroidectomy depend upon the indication for operation and the amount of gland removed.

B The entire thyroid gland is usually removed (total thyroidectomy) only for cancer. If the lymph glands around the thyroid contain cancer, they are removed along with the gland. This more extensive operation increases the probability of complications following operation.

C Two nerves on each side of the neck lie next to the thyroid gland. One (the superior or upper-laryngeal nerve) controls the fine tuning of the voice, and its damage or absence is noticed only by singers. It is occasionally sacrificed during thyroidectomy. The other much more important nerve controls the vocal cord, and its damage leads to hoarseness. Its sacrifice is more probable (3–4% of the time) if thyroidectomy is performed for cancer. Hoarseness, due to damage of these nerves, usually disappears within one to two weeks following operation if the nerves have not been cut.

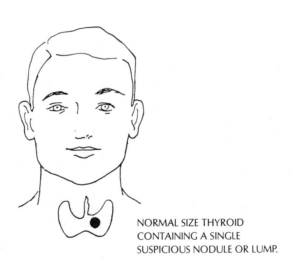

NORMAL SIZE THYROID
CONTAINING A SINGLE
SUSPICIOUS NODULE OR LUMP.

Thyroidectomy

D Two tiny parathyroid glands lie on each side of the thyroid in the neck. Although very small and difficult to identify, they control the use of calcium throughout the body. They are more likely to be injured or even entirely removed when the whole thyroid gland is taken out because of cancer.

The chance of having decreased parathyroid function following thyroidectomy is:

Total thyroidectomy: temporary 3%; permanent, 7%
Subtotal thyroidectomy: temporary, 4%; permanent, 0.2%

E When the thyroid gland is removed for overactivity (hyperthyroidism) the surgeon faces a dilemma. If he takes out too little gland, he will not totally cure the patient and

THYROID GLAND
CONTAINING SEVERAL LUMPS
IN BOTH LOBES OF THE GLAND.

FOLLOWING OPERATIVE REMOVAL
OF ONE LOBE OF THE THYROID.

some degree of overactivity (hyperthyroidism) will persist. If he removes too much gland, thyroid activity will be below normal (hypothyroidism), and the patient will have to take thyroid extract as an oral medicine for the rest of his life. No surgeon can guarantee he will be able to guess exactly how much gland to remove. Because it is so safe and simple to take thyroid extract, it is wiser for the surgeon to take out more rather than less thyroid tissue. This is why the likelihood of low thyroid function following thyroidectomy ranges from 5–42% and why 10% of patients may have some remaining thyroid toxicity (hyperthyroidism). This latter condition can be treated by further operation or by drugs that will decrease thyroid activity.

F The chance of thyroid cancer recurrence is discussed in "Thyroid Cancer," page **62.**

G The probability of finding cancer in the removed thyroid gland depends on the indications for the operation. Since an indication for thyroidectomy is often suspicion of cancer in a thyroid nodule, it is not surprising that between 10–20% of the lumps removed actually are cancerous.

H Other rare (less than 5 per thousand) complications of thyroidectomy include: wound breakdown, unsightly scar, or need for emergency reoperation for bleeding or swelling around the airway.

12. Lip Cancer

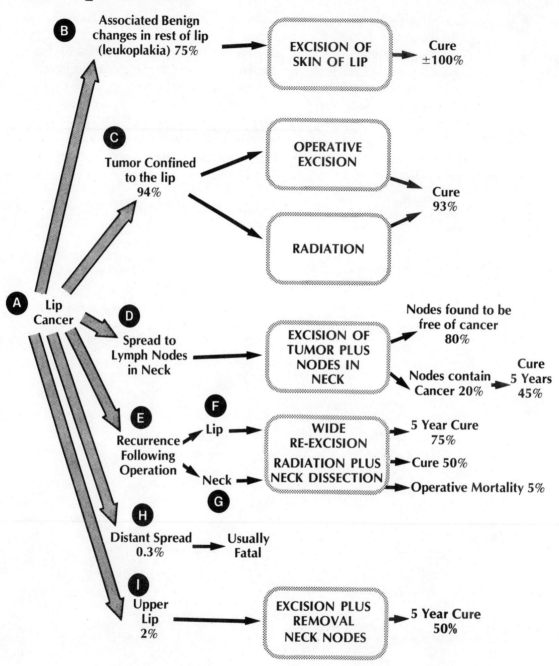

B Associated Benign changes in rest of lip (leukoplakia) 75% → EXCISION OF SKIN OF LIP → Cure ±100%

A Lip Cancer

C Tumor Confined to the lip 94% → OPERATIVE EXCISION / RADIATION → Cure 93%

D Spread to Lymph Nodes in Neck → EXCISION OF TUMOR PLUS NODES IN NECK → Nodes found to be free of cancer 80% / Nodes contain Cancer 20% → Cure 5 Years 45%

E Recurrence Following Operation → **F** Lip → WIDE RE-EXCISION → 5 Year Cure 75%

G Neck → RADIATION PLUS NECK DISSECTION → Cure 50% / Operative Mortality 5%

H Distant Spread 0.3% → Usually Fatal

I Upper Lip 2% → EXCISION PLUS REMOVAL NECK NODES → 5 Year Cure 50%

A In some people, a cancer may develop on the lower lip, after many years' exposure to the sun.

B The first evidence of pre-cancerous change is a rough scale (leukoplakia) that forms over much of the lower lip. Seventy-five percent of patients with lip cancer will have leukoplakia on the rest of the lip. If leukoplakia persists, the skin of the lip is removed by an operation called "lip shave" to prevent the roughened skin over the lip from becoming cancerous. It leaves only a very slight lip deformity.

C The most common form of lip cancer is a small sore or ulcer that fails to heal. Both radiation and operative excision of a localized lip cancer have the same chance of cure (93%), and both leave about the same type of scar on the lip.

D Lip cancers can spread to lymph nodes below the jaw, but only in 6% of lip cancers are the node sufficiently suspicious to warrant operative excision at the time of removing the lip cancer. Even when these suspicious nodes are removed, cancer will actually be found in only 20%.

E Recurrences appear with equal likelihood in the lip at the site of the original tumor or in the lymph nodes in the neck.

F Recurrences in the lip appear within two years in 30% of the cases, indicating the slow growth rate of these cancers. When they occur, treatment by wide excision of the recurrence with all surrounding involved tissue provides a 90% chance of cure.

G When cancer recurs in the neck, 50% will show up within five years. Such recurrence is treated by removing all the lymph nodes on one side of the neck (see "Radical Neck Dissection," page 70), plus radiation. This operation may also require removal of part of the jawbone and floor of the mouth if the tumor invades these areas. Expected death rate in this operation is 5%, and the complication rate is 20%. The chance of cure is 50%, however, even of this recurrent tumor.

H In about 3 of every 1,000 patients with lip cancer, there is spread of the tumor to the lungs. When this happens, death usually occurs within a year.

I Cancer of the upper lip is rare (2% of lip cancers), but when it occurs, it is likely (50% of the time) to involve the lymph nodes in the neck. Excision or radiation of this rare type of lip cancer, combined with removal of the lymph nodes in the neck, gives a 50% chance of cure.

13. Radical Neck Dissection

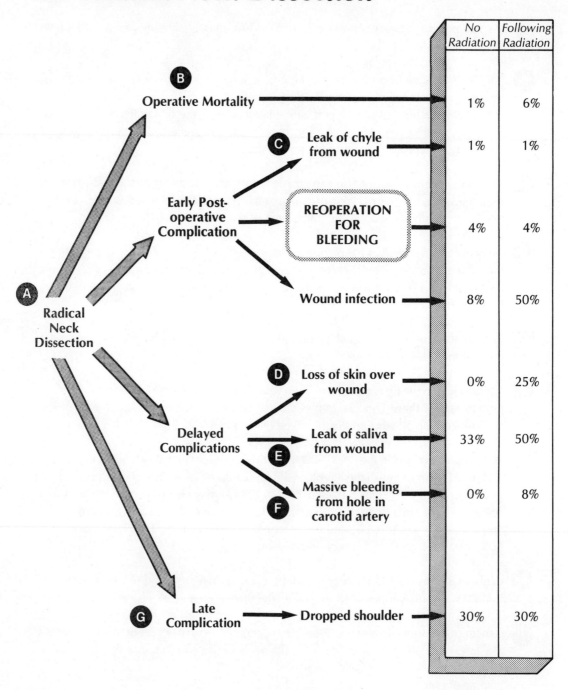

	No Radiation	Following Radiation
Operative Mortality	1%	6%
Leak of chyle from wound	1%	1%
REOPERATION FOR BLEEDING	4%	4%
Wound infection	8%	50%
Loss of skin over wound	0%	25%
Leak of saliva from wound	33%	50%
Massive bleeding from hole in carotid artery	0%	8%
Dropped shoulder	30%	30%

A — Radical Neck Dissection

B — Operative Mortality

Early Post-operative Complication

C — Leak of chyle from wound

Delayed Complications

D — Loss of skin over wound

E — Leak of saliva from wound

F — Massive bleeding from hole in carotid artery

G — Late Complication — Dropped shoulder

A This operation, which removes all the lymph nodes along the side of the neck, is usually performed to remove cancer that has spread to these nodes from tumors that arise in the head and neck. The operation requires general anesthesia and hospitalization of about ten days.

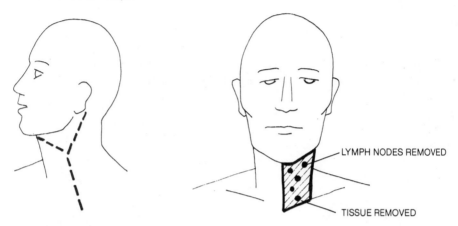

LYMPH NODES REMOVED

TISSUE REMOVED

SKIN INCISION *(Left)* AND TISSUE REMOVED *(Right)* IN RADICAL NECK DISSECTION

B Serious complications following neck dissection are usually not the result of removing the lymph nodes, but are associated with removing the main tumor in the tongue or voice box (larynx).

C A thin-walled tube empties lymph from the intestine into the large veins at the base of the neck. Rarely (about 1% of the time) this duct is damaged by neck dissection and leaks lymph fluid for a week or two. Except in rare instances, it ultimately closes spontaneously.

D It is necessary to free a broad area of skin to remove all the lymph nodes in this operation. Particularly following previous x-radiation, this may result in loss of some blood supply to the skin, which then may not heal properly. The defect in the wound usually closes within a few weeks. If it does not, skin from the chest can be brought up as a flap to cover the defect.

E Saliva may leak out of a wound from the back of the mouth when this area forms one boundary of the operative field. It usually closes without the need for reoperation, but may require several weeks to do so.

Radical Neck Dissection

F One possible cause of death after neck dissection is torrential bleeding resulting from a hole developing in the big artery in the neck that supplies the brain (carotid artery). Such a complication is more likely if there has been radiation of the tumor area before the operation.

G A large nerve (XI) controlling one of the muscles that elevates the shoulder runs through the tissue that is usually removed in this operation. In 30% of these operations, this nerve is removed to insure a better chance for curing the tumor. This produces some weakness, which can be compensated for somewhat by exercises.

IV
Chest

1. Nodule in the Lung

(SOLITARY PULMONARY NODULE)

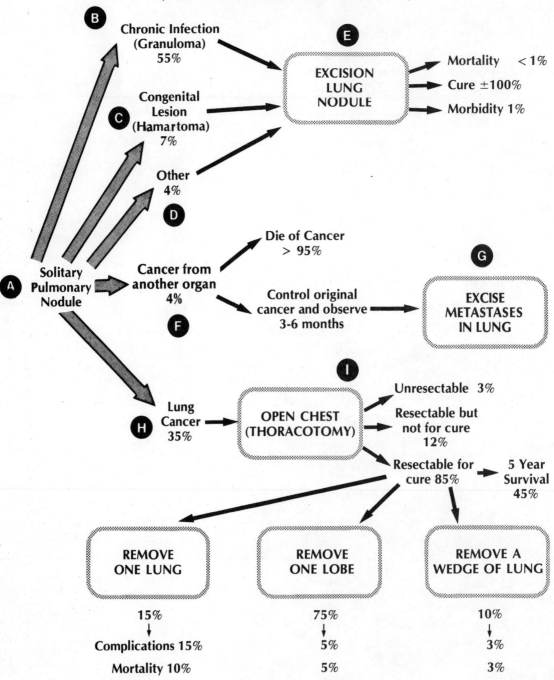

B Chronic Infection (Granuloma) 55%

C Congenital Lesion (Hamartoma) 7%

D Other 4%

A Solitary Pulmonary Nodule

E EXCISION LUNG NODULE
- Mortality < 1%
- Cure ±100%
- Morbidity 1%

F Cancer from another organ 4%
- Die of Cancer > 95%
- Control original cancer and observe 3-6 months

G EXCISE METASTASES IN LUNG

H Lung Cancer 35%

I OPEN CHEST (THORACOTOMY)
- Unresectable 3%
- Resectable but not for cure 12%
- Resectable for cure 85% → 5 Year Survival 45%

REMOVE ONE LUNG
15%
↓
Complications 15%
Mortality 10%

REMOVE ONE LOBE
75%
↓
5%
5%

REMOVE A WEDGE OF LUNG
10%
↓
3%
3%

A What can a person look forward to when the startling news is given him that a routine chest X-ray examination shows a spot on the lung? No previous symptoms, no problems, just a spot on the lung on the X-ray film. The main questions that arise are, "Is it cancer?", "Should it be removed?", and "Is it curable?"

The incidence of each of the several diseases that can produce such a lesion in the lung depends heavily on factors such as the age and past history of the patient, his smoking history, whether he has lived in areas where certain fungus disease are common, etc. The figures given on the diagram are averages for all adults living in the United States, most of whom smoke.

Many diagnostic tests are usually performed on a patient with a solitary pulmonary nodule. But in a large percentage of cases, the chest is opened and the nodule removed with a rim of lung tissue around the mass. Microscopic examination of the tissue gives the exact diagnosis.

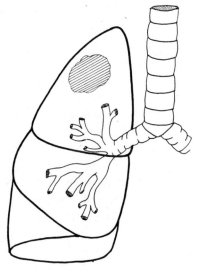

NODULE IN UPPER PART OF RIGHT LUNG

B Chronic lung infections by tuberculosis and two fungus diseases (histoplamosis and coccidiomycosis) are common in certain parts of the United States. Each of these three infections are likely to produce a solitary nodule in the periphery of the lung. However, the X-ray shadows of the lesions due to these infections often contain flecks of calcium and occasionally have a hole or cavity in the center, signs that occur in only about 4% of lung cancers. If the nodule is tuberculosis, the patient is placed on anti-tuberculosis drugs for a year after operation. There is less than a 1% chance of spread or progression of the tuberculosis.

Nodule in the Lung

C A fraction (7%) of such lesions will turn out to be normal lung cells packed together in an abnormal fashion. This is called a hamartoma and is *not* cancer. Once excised, these hamartomas are cured.

D A variety of cysts, abnormal formations of blood vessels, and blood clots can occasionally appear on a chest X-ray examination as spots on the lung. If excised, they too are cured.

E The operation removing these benign (non-cancerous) lesions requires general anesthesia and a hospital stay of five to ten days. It seldom has any mortality. The likelihood of complication is actually less than in opening the abdomen.

F Cancers from other organs often spread through the blood stream to the lung, where they usually grow very quickly. These are called pulmonary (lung) metastases.

G Occasionally, after all of a tumor from the rectum, breast, or uterus has been removed, only a single nodule will appear on the X-ray film of the lung. Usually, more tumor will show up within a few weeks, but if after three to six months no more tumor appears, it is justified to remove the solitary tumor nodule. There is a 30–50% chance that this may be curative in these highly selected circumstances.

H The great concern before operation is whether the spot on the X-ray film represents lung cancer. The chances are 33% that there will be certain features of the nodule on the X-ray film that are characteristic of cancer, but no one can be certain of the diagnosis until the nodule is removed. These nodules are in the periphery of the lung and usually are not able to be seen through a bronchoscope nor have a piece taken from them for a biopsy examination. Roughly 35% of the time, however, cells loosened from the tumor and recovered from washings from that area of the lung can be recognized as cancer when examined under the microscope. In some peripheral lung lesions (about 50%), a needle can be stuck through the chest wall into the tumor and a specimen obtained for diagnosis. This procedure has a 10% risk of minor complication.

I Even if the suspicious nodule turns out to be lung cancer, there is a 90% chance that in this favorable location, away from the center of the lung, the tumor will be localized in that part of the lung and, therefore, resectable for cure. Such peripheral lung cancers have a five times better chance for cure than tumors located near the central part of the lung. How much lung must be removed (segment, lobe, or the entire lung) depends on the location and size of the tumor, but removing one lobe is adequate in 75% of patients. Almost half (45%) of the patients with lung cancers discovered on routine chest X-ray studies as a symptomless nodule are alive without disease five years later.

2. Lung Cancer

A Lung cancer is the commonest cancer and the most common cancer causing death in the United States. Its relationship to smoking is beyond challenge. Less than 5% of patients who develop lung cancer will be alive five years later.

B In over one-half (55%) of these patients, the tumor will have spread so widely at the time the tumor is first diagnosed that it is clearly incurable. Many procedures are used to diagnose lung cancer, including many types of X-ray examinations and studies of cells in the sputum or from the lungs. Each of these studies is helpful, but none, of course, is infallible, either in precisely identifying cancer or ruling it out.

LOOKING AT TUMOR IN RIGHT LUNG THROUGH A
BROCHOSCOPE

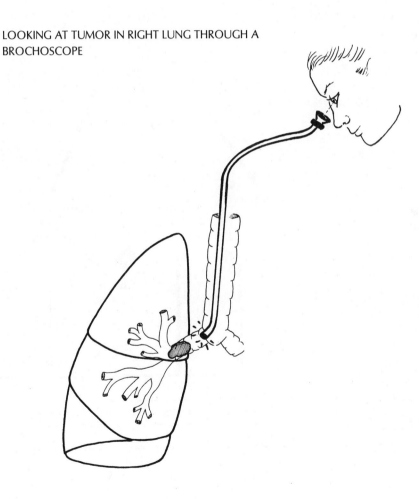

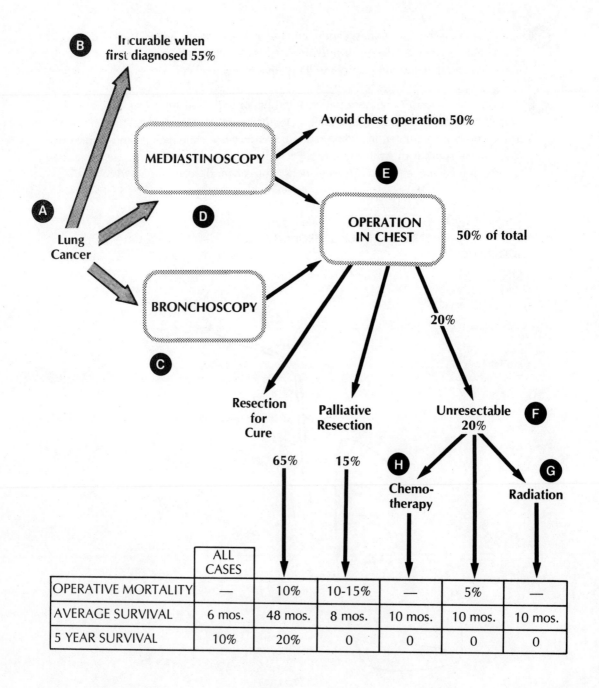

	ALL CASES	65%	15%		20%	
OPERATIVE MORTALITY	—	10%	10-15%	—	5%	—
AVERAGE SURVIVAL	6 mos.	48 mos.	8 mos.	10 mos.	10 mos.	10 mos.
5 YEAR SURVIVAL	10%	20%	0	0	0	0

C Key to diagnosis is bronchoscopy, which consists of looking down the windpipe (trachea) into the lung with a flexible, lighted tube. Such a procedure identifies about 80% of lung cancers.

D A similar procedure (mediastinoscopy) involves passing a lighted tube under the breastbone (sternum) to determine if the tumor has spread beyond the lung into the central part of the chest. If a tumor is found in the mediastinum, it greatly reduces the chance of cure. Mediastinoscopy avoids the need to open the chest in almost one-half of the cases.

E The chest is opened (thoracotomy) in about half of all patients in whom lung cancer is suspected. Of these, 20% have such a wide extension of the tumor at the time of thoractomy that all of it cannot be removed. Fifteen percent have spread, but it is thought prudent to remove part of the tumor to provide relief from painful symptoms. In 65% of patients, the lung containing all visible tumor can be removed. These patients are considered resectable for cure.

F Those with unresectable tumors live an average of ten months. None survive five years.

G Radiation will make most lung cancers temporarily shrink in size. It may not prolong survival, but X-ray therapy can often give relief from pain due to tumor or open up airway passages in the lung blocked by tumor. It makes life more pleasant for the weeks that remain.

H Combinations of drugs that are toxic to the tumor have temporarily benefited up to 45% of patients with lung cancer. But the average survival in unresectable tumors given these drugs is only between three and seven months.

3. Pulmonary Lobectomy

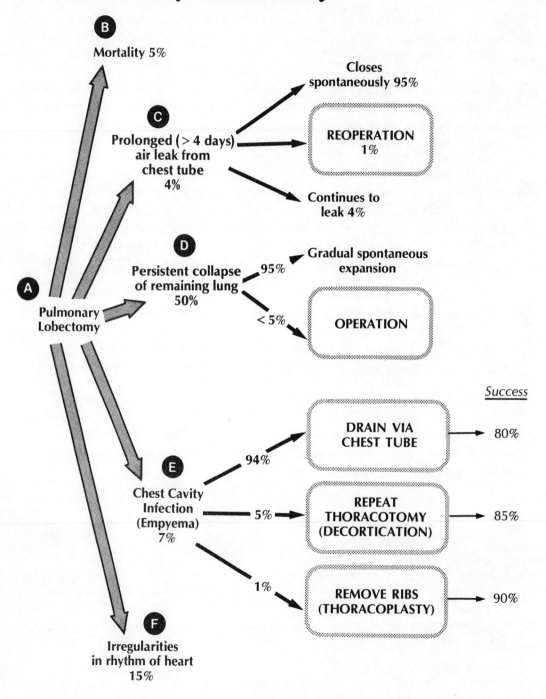

B Mortality 5%

C Prolonged (> 4 days) air leak from chest tube 4%

Closes spontaneously 95%

REOPERATION 1%

Continues to leak 4%

A Pulmonary Lobectomy

D Persistent collapse of remaining lung 50%

Gradual spontaneous expansion 95%

OPERATION < 5%

Success

E Chest Cavity Infection (Empyema) 7%

DRAIN VIA CHEST TUBE 94% → 80%

REPEAT THORACOTOMY (DECORTICATION) 5% → 85%

REMOVE RIBS (THORACOPLASTY) 1% → 90%

F Irregularities in rhythm of heart 15%

A Each of the two lungs in a human being is divided into lobes: two on the left, three on the right. A lobe can be removed (lobectomy) without injuring the remaining lobes of the lung. Tumor or persistent infections are the usual indication for such lobectomy. A normal person has a great deal more lung tissue than he needs for normal activity, so removal of a lobe usually will not produce any difficulty in breathing, even with moderate exercise. Cigarette smokers often destroy more than one lobe's worth of lung over a period of twenty to thirty years.

B The chance of dying from lobectomy averages about 5%, but varies with the age and general condition of the patient and the reason—such as infection or tumor—for which the lobe was removed. Heart disease impairs the ability of a person to tolerate lobectomy.

C Following lobectomy, a tube attached to a water bottle is usually left in the chest for a few days to drain air and fluid. For a day or two, it is expected that some blood-tinged fluid and air will drain out the tube into the bottle. Sometimes, the leak continues and the tube cannot be removed so soon. In 95% of cases, the leak gradually decreases and stops without need for other treatment. In an occasional case (about 1%), the leak is so large that within the first few days the surgeon chooses to reopen the chest and tries to reclose the leaking airway or resect more lung tissue. Chances of success are slim (roughly 20%).

D Within a few days after one lobe is removed, the remaining lung expands and fills the space left by the excised tissue. In about 5% of cases, this may not occur, requiring prolonged drainage. Clearing out the airway through a tube placed from the mouth into the lung (bronchoscope) may be helpful. In at least 5% of cases, a second operation is necessary to expand the lung or stop a leak of air that prolongs lung collapse.

E If the lung does not expand to fill the chest cavity, or if air continues to leak through the remaining lung, an infection (empyema) will develop within the chest.

F Removing a lobe from the lung requires operating around the nerves that help control heart rate and rhythm. In about 30% of cases, irregularities in heartbeat occur in the first few days after operation. Except in the elderly, these are of little consequence and can usually be controlled by drugs that specifically affect the rate and rhythm of heartbeat.

4. Cancer of the Esophagus

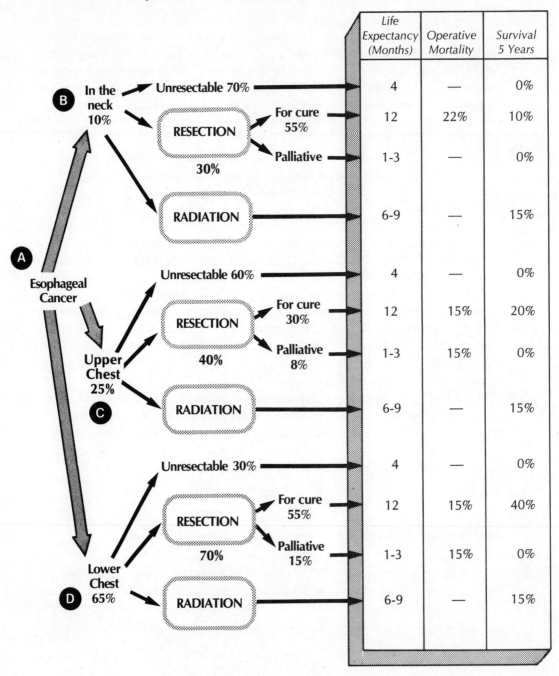

	Life Expectancy (Months)	Operative Mortality	Survival 5 Years
B — In the neck 10%			
Unresectable 70%	4	—	0%
RESECTION 30% — For cure 55%	12	22%	10%
RESECTION — Palliative	1-3	—	0%
RADIATION	6-9	—	15%
Upper Chest 25% (C)			
Unresectable 60%	4	—	0%
RESECTION 40% — For cure 30%	12	15%	20%
RESECTION — Palliative 8%	1-3	15%	0%
RADIATION	6-9	—	15%
Lower Chest 65% (D)			
Unresectable 30%	4	—	0%
RESECTION 70% — For cure 55%	12	15%	40%
RESECTION — Palliative 15%	1-3	15%	0%
RADIATION	6-9	—	15%

A — Esophageal Cancer

A The esophagus is a muscular tube that carries food from the mouth down the neck and through the chest to the stomach. Typical symptoms of esophageal cancer are pain and difficulty in swallowing. It frequently occurs in alcoholics and smokers. Esophageal cancers are arbitrarily classified by their location; those in the neck (upper third), those within the chest (middle third), and those low in the chest near the entrance of the

TUMOR AT LOWER END OF ESOPHAGUS

esophagus into the stomach. Regardless of location or method of treatment, the chances for cure are poor compared to most diseases or even most tumors.

B The 10% of cancers in the neck (upper third) are mostly (70%) inoperable when first identified, usually because they have grown into nearby organs that cannot be removed. Radiation given over four to six weeks provides moderate relief from pain in 60% of patients for the six to nine months of life that remains. There is an occasional reported five-year cure in these cancers.

C Sixty percent of middle-third esophageal cancers have spread beyond chance of cure when first recognized. But in the other 40%, the tumor appears to be still limited to the esophagus, and an attempt at operative removal of the tumor is justified. If the tumor can be removed, a variety of procedures can be used to bring the stomach or various segments of intestine up into the chest to carry food across the area of the removed esophagus. These are major operations and have both a high operative mortality (about 15%) and a considerable chance for complication (about 20%). This is a big price to pay for a slim chance (10-15%) of cure, but one that many patients want to take. As with upper-third esophageal cancers, radiation is helpful in relieving symptoms, either with or without operation.

D Most esophageal cancers (about 65%) are in the lower third of the chest, just above where the esophagus joins the stomach. Seventy percent of these esophageal cancers appear not to have spread when first diagnosed at operation. About one-half of these tumors are resectable, and of these, 15–40% of patients will survive five years. After removing the lower part of the esophagus containing the cancer, the stomach is brought into the chest and connected to the esophagus. The chances of complications after operation in a lower-third lesion are about 10%. Hospitalization is usually two to three weeks.

5. *Esophagitis*

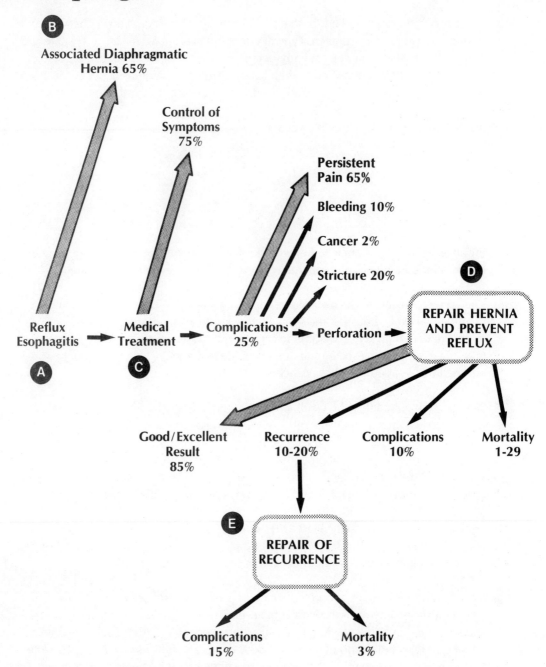

A The path from the esophagus into the stomach is supposed to be a one-way street. Food and stomach contents are normally kept from reversing direction and coming back up into the esophagus by a delicate one-way valve mechanism that protects the pristine lining of the esophagus from corrosive stomach contents. When this valve goes awry,

INFLAMATION AT LOWER END OF
ESOPHAGUS

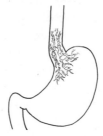

the lower esophagus becomes bathed in irritative acid secretion that refluxes or regurgitates from the stomach. Such inflammation of the esophagus is called esophagitis. It causes discomfort in the lower chest (heartburn), particularly in fat people who lie down after eating large meals or drinking a lot of alcohol.

B In two-thirds of the patients suffering from esophagitis, the protective sphincter mechanism (there really isn't a visible valve) is destroyed because the stomach slips through an enlarged hole or hernia in the diaphragm into the chest where it does not belong. Treatment of esophagitis is principally directed to restoring the mechanism to stop reflux of stomach contents into the esophagus and to repair the diaphragmatic hernia that encourages reflux.

C Three-quarters of the patients with symptoms of esophagitis can be controlled by non-operative means such as losing weight, eating small meals, not lying down after meals, and taking certain medicines. But in the remaining 25%, the symptoms persist and are so severe that operation is required.

D Operations to cure both the hiatus hernia and the related reflux esophagitis can be performed either through the chest or through the abdomen. They differ in detail, but have in common 1) preventing the return or reflux of stomach contents into the esophagus by 2) restoring the one-way valve mechanism and 3) repairing the hernia defect in the diaphragm. Mortality is very low (1% or less) and good to excellent relief of symptoms can be expected in 85% of cases. Recurrence of symptoms occurs in about 15% of patients after operation.

E Reoperation for recurrence of esophagitis is a good deal more difficult than the original procedure, and the chance of technical complication a great deal higher—about 15%.

Esophagitis

After prolonged irritation and inflammation, scars will develop around the lower end of the esophagus, narrowing (or stricturing) this normally soft, pliable, muscular tube. Gradually, a firm scar constricts the esophagus and stops the passage of bulky food, such as chunks of meat.

The longer esophagitis goes untreated the greater the likelihood of developing a stricture. Short strictures may resolve if an operation stops regurgitation. But a tight scar, 5 centimeters or more in length, will never resolve and requires operative repair. Various types of operations are available to relieve the obstruction. They have about a 90% chance of giving relief of obstruction and about the same likelihood of relieving pain. There is a 50% chance that the patient will have some residual discomfort, even though the obstruction from the stricture has been relieved.

6. Pulmonary Embolus

A Following an operation, the normally liquid blood develops a tendancy to form clots throughout the entire body, not just in the operative wound. In about 3% of patients, clots will form in the leg veins, causing swelling and tenderness of the calf. This is called thrombophlebitis (see "Postoperative Thromobophlebitis" page 150). In fact, various complicated tests can detect small clots in 25% of patients following a big operation, but symptoms appear in only about 3%. The immediate danger of such a clot is that a part might break loose from the leg and be swept up the veins to the heart and then out into the lung. Such a pulmonary (lung) embolus can block one of the big arteries in the lung.

B There is a 15% chance that a patient with thrombophlebitis will throw a pulmonary embolus. A pulmonary embolus occurs following 0.5% of all major operations. All the same factors that tend to produce thrombophlebitis—obesity, length of immobilization in bed, advanced age, cancer, operations on the legs and hip, and heart disease—also increase the chance of a pulmonary embolus.

C A pulmonary embolus usually causes sudden pain in the chest and the coughing up of a little blood. However, about 10% of the time there are no warning symptoms of embolism until the patient has sudden chest pain and dies within minutes, before any treatment can be begun.

D If a patient recovers from the first pulmonary embolus, there is a 30% chance that he will develop another if not treated with anticoagulants. There is a 20% chance of death with this second embolus.

E When because of obesity, heart disease, and other factors, a patient is at high risk for thrombophlebitis and pulmonary embolus after operation, it sometimes is thought prudent to give small doses of the anticoagulant heparin before any symptoms of clots in the leg or embolus to the lung develop. Prophylactic or preventive treatment decreases the tendency of blood to clot, providing some protection against thrombophlebitis, but not interfering with the clotting necessary to prevent bleeding from the operative wound. Such small doses of heparin will diminish the likelihood of thrombophlebitis from 3% to 1% and, similarly, decrease the chance of pulmonary embolus from 0.5% to 0.2%. The risks of this preventive treatment are so low that the partial protection against thrombophlebitis and pulmonary embolus are often worthwhile.

There are few instances in medicine where an accepted course of treatment so clearly depends on the probabilities of benefit with and without use of a drug.

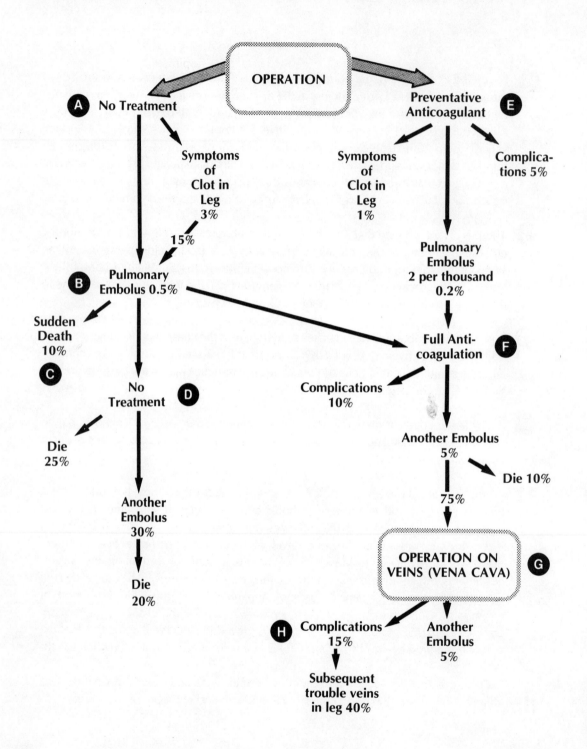

OPERATION

A No Treatment

Symptoms of Clot in Leg 3%

15%

B Pulmonary Embolus 0.5%

Sudden Death 10%

C

No Treatment **D**

Die 25%

Another Embolus 30%

Die 20%

Preventative Anticoagulant **E**

Symptoms of Clot in Leg 1%

Complications 5%

Pulmonary Embolus 2 per thousand 0.2%

Full Anti-coagulation **F**

Complications 10%

Another Embolus 5%

Die 10%

75%

OPERATION ON VEINS (VENA CAVA) **G**

H Complications 15%

Another Embolus 5%

Subsequent trouble veins in leg 40%

F Once a pulmonary embolus develops, the patient usually is given larger doses of heparin immediately. The 10% chance of increased bleeding that occurs is worth the comparative protection that is afforded against developing another often fatal pulmonary embolus. The chance of a second pulmonary embolus developing in an untreated patient who has had one pulmonary embolus is 30%; if treated will full doses of heparin, the risk is 5%.

G If such a pulmonary embolus occurs despite good anticoagulant drug treatment, about 75% of patients would be well advised to have the large vein in the abdomen (vena cava) interrupted by one of several types of operations. This prevents clots that have formed in the leg veins from reaching the lungs. In the other 25% change in drug regime is judged to be safer than operation.

H None of the operations designed to block the vena cava (application of clips, tying the vein, or placing an umbrella device within the vena cava) absolutely guarantees that still another embolus will not occur, but it clearly cuts the risk. In this high-risk group, where two pulmonary emboli already have occurred, only 5% will develop a third after interrupting the vena cava. Following operation, there is about a 40% chance that a patient will have some swelling of the legs, due to interruption of the vein that returns blood from the lower part of the body to the heart. These complications are the small price paid for a life-saving procedure to prevent further pulmonary emboli.

V
Heart

1. Irregular Heartbeat

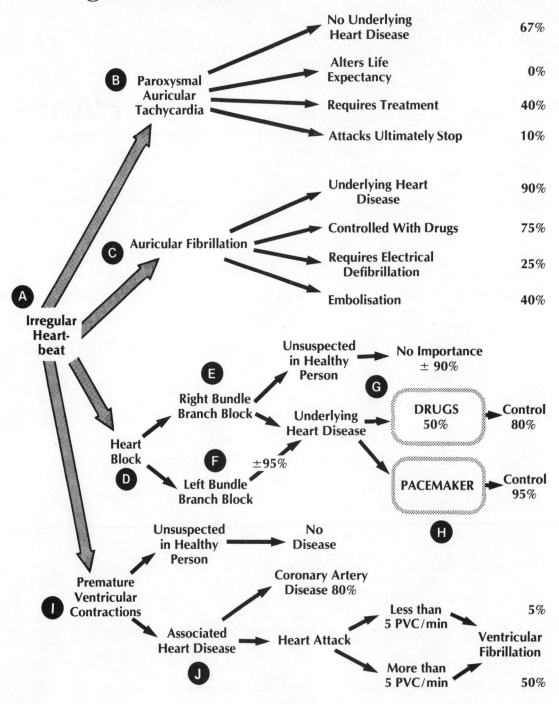

A Irregular Heartbeat

B Paroxysmal Auricular Tachycardia
- No Underlying Heart Disease — 67%
- Alters Life Expectancy — 0%
- Requires Treatment — 40%
- Attacks Ultimately Stop — 10%

C Auricular Fibrillation
- Underlying Heart Disease — 90%
- Controlled With Drugs — 75%
- Requires Electrical Defibrillation — 25%
- Embolisation — 40%

D Heart Block
E Right Bundle Branch Block
- Unsuspected in Healthy Person → No Importance ± 90%
- Underlying Heart Disease
F Left Bundle Branch Block — ±95%
G DRUGS 50% → Control 80%
H PACEMAKER → Control 95%

I Premature Ventricular Contractions
- Unsuspected in Healthy Person → No Disease
J Associated Heart Disease
- Coronary Artery Disease 80%
- Heart Attack
  - Less than 5 PVC/min → Ventricular Fibrillation 5%
  - More than 5 PVC/min → 50%

A The heart normally contracts with a regular rhythm about sixty to one hundred times per minute. This constant beat can be felt as a pulse at the wrist. With exercise, the *rate* speeds up, but the rhythm remains regular. With certain abnormal conditions, the rhythm becomes irregular.

B In paroxysmal atrial tachycardia, there is a sudden onset of a quickening of the heart rate, frequently occurring without any known stimulation in young and middle-aged people. Two-thirds of the time, it does not signal any underlying heart disease, nor does it threaten life or shorten life expectancy. It is more a nuisance than a threat. Attacks usually last a few minutes to a few hours if untreated and then suddenly stop. Pressure on the neck, just beneath the jaw, will stop about 60% of attacks. After one attack, there is a 90% likelihood of having others. It is impossible to predict how often they will occur. About 40% of patients will require medication (80% effective) to stop or prevent these bothersome attacks. Hospitalization, except for diagnosis, is needed in only 5% of cases. The attacks gradually disappear in about 10% of cases, usually within two to five years.

C Atrial fibrillation involves a completely irregular beat of the atria. This causes an irregular contraction of the ventricle and the pulse, as felt at the wrist or over the chest. Ninety percent of people with atrial fibrillation have some underlying heart problem: 10%, congenital heart disease, 40%, rheumatic fever, and 50%, coronary arterio–sclerosis. A diseased mitral valve from rheumatic heart disease often leads to atrial fibrillation (see "Mitral Valve Insufficiency," page 113). About 15% of people who have had heart attacks develop atrial fibrillation. Atrial fibrillation seldom spontaneously disappears (less than 5% of total cases).

There is a 40% chance that a person with chronic atrial fibrillation, on the basis of mitral valve disease, will throw off a clot from the heart that will lodge in an artery and block circulation to a leg, the brain, or some vital organ. Treatment with the anticoagulant drug coumadin will reduce this risk to less than 5–10%.

Treatment of atrial fibrillation with drugs, such as quinidine or digitalis, successfully converts or slows the pulse to normal in about 75% of cases, depending on the severity of the underlying disease. Shocking the heart with an electrical defibrillator to stop the irregular beat is indicated in about 25% of cases and is successful about 90% of the time. Repeat defibrillation is required in about 25% of cases. Such treatment requires hospitalization for several days.

In about 10% of patients with atrial fibrillation, there is no known underlying heart disease. Attacks last for several minutes to three days before ending spontaneously. About 60% of these patients will have no further problems, while about 5% will develop chronic artrial fibrillation and will require drug therapy.

D Occasionally, a patient unaware of any heart problem is told by his physician, after an examination, that he has heart block. This means that there is a block or delay of some kind in the normal transmission of the nerve impulse from the top part of the heart (the atria) to the lower part of the heart (the ventricle) where the blood is propelled to the periphery. Such a block is like a delay in transmission of a message along a telegraph line. The pulse rate may also become abnormally slow.

E The cord of nerves (main bundle) that signals the ventricles to contract and pump blood divides near the top of the heart, sending one branch to the right side of the heart (the right bundle) and the other to the left ventricle (the left bundle). Interference in transmission of the right bundle (right bundle branch block) is usually of little significance or threat to the patient. This is particularly true if the finding of block is made on a routine physical examination in a patient who has no symptoms of heart disease. Two percent of blacks and 0.5% of whites inherit such a disorder and are usually unaware of it. It does not interfere with good health.

F Block of the nerves to the left ventricle (left bundle branch block) is usually much more serious. About 95% of patients will have some underlying heart disease, such as rheumatic fever (25%), arteriosclerosis (50%), or an infectious disease (15%). It is a common complication of certain types of heart attacks, such as myocardial infarctions (see "Heart Attack," page 99).

G About 50% of patients with moderate block of the left bundle will require treatment with drugs, such as atropine or isoproterenol, that effect transmission along the special nerves in the heart. This will control the block in about 80% of patients.

H About 10% of the time, the block will cause such a slow and irregular heart rate and rhythm that it will cause dizzy or black-out spells. These may last up to twenty seconds. During this time, the heart either does not beat at all or does so ineffectively. Since about 60% of such episodes are fatal within a year if untreated, such patients will require the immediate insertion of an electronic pacemaker to sustain a normal heartbeat. This procedure is successful about 90% of the time (see "Cardiac Pacemaker," page 107).

I A premature (early) ventricular contraction (known by the acronym PVC) is a sudden extra beat of the heart that interrupts its normal, stately, steady rhythm. This occurs several times a day in almost everyone and goes without notice, unless someone happens to be taking an electrocardiogram (EKG) reading. It is obviously the most common arrhythmia or heart irregularity. It is often precipitated by drinking too much coffee, by smoking cigarettes, or by being excessively fatigued. Such PVCs often go away when the stimulant is stopped. Such occasional PVCs occurring in otherwise healthy people must be differentiated from those resulting from serious heart disease.

J Premature ventricular contractions (PVCs) occuring after a heart attack or in a patient with angina pectoris (see "Angina Pectoris," page 96) are serious. Of these patients, 80% have coronary artery disease with or without evidence of a recent heart attack. If after a heart attack, there are less than five PVCs per minute as registered on the electrocardiogram (EKG), there is about a 10% chance of developing a life-threatening ventricular fibrillation. If there are more than five per minute, the chances are 50%.

Treatment with drugs, such as intravenous Xylocaine, effectively reduces this risk to about 5%. PVCs are one of the abnormalities treated very successfully in a coronary care unit after a heart attack.

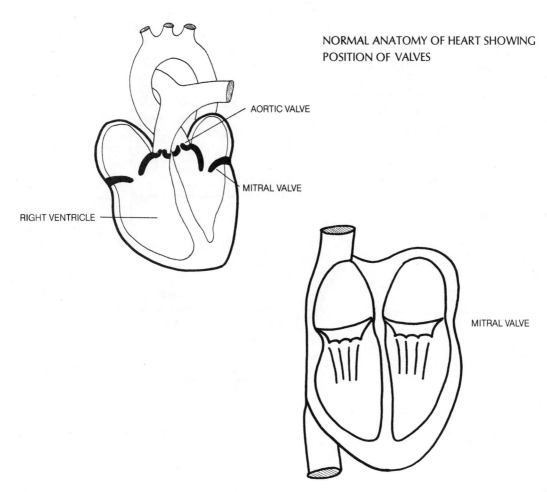

NORMAL ANATOMY OF HEART SHOWING POSITION OF VALVES

AORTIC VALVE

MITRAL VALVE

RIGHT VENTRICLE

MITRAL VALVE

2. Angina Pectoris

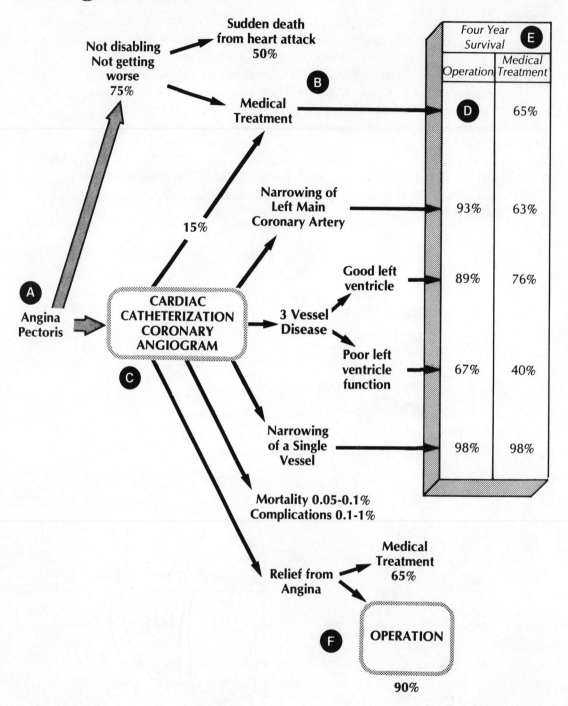

Four Year Survival

	Operation	Medical Treatment
Medical Treatment	D	65%
Narrowing of Left Main Coronary Artery	93%	63%
Good left ventricle	89%	76%
Poor left ventricle function	67%	40%
Narrowing of a Single Vessel	98%	98%

Sudden death from heart attack 50%

Not disabling Not getting worse 75%

A — Angina Pectoris

B

CARDIAC CATHETERIZATION CORONARY ANGIOGRAM

C

15%

3 Vessel Disease

Mortality 0.05-0.1%
Complications 0.1-1%

E

Relief from Angina

Medical Treatment 65%

F — OPERATION

90%

A In cold weather, a middle-aged jogger sometimes gets cramps if the blood supply to his leg muscles is inadequate. When he stops and rests, the discomfort soon goes away. The same thing may happen to his overactive heart muscle if its blood supply through the coronary arteries cannot furnish the energy it needs. Pain in the heart muscle is called angina pectoris and is usually due to narrowing of the coronary arteries by arteriosclerosis. In addition to being very unpleasant, angina serves as a warning that there is disease in the coronary arteries, which may lead to a heart attack (see "Heart Attack," page 99).

B Angina will stabilize for a time, getting no worse nor better in about 75% of patients. Treatment is then by rest, limitation of exercise, and drugs that decrease the work of the heart. Once angina has begun, mortality on medical treatment is 5% per year. A heart attack occurs as the first indication of coronary artery disease before any symptoms of angina in 50% of patients.

C Before considering an operation to control angina, a special X-ray study (coronary angiogram) is performed to visualize the condition of each of the major arteries nourishing the heart and to measure the heart function. This requires either an incision over the artery in the arm or a puncturing of the artery in the groin and the passage of a catheter up the artery to the base of the heart, opposite the openings of the coronary arteries. The procedure has its risks (see "Cardiac Catheterization," page 102). In about 15% of cases, no operation will be advisable after the studies have been completed.

D Coronary artery bypass is now one of the most common operations performed in the United States. With heart-lung machine support for one to three hours (see "Cardio-Pulmonary Bypass," page 104), a length of vein from the leg is sewn between the aorta and a coronary artery beyond the point of narrowing or block. From one to five such grafts may be used. The new bypass graft delivers a good supply of blood to the heart muscle, which before operation was working without adequate nutrition and, like the jogger's calf muscles, was developing cramps (angina). The chances of operative mortality from aorto-coronary bypass are 1–3%, and the likelihood of a heart attack in the early days following operation is about 5%. Hospitalization is for one to three weeks. The vein grafts can be expected to remain open for over five years in about 85% of cases.

E There is still some disagreement as to when coronary artery bypass should be advised. With narrowing or occlusion of the left main stem coronary artery, four-year survival on medical treatment is 63%. After coronary artery bypass, equivalent survival is

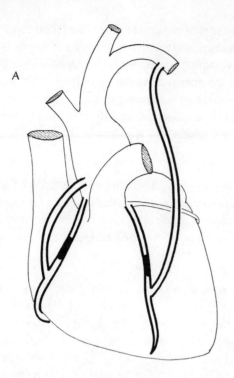

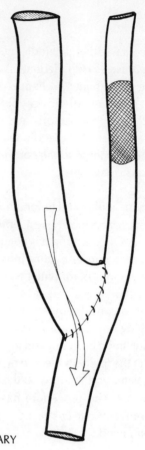

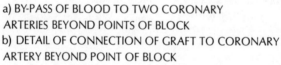

a) BY-PASS OF BLOOD TO TWO CORONARY
ARTERIES BEYOND POINTS OF BLOCK
b) DETAIL OF CONNECTION OF GRAFT TO CORONARY
ARTERY BEYOND POINT OF BLOCK

increased to 93%. There can be little doubt that in this situation the bypass operation increases the expected longevity. The evidence of benefit by operation is slightly less when performed for disease in three coronary arteries (89%, four-year survival with operation as opposed to 76% without). There is no appreciable benefit in survival if only one coronary artery is involved with disease.

F Even when life is not prolonged by coronary artery bypass, the operation usually dramatically decreases the crippling discomfort of angina. About 60% of patients after operation are completely free of discomfort, and in another 30% the pain is greatly diminished. Only in about 10% is there no benefit. With the best non-operative drug treatment and restriction of exercise, 30% of patients still have angina. After operation, only 10% of patients may have no improvement in their anginal attacks. If for no other reason, many think these statistics are sufficient to recommend the operation.

3. Heart Attack

A What is popularly known as a heart attack is in fact narrowing of a coronary artery to a point where the needs for blood in that area of heart muscle suddenly cannot be met. This results in severe irregularities in heartbeat. In almost half the patients, this is fatal before they can be taken to a hospital. Ambulance technicians can occasionally save a patient by restoring a good heartbeat.

If the patient survives the immediate irregularities in heartbeat, there is usually an area of heart muscle that has a precarious blood supply. If some of the heart muscle fibers die, the condition is called an infarct.

B With prompt treatment with oxygen, with morphine given to relieve pain, and with intravenous fluids, 85% of patients with a heart attack (myocardial infarct) will quickly respond, and 40% will get well with a relatively uncomplicated hospital course. An occasional patient (about 1%) will have a second sudden infarct without warning while in the hospital and die.

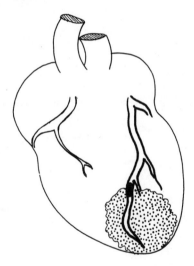

DEAD HEART MUSCLE BEYOND BLOCK
IN A CORONARY ARTERY

C Hospitalization for those with an uncomplicated course is one to three weeks. Thereafter, with good medical care, the mortality from heart trouble is 6% in the first six months and then 6% per year thereafter.

Other expected complications after an infarct are angina in 50% of cases, heart failure in 15%, and a swelling (aneurysm) of the previously softened (infarcted) part of the heart muscle in 5%.

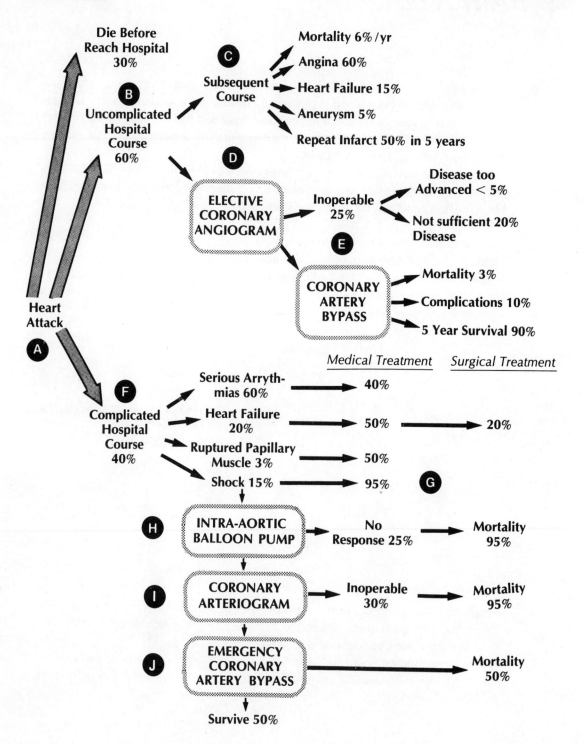

**Die Before
Reach Hospital
30%**

C **Subsequent
Course**

Mortality 6% / yr

Angina 60%

Heart Failure 15%

Aneurysm 5%

Repeat Infarct 50% in 5 years

B

**Uncomplicated
Hospital
Course
60%**

D

**ELECTIVE
CORONARY
ANGIOGRAM**

Inoperable
25%

Disease too
Advanced < 5%

Not sufficient 20%
Disease

E

**CORONARY
ARTERY
BYPASS**

Mortality 3%

Complications 10%

5 Year Survival 90%

**Heart
Attack**

A

Medical Treatment   *Surgical Treatment*

F

**Complicated
Hospital
Course
40%**

Serious Arryth-
mias 60% — 40%

Heart Failure
20% — 50% — 20%

Ruptured Papillary
Muscle 3% — 50%

Shock 15% — 95% **G**

H

**INTRA-AORTIC
BALLOON PUMP**

No
Response 25% — Mortality
95%

I

**CORONARY
ARTERIOGRAM**

Inoperable
30% — Mortality
95%

J

**EMERGENCY
CORONARY
ARTERY BYPASS**

Mortality
50%

Survive 50%

D Six weeks or more after the heart attack, selected patients should undergo visualization of the coronary arteries by a special X-ray examination (coronary arteriogram, see "Cardiac Catheterization," page 102) to determine whether an operation on the coronary arteries is advisable. In about 85% of the cases, it is.

E Coronary artery bypass operation is done through an incision in the chest and the use of an artificial heart-lung machine (see "Cardio-Pulmonary Bypass," page 104). Mortality of the operation in the patient who has had a previous heart attack is about 3%, and the complication rate 10%. Once the patient has left the hospital, the expected five-year survival is about 80%.

F The hospital course is complicated in about 60% of patients following a heart attack. Irregularities in heart rhythm can be recorded in almost every such patient, but serious ones that threaten life occur in about 60%. Of these with life-threatening irregularities, 40% will die. Treatment in a coronary care unit can save the lives of some patients who develop such cardiac arrhythmias. Heart failure occurs in 15–30% of patients following a heart attack, the wide variance depending on the size of the original infarcted area of heart muscle. Mortality with this complication is 30%.

G In about 10–15% of patients with a heart attack, there will be no immediate response to good emergency-department treatment. The patient will remain in shock (low blood pressure) despite all treatment. Without extraordinary methods of treatment, over 95% of these patients will die within a few hours.

H A device called an intra-aortic balloon pump is now used in such desperately ill and all-but-doomed persons. It quickly improves the condition in 75% of such patients. This procedure consists of threading a large caliber catheter from an artery in the groin up toward the heart. A balloon at the end of the catheter inflates inside the aorta with each beat of the heart and improves heart function. This device can be used to support a patient for a week or more if necessary.

I If a patient in cardiogenic shock after a myocardial infarct responds to intra-aortic balloon assist, he then can be taken to the X-ray unit, where an emergency coronary arteriogram can be performed to determine whether emergency coronary artery surgery is advisable. In 70% of cases, it is.

J Emergency coronary artery bypass (see E above) has a 40–50% chance of saving these desperately ill patients who otherwise would have essentially no other likelihood for survival.

4. Cardiac Catheterization

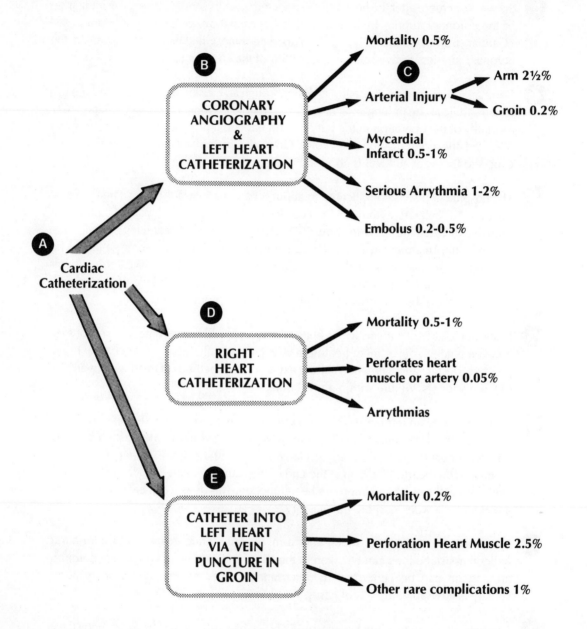

A Cardiac Catheterization

B CORONARY ANGIOGRAPHY & LEFT HEART CATHETERIZATION

Mortality 0.5%

Arterial Injury

C Arm 2½%

Groin 0.2%

Mycardial Infarct 0.5-1%

Serious Arrythmia 1-2%

Embolus 0.2-0.5%

D RIGHT HEART CATHETERIZATION

Mortality 0.5-1%

Perforates heart muscle or artery 0.05%

Arrythmias

E CATHETER INTO LEFT HEART VIA VEIN PUNCTURE IN GROIN

Mortality 0.2%

Perforation Heart Muscle 2.5%

Other rare complications 1%

A Until a few years ago, the doctor had to guess what was going on inside the heart by trying to interpret the sounds he heard through a stethoscope and looking at the shadows thrown by the heart on a photographic film by X-rays. Often, he was wrong. Then came cardiac catheterization, and with it, the highly developed art of diagnosing heart disease changed to a science. This technique consists of passing a small tube or catheter from an artery or vein in the arm or leg into the heart. It provides four kinds of information:

- Abnormal holes can be probed and identified under X-ray visualization
- Pressures can be studied in all parts of the heart, detecting abnormal changes and measuring heart function
- Blood samples can be withdrawn to determine concentrations of oxygen, which may indicate abnormal openings within the heart.
- The catheter can be used for injecting dye, which shows up on X-ray examination.

Catheterization takes from a half to three hours and can be done under local anesthesia. The patient is usually kept in the hospital for several days.

B Coronary angiography is a technique to photograph and study the coronary arteries that feed blood to the heart muscle. The catheter is passed to the base of the heart as in any cardiac catheterization. Dye that shows up on X-ray examination is then injected into the openings of the coronary arteries and the outlines of the arteries photographed. The outlines of the cavities of the heart can also be demonstrated to measure the pumping function of the heart.

C There is a 2% likelihood of some complication associated with cardiac catheterization. This includes a 0.2–2.5% chance of damaging the small artery at the point where the catheter is inserted, a 1–2% likelihood of producing irregularities in heart rhythm, and a 1% chance of some actual damage to the heart muscle. Other rare injuries include reaction to the drug.

D The right side of the heart can easily be catheterized by passing the catheter into the heart from a vein in the arm or in the groin. Possible complications include irregularity in heartbeat and actual perforation of the heart muscle by the catheter. The hole is so small that this usually causes no difficulty and rarely requires treatment.

E In very small infants, it occasionally is judged safer to pass a catheter into the left side of the heart from the right side. The catheter is passed into the right atrium from a simple intravenous approach. When the catheter is correctly positioned under X-ray visualization, it is pushed through the muscular wall or septum into the left heart and the study is performed.

5. Cardio-Pulmonary Bypass (Heart-Lung Machine)

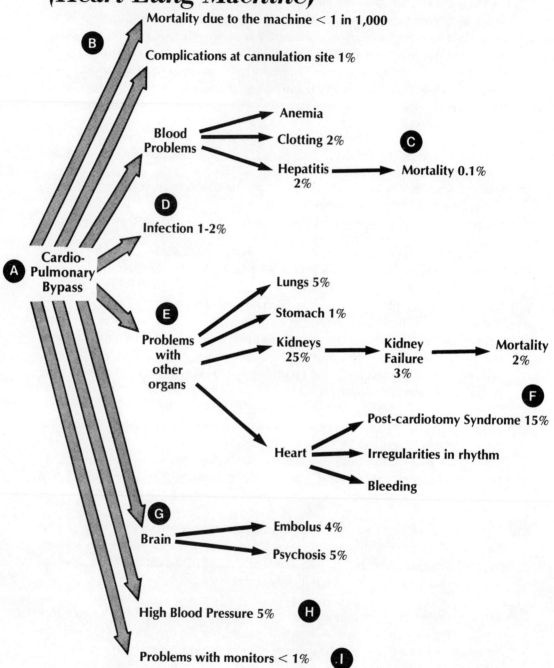

B Mortality due to the machine < 1 in 1,000

Complications at cannulation site 1%

A Cardio-Pulmonary Bypass

Blood Problems → Anemia

Blood Problems → Clotting 2%

Blood Problems → Hepatitis 2% → **C** Mortality 0.1%

D Infection 1-2%

E Problems with other organs → Lungs 5%

Problems with other organs → Stomach 1%

Problems with other organs → Kidneys 25% → Kidney Failure 3% → Mortality 2%

F

Problems with other organs → Heart → Post-cardiotomy Syndrome 15%

Heart → Irregularities in rhythm

Heart → Bleeding

G Brain → Embolus 4%

Brain → Psychosis 5%

High Blood Pressure 5% **H**

Problems with monitors < 1% **I**

A The heart-lung machine (or cardio-pulmonary bypass) is a mechanical device that assumes the function of both the heart and lungs for the one to four hours needed for open-heart surgery.

The heart is primarily a pump. The lungs add oxygen to the blue venous blood, turning it red. The pump oxygenator performs both functions, providing enough oxygenated blood to support the body while the heart is stopped and excluded from the circulation. This provides the surgeon a bloodless field in which to work inside the heart.

This device is complicated, and as with any machine, there is a small but definite risk in its use. The rare death during open-heart operation is almost never (less than 0.1%) due to a malfunction or a complication of the machine.

B Blood is withdrawn through a tube (cannula) placed in the big veins leading to the heart, and after oxygenation, the blood is reintroduced into an artery in the groin or the chest. The sites of cannulation may, in about 1% of the operations, either leak or complicate blood flow to the leg into which the tubes are placed.

C The machine is filled with about two liters of blood or a salt solution before being attached to the patient. There is always a risk that some of the blood used to prime the machine may contain the virus that causes hepatitis, just as it occasionally does after any blood transfusion. The chance of getting hepatitis is about 2%. The pump and the oxygenator both tend to destroy tiny fragments in the blood called platelets, which are important in blood clotting. The likelihood of this being of any clinical importance is about 2%.

D Infection occurs in less than 1% of the cases, but is always a threat, particularly when the pump oxygenator must be used for long periods.

E Pumping for over four hours leads to some difficulty in breathing after operation in 5% of patients. Most patients, after open-heart surgery and pump oxygenator support, are kept on a mechanical ventilator for one to four days after operation. Occasionally (less than 1%) these patients bleed from a "stress" stomach ulcer following the surgery.

F One to five weeks following operation, 15% of patients may develop fever and feel generally ill. The exact cause of this syndrome (called the post-cardiotomy syndrome) is unknown, but seems related to opening the sac (pericardium) that surrounds the heart and not to the use of a pump oxygenator. The symptoms go away within a few weeks, but meanwhile are a nuisance.

Cardio-Pulmonary Bypass

G During the operation, clots or bubbles of air can very rarely (less than 1% of the time) be thrown off from the machine to lodge in the brain where they may damage some nerve cells. Usually the signs of such a complication soon clear without treatment.

Patients may become temporarily psychotic following operation, particularly if they have to remain long in the intensive care unit where constant nursing attention may interfere with uninterrupted sleep. This is probably not associated with the heart-lung machine, but rather with the post-operative environment.

H High blood pressure, for a few hours, occurs in about 5–10% of patients after the use of the pump oxygenator. Its exact cause is unknown, but usually it goes away spontaneously.

I Following operation the surgeon has to keep watch over many aspects of heart, kidney, and lung function in order to anticipate and treat complications. But with the introduction of each tube or cannula or monitoring wire goes a slight risk of infection, bleeding, introduction of air, having the cannula break off in the blood vessel, or even an electrical shock from a short-circuited wire. The likelihood is small (less than 1%) but significant.

6. Cardiac Pacemaker

A Each muscle fiber of the heart is like a tiny spring that contracts every time it receives a pulse of electric current. Normally, this occurs eighty to ninety times a minute. The normal heart regulates its own best rate of beating. A number of diseases, however, may so interfere with the heart rate that its pumping action fails and life is threatened. When this occurs, an electrical wire attached to a small electronic pacemaker may be used to stimulate the heart to beat at a regular, predetermined rate. For periods of up to three weeks, pacemakers using a power source outside of the body can be used. But for prolonged pacing, a sterile electronic unit about the size of a package of cigarettes is placed under the skin of the chest. The pacemaker contains small long-life batteries and a generator, which sends a pulse of electric current through wires to the heart muscle eighty times a minutes. This stimulates the heart to contract in a regular fashion. The operation itself is performed in a hospitalized patient under local or general anesthesia and usually takes about a half to one-and-a-half hours.

B Earlier pacemaker batteries had to be replaced every few months. Current lithium batteries have a projected life of up to fifteen years, and atomic (plutonium) devices, a theoretical life of thirty-five years.

C Minor irregularities in heart rate and rhythm (arrhythmias) occur in almost all patients during insertion of the wires and when the heart begins to be paced artificially. All but about 10% of such irregularities subside within three to four days, and the heart settles down to the rate and rhythm supplied by the electrical unit.

D Infection occurs in about 5% of cases where the wires are passed into the heart through the veins (transvenous pacemaker). When the wires are sewn directly onto the heart muscle (epicardial leads) at operation, the infection rate is less than 1%, both upon original insertion of the wires and when the generator has to be replaced.

E Sterile fluid accumulates around many foreign substances placed under the skin, and the bulky pacemaker packs are no exception. The probability of effusion depends upon whether the wires are passed into the heart cavity (endocardial leads), where the effusion rate is 2%, or if the wires stop on the surface of the heart at operation (epicardial leads), where the chance of effusion is 20%.

F As with any mechanical device, there can be failures. Rarely (less than 5% of the time), it is with the generator itself. More frequently, a wire breaks, becomes dislocated, or builds up a scar and interferes with electrical transmission of the impulse at the point

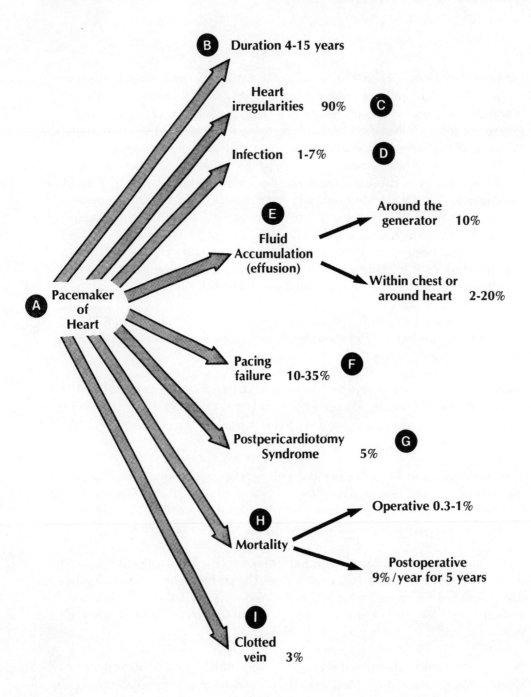

B Duration 4-15 years

Heart
irregularities   90%   C

Infection   1-7%   D

E

Fluid
Accumulation
(effusion)

Around the
generator   10%

Within chest or
around heart   2-20%

A Pacemaker
of
Heart

Pacing
failure   10-35%   F

Postpericardiotomy
Syndrome   5%   G

H

Mortality

Operative 0.3-1%

Postoperative
9%/year for 5 years

I

Clotted
vein   3%

where the wire connects with heart muscle. When these complications occur, it is usually necessary to replace the wire.

G Two to ten weeks following any kind of operation on the heart, the patient may become sick, have a slight fever, and develop some fluid around the heart. No one knows what causes the condition, which is called the postpericardiotomy syndrome. It occasionally occurs after pacemaker insertion and may take weeks to disappear, but ultimately it does.

H Pacemakers are put into people who have sick hearts and have a chance of dying during the manipulation. Chance of mortality at the time of insertion is about 0.3–1%. The 9% per year mortality rate thereafter reflects the underlying heart condition and rarely is due to the pacemaker itself.

I When the wire is passed into the heart through a vein beneath the collarbone, there is a 3% chance the vein will clot. Sometimes, this will require removal of the wire; usually not.

7. *Mitral Valve Stenosis*

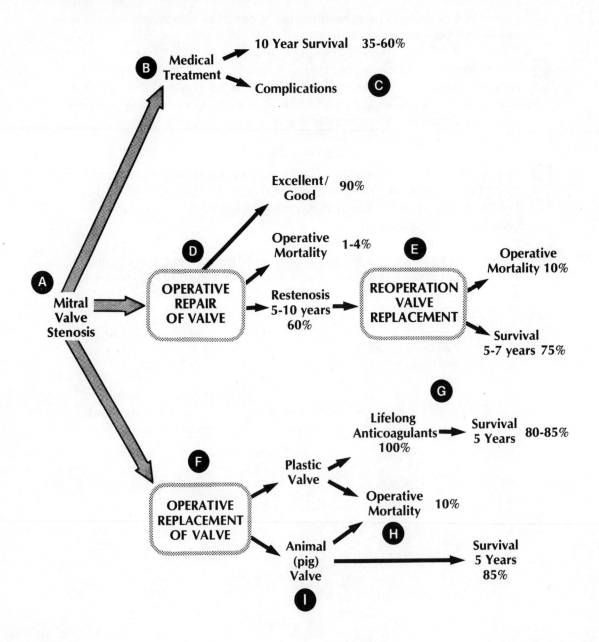

A The mitral valve guards the entrance to the left ventricle. Like electronically operated double doors, it swings open, allowing almost unimpeded entrance of blood to the left ventricle. When the ventricle contracts, the blood catches the doors and slams them shut with a snap, stopping blood from going back toward the lungs and forcing it out the aortic valve to the organs of the body. When the valves become involved with rheumatic fever or arteriosclerosis, the valve opening may narrow and block free blood flow into the left ventricle. Like crowds trying to get out of a theater, there is congestion behind the narrow door, as everyone tries to crowd through the constriction. Behind a constricted (stenotic) mitral valve, blood cells back up and congest the lung.

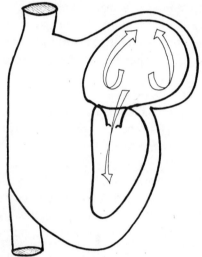

OBSTRUCTION TO BLOOD FLOW FROM LEFT AURICLE DUE
TO MITRAL STENOSIS

B A person with symptoms of mitral stenosis has a 60% chance of living ten years if treated by drugs and restriction of exercise, but the worse the stenosis, the shorter the expectancy. For example, in minimal mitral stenosis (Grade 1) the chance of living ten years is 84%, while it is only 15% in those with tight stenosis (Grade III). Cause of death with mitral stenosis is heart failure in 60% of patients and from a blood clot loosened from the heart in 25%.

C Expected complications during medical treatment of mitral stenosis over a ten-year period include:

- Abnormal heart rhythm (fibrillation): 15%
- Heart failure: 25%
- Coughing up blood: 10%
- Blood clot thrown to brain or other organ: 10%

D The narrowed valve can be repaired under direct vision, using a heart-lung machine (see "Cardio-Pulmonary Bypass," page 104). This is called open valve repair. Closed repair does the same thing, without the use of the pump oxygenator during the operation. Hospital mortality for the two techniques is about equal (0–2%) depending more on the severity of the heart disease than on the operative technique. The likelihood of the mitral valve again growing too narrow is less than 5% if the original operation is done with a pump-oxygenator, compared to the much greater 60% chance of restenosis (recurrent stenosis) following an original closed repair. Which technique is first used depends a good deal on the patient's age.

E There is a 60% chance of restenosis within ten years after mitral valve repair. If the valve is again repaired rather than replaced, there is about a 10% chance of operative mortality, the actual risk depending on the severity of the heart disease. Expectancy for ten-year survival after this second repair for mitral stenosis varies from 50–90%.

F Ultimately, the mitral valve usually becomes so diseased that it cannot be repaired, and it must be replaced with one or several types of available plastic or metal prosthetic valves. An alternative is to substitute a specially processed pig-heart valve. Both operations require pump-oxygenator support while the new valve is sewn in place.

G When a plastic or metal valve is used, the patient must, for the rest of his life, take a drug that slows blood coagulation or clotting (anticoagulant). Taken by mouth, this drug prevents a clot from forming on the plastic valve.

H Operative mortality for mitral valve replacement varies from 5–25%, depending primarily on the condition of the heart.

I When a pig valve is used as a mitral valve replacement, the chances of a clot forming are slight (about 5%). Some surgeons are willing to balance this risk against the 20% threat of bleeding if anticoagulants are used to prevent such clotting. It is the judgment of others that anticoagulants should be used on all patients when any valve substitute is inserted for the mitral valve.

8. Mitral Valve Insufficiency

A The normal, pliable leaflets of the mitral valve flap open to allow blood free entry to the left ventricle. When the heart contracts, they snap shut, stopping blood from going back the wrong way. If the leaflets become thick, stiff, or shortened, they cannot totally close, and blood leaks back through the valve opening. Such a leaky valve is referred to as mitral insufficiency.

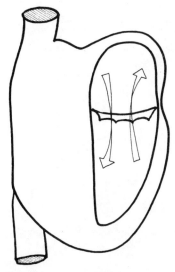

TWO WAY BLOOD FLOW THROUGH A DAMAGED
(INSUFFICIENT) MITRAL VALVE

B Half of patients even with moderate mitral insufficiency can be managed by non-operative means. They have a ten-year survival expectancy of about 20%. People withstand a leaky insufficient valve better than they do one that is narrowed (stenotic, see "Mitral Valve Stenosis," page 110).

C In certain cases, the insufficient valve can be repaired rather than replaced. This is done with the heart open using the pump-oxygenator ("Cardio-Pulmonary Bypass," page 104). The various techniques for repair may involve tightening the ring in which the valve is seated, fixing the diseased leaflets, or repairing the cords that control the spinnakerlike valve leaflets.

D Such valve repair will improve function in 80% of cases. In about 25%, insufficiency will gradually recur and the valve will ultimately have to be removed and replaced.

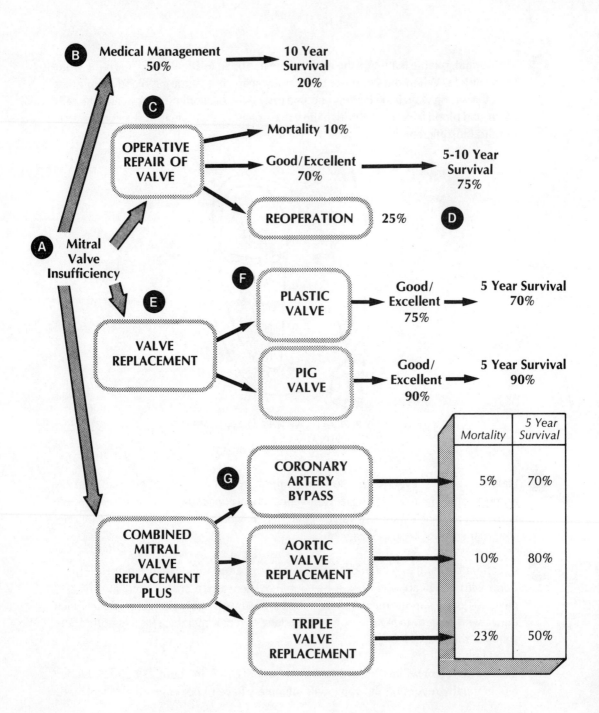

E About 80% of insufficient mitral valves that require operation must be removed and replaced at the first operation. Several kinds of artificial valves are available for replacement. Operative mortality and complication rate are about the same as for valve replacement for stenosis (see "Mitral Valve Stenosis," page 110). Good to excellent results can be expected in 75–90%, with an average five-year survival of about 80%.

F When plastic valves are used, the patient must be maintained the rest of his life on anticoagulants to avoid clot formation on the prosthetic. If a pig valve is inserted, the chances of clotting are much less, but most surgeons now also use anticoagulants. No immunosuppressive drugs are needed.

G An increasing number of older people with mitral valve disease are found to have significant coexisting coronary artery disease at the time the valve is replaced. Adding an additional aorta coronary-artery bypass to improve heart function at the time of replacing the mitral valve causes little additional risk to the operation.

9. Aortic Valve Disease

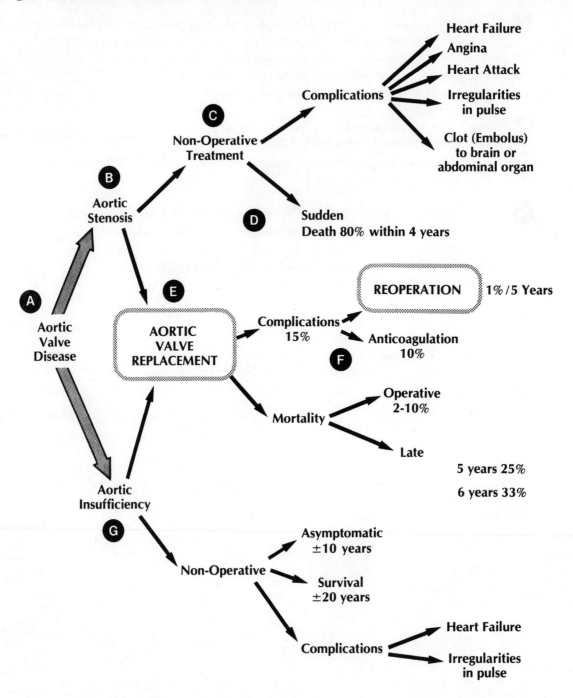

Heart Failure

Angina

Heart Attack

Irregularities in pulse

Clot (Embolus) to brain or abdominal organ

Complications

C Non-Operative Treatment

B Aortic Stenosis

D Sudden Death 80% within 4 years

A Aortic Valve Disease

E AORTIC VALVE REPLACEMENT

Complications 15%

REOPERATION 1%/5 Years

Anticoagulation 10%

F

Mortality

Operative 2-10%

Late

5 years 25%

6 years 33%

Aortic Insufficiency

G Non-Operative

Asymptomatic ±10 years

Survival ±20 years

Complications

Heart Failure

Irregularities in pulse

A The aortic valve lies at the exit of the heart where the blood leaves the left ventricle under high pressure and starts its passage to the organs of the body. The all-important openings to the two coronary arteries are immediately adjacent to this valve. This valve permits blood to squirt out of the heart into the aorta when the heart contracts. But the moment the heart relaxes between each beat, the thin cusps of the aortic valve snap shut with a click and stop blood from backing up into the relaxed left ventricle, resting and gathering itself for the next contraction about three-fourths of a second later. If this crucial valve becomes narrowed (aortic stenosis), it places an abnormal strain on the ventricle. If it does not snap shut when the heart relaxes between beats, a jet of blood will stream back into the left heart during the period it is supposed to be resting. Aortic valve disease may be inherited (congenital) or result from rheumatic fever or arteriosclerosis.

B When the aortic valve opening is narrowed, it is said to be stenotic. This not only puts a strain on the heart muscle trying to push blood through the narrow opening, but it also decreases blood flow to the coronary arteries and to the brain, both of which can have disastrous effects.

C Non-operative treatment of significant aortic stenosis is dangerous. Heart failure is often the first symptom of stenosis in the elderly, and 5% of sudden deaths in old people are due to aortic stenosis. The average life span after the left side of the heart begins to fail because of aortic stenosis is about two years; with right-sided heart failure, death is usually within one year.

D As the stenosis is a silent threat, death may come suddenly without previous warning, due either to an irregularity in the heart rhythm or to a heart attack (see "Heart Attack," page 99) caused by poor coronary artery blood flow. The threat can only be measured accurately by determining the actual size of the aortic valve opening by cardiac catheterization (see page 102).

E Because of this threat, most patients with tight aortic valve stenosis require valve excision and replacement. The operation is performed through an incision in the chest and requires pump-oxygenator support (see "Cardio-Pulmonary Bypass," page 104) for one to two hours. The risk of operative mortality depends mostly on the state of the heart muscle and whether there is coexisting coronary artery disease. In about 15% of patients, coronary artery bypass is also performed at the time of aortic valve replacement. Mortality without coronary artery bypass varies from 2% to 5%. In those who also require bypass, mortality is about 10%. Hospitalization is usually one to three weeks.

F Replacing the aortic valve has the usual risks of any open-heart operation, such as bleeding, infection, myocardial infarct, etc. There is also a 1–3% chance that during the operation a small clot (or embolus) might break loose from the diseased valve site and be swept to the brain. When a plastic or metal valve is used for replacement, the patient must be kept on an anticoagulant for the rest of his life to prevent a clot from forming on the valve. The use of a pig valve reduces the risk of clotting and leads many surgeons not to use anticoagulants.

G The normal aortic valve allows blood to flow only one way. When diseased, it may become insufficient, permitting blood to back up or regurgitate from the aorta into the heart. This is aortic insufficiency (or aortic regurgitation). A person can tolerate aortic regurgitation much better than he can aortic stenosis. The expected ten-year survival of a person with aortic insufficiency treated without operation is 85–95%. When heart failure results from an incompetent aortic valve, the valve should be replaced. The risks and complications of valve replacement are the same as for aortic stenosis.

10. Atrial Septal Defect

A The atrium was the name given to the first room one came to in entering a Roman home. It was the equivalent to the front hall (or mudroom) in a modern home. The atrium of the heart is the first chamber blood gets to as it enters the heart. The atria on each side opens into the ventricles. Ordinarily, there is no connection between the right and left side of the heart. Like a duplex apartment, they lie side by side but without any connecting passages. Certainly, none exists between the atria. In the early stages of embryonic development, the two atria are fused into one chamber. As the fetus develops, a sheet of tissue (septum) grows between the atria separating the right from the left. When this septum does not completely close, a hole connects the two atria,

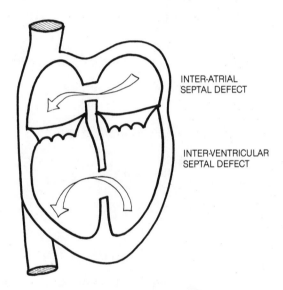

INTER-ATRIAL
SEPTAL DEFECT

INTER-VENTRICULAR
SEPTAL DEFECT

and the infant has an atrial septal defect. Blood then passes from the left atrium to the right, shunting an abnormal amount of blood into the right heart and through the lungs. Atrial septal defect is relatively common, forming about 10% of all congenital heart disease.

B Ninety percent of atrial septal defects are of the uncomplicated type and have few associated defects *outside* of the heart. Mental retardation is rare. About 30% of simple atrial septal defects have associated defects *within* the heart.

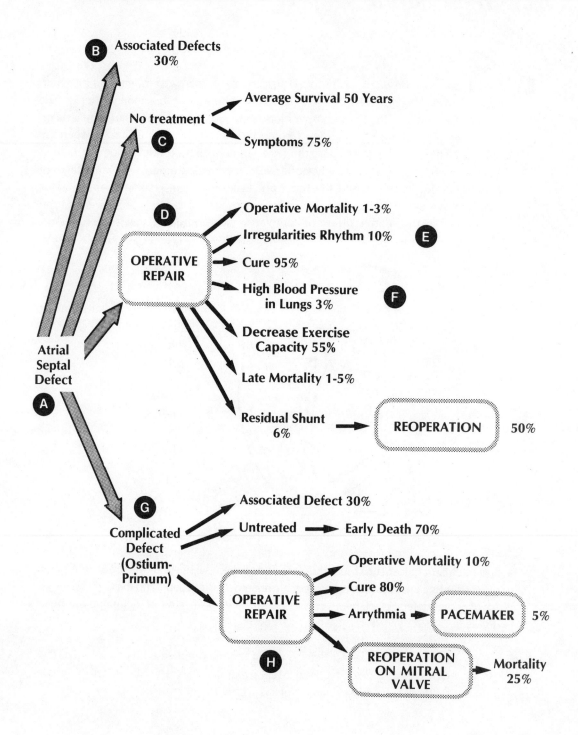

B Associated Defects 30%

No treatment
C
→ Average Survival 50 Years
→ Symptoms 75%

Atrial Septal Defect
A

D
OPERATIVE REPAIR
→ Operative Mortality 1-3%
→ Irregularities Rhythm 10% E
→ Cure 95%
→ High Blood Pressure in Lungs 3% F
→ Decrease Exercise Capacity 55%
→ Late Mortality 1-5%
→ Residual Shunt 6% → REOPERATION 50%

G
Complicated Defect (Ostium-Primum)
→ Associated Defect 30%
→ Untreated → Early Death 70%
→ OPERATIVE REPAIR
H
→ Operative Mortality 10%
→ Cure 80%
→ Arrythmia → PACEMAKER 5%
→ REOPERATION ON MITRAL VALVE → Mortality 25%

C Untreated patients with small atrial defects live reasonably well until as adults they may develop high blood pressure in the lungs that causes difficulty in breathing and heart failure. Operative repair of an atrial septal defect is a satisfying procedure with a low mortality rate (1–3%) and an excellent chance of cure (about 95%). With the patient supported by a pump-oxygenator, the heart is opened and the hole between the atria sewn shut. Hospitalization is about a week, and operative mortality approaches zero in uncomplicated lesions.

About 95% of these patients are totally cured. Sophisticated studies of subsequent exercise tolerance may show some change in about half of these patients, but none in the remainder.

E Temporary irregularities in heart rhythm are common after the operation, due to manipulation of the heart muscle near the area where the nerves pass that control the heartbeat. Rarely (less than 5% of the time) will the irregularities be permanent and require the prolonged use of a pacemaker (see "Cardiac Pacemaker," page 107).

F All the blood that goes through the atrial septal defect to the right side of the heart must circulate for a second time through the lungs. After years of this constant overload, 3% of patients will develop permanent changes in the blood vessels of the lung, which may not reverse when the hole in the heart is closed. This strains the heart and is the main cause of symptoms.

G One in ten patients with a hole in the atrial septum will have a complicated lesion called an ostium primum defect. This involves not only the septum but the nearby mitral valve and the nerves that control heart rate and rhythm. Eight percent of these infants are also mentally retarded. The indications for operation and the mental status of the child must be carefully considered before undertaking operation on these children. Untreated, 70% of such patients with an ostium primum defect die in childhood.

H There is a 10% anticipated operative mortality and a 20% expected complication rate after operative closure of these complicated defects. A pacemaker is required in about 50% of these patients because of heart irregularities after operation. In about 15% of such patients, a second later operation may be required to fix or replace the mitral valve, which always is involved in this complicated lesion.

11. *Patent Ductus Arteriosus*

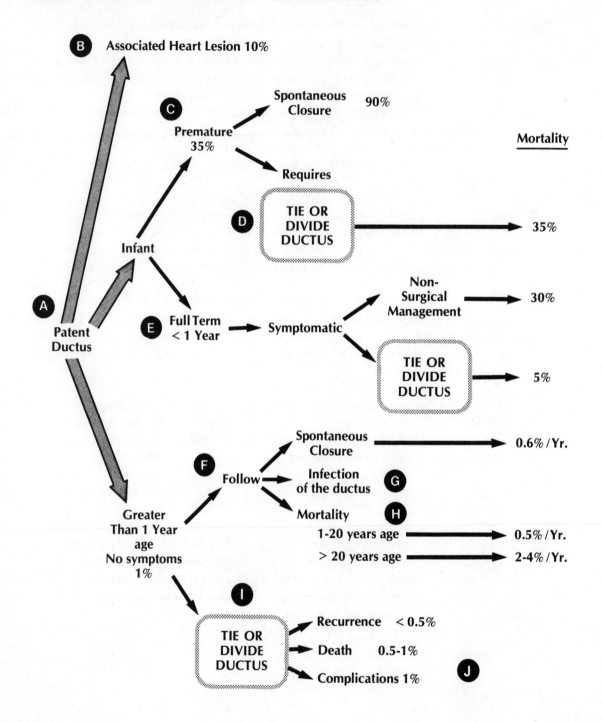

B Associated Heart Lesion 10%

C Premature 35%

Spontaneous Closure 90%

Requires

Mortality

D TIE OR DIVIDE DUCTUS → 35%

A Patent Ductus

Infant

E Full Term < 1 Year → Symptomatic

Non-Surgical Management → 30%

TIE OR DIVIDE DUCTUS → 5%

F Follow

Spontaneous Closure → 0.6% / Yr.

Infection of the ductus **G**

Mortality **H**

Greater Than 1 Year age No symptoms 1%

1-20 years age → 0.5% / Yr.

> 20 years age → 2-4% / Yr.

I TIE OR DIVIDE DUCTUS

Recurrence < 0.5%

Death 0.5-1%

Complications 1%

J

A Before birth, when the lungs are of no use to the fetus in oxygenating blood, a short thick vessel (the ductus arteriosus) bypasses the lungs, short-circuiting blood directly from the heart to the aorta. At birth, this vessel begins to close, almost with the newborn infant's first breath; by the end of a month, it is closed in 90% of infants. Sometimes, however, the ductus remains open (patent) and maintains an abnormal bypass around the lungs. Sooner or later, this will cause heart failure.

B As with many congenital heart defects, a child with a patent ductus has about a 10% chance of having another congenital abnormality.

C Thirty-five percent of infants born prematurely have an open ductus arteriosus, but about 90% will close spontaneously within a few months.

D In less than 10% of such prematures, the ductus will have to be closed surgically in order to relieve the extra work load that it throws on the heart. The high anticipated death rate (about 35%) comes almost solely from the changes that occur in the lungs with this defect or from heart failure, not due to the operation itself.

E Operative mortality is about 5% in the occasional full-term infant with a patent ductus. This is one-seventh that in prematures.

F If the ductus is still open at the end of a year, the chances of its closing are about 0.6% per year. At the end of ten years, about 6% will be closed, but the open ductus takes its toll, and the average length of expected life in a person with an untreated ductus is only thirty-seven years. It is, therefore, wise to operate on a child with a patent ductus in order to prevent future trouble, even though the condition is not causing symptoms at the time.

G There is a 0.5% chance per year that an infection called bacterial endocarditis will develop on a neglected patent ductus. Untreated, such an infection is almost universally fatal. Surgical treatment must include cutting the artery in two, not only tying it, when infection is present. Under these circumstances, there is 5–10% chance of death as a result of the disease and the operation. This provides another reason to ligate a ductus before it becomes symptomatic.

H Untreated, the mortality rate is 0.5% per year for the first twenty years of life, but increases to 2–4% per year thereafter. In adults over thirty, ligation of the ductus may itself become more hazardous.

Patent Ductus Arteriosus

I Except in the presence of infection, there is little difference between the ultimate benefit of simply tieing the ductus and cutting it in two between ties.

J In about 1% of the cases, the nerve to the left vocal cord can be injured in ligating a ductus. This will result in hoarseness.

VI
Vascular

1. Little Stroke

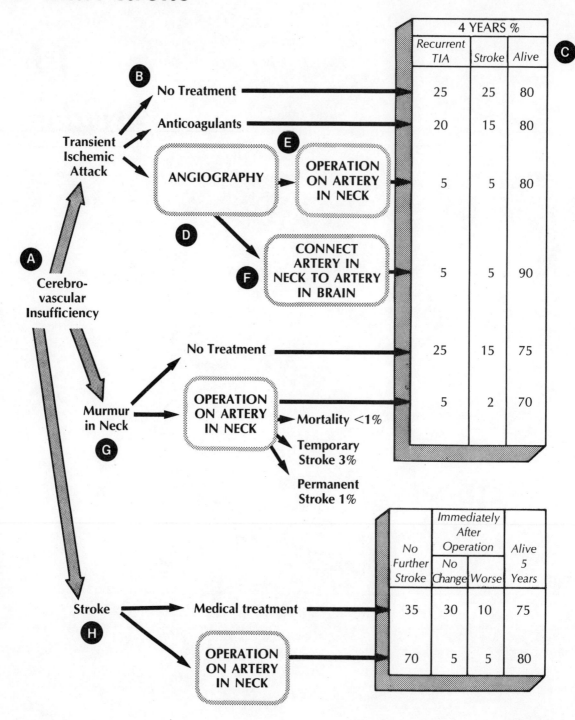

	4 YEARS %		
	Recurrent TIA	Stroke	Alive
No Treatment	25	25	80
Anticoagulants	20	15	80
OPERATION ON ARTERY IN NECK	5	5	80
CONNECT ARTERY IN NECK TO ARTERY IN BRAIN	5	5	90
No Treatment	25	15	75
OPERATION ON ARTERY IN NECK	5	2	70

A Cerebro-vascular Insufficiency

B Transient Ischemic Attack

C

D ANGIOGRAPHY

E OPERATION ON ARTERY IN NECK

F CONNECT ARTERY IN NECK TO ARTERY IN BRAIN

G Murmur in Neck

Mortality <1%

Temporary Stroke 3%

Permanent Stroke 1%

H Stroke

	No Further Stroke	Immediately After Operation		Alive 5 Years
		No Change	Worse	
Medical treatment	35	30	10	75
OPERATION ON ARTERY IN NECK	70	5	5	80

A The brain is extraordinarily sensitive to any decrease in its blood supply. If oxygen or blood flow is shut off even for a minute or two, the person faints. If blood flow stops too long, brain cells begin to die, and when the person recovers consciousness, he may have permanent loss of function in some part of his body. This is a stroke. Sometimes, brain cells are injured but not totally dead after such an episode, resulting in only temporary weakness in a particular part of the body, such as an arm or one leg. This is a transient (temporary) ischemic (bloodless) attack (TIA), or a little stroke. Such decreased blood flow to the brain can result from a narrowing of the big arteries in the neck (carotid arteries) that nourish the brain or from tiny bits of debris thrown off from the roughened or ulcerated lining of the narrowed carotid arteries in a person with arteriosclerosis (hardening of the arteries).

PARTIAL BLOCK OF CAROTID ARTERY SUPPLYING THE BRAIN
INSERT: SHOWS DEBRIS FROM THE LESION BEING SWEPT
TOWARD THE BRAIN

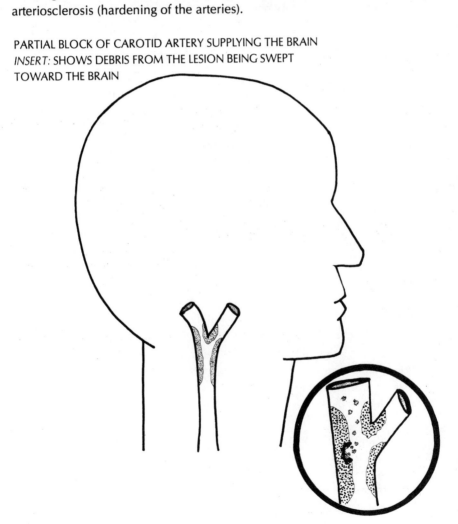

Little Stroke

B Once a person has had an untreated TIA, he has a 25% chance of having another. The chances are 25% that such a stroke will leave him with permanent paralysis within three to five years. Anticoagulants (drugs that slow blood clotting) decrease the likelihood of recurrent TIAs, but these drugs will not increase life expectancy.

C Little strokes are a local symptom of arteriosclerosis, and treatment of the blood vessels in the head and neck does not, of course, alter symptoms or progression of disease elsewhere. At least one-half of those with TIAs have evidence of arteriosclerosis in the coronary arteries, in arteries of the kidney, or in the blood vessels nourishing the legs. Within five years, heart attacks and high blood pressure will have caused 80% of the ultimate deaths of patients who have recovered from successful operation on the carotid arteries for TIAs.

D TIAs can be produced by many diseases other than those of the carotid artery. A series of tests must, therefore, be done on a person who has had a TIA to determine whether the problem is in this artery, and if so, the extent of the disease. One important test involves injecting a dye that outlines on X-ray film the profile of the arteries going to the brain. This study is called an arteriogram or angiogram (see "Cardiac Catheterization," page 102). Other special studies measure blood flow and pressure of blood going to the brain.

E Operation on the carotid artery (carotid endarterectomy) consists of opening the artery and removing the material that has built up on its lining and blocked the free flow of blood. There is about a 95% chance the operation and five to seven day period of hospitalization will be entirely uncomplicated.

The expected death rate from the operation is about 1%. In about 3% of patients, the operation will produce a temporary stroke—similar to the original TIA—which usually clears within a few days. Occasionally after operation, (in less than 5% of patients), there will be some type of permanent paralysis, i.e., a completed stroke. Although this operation decreases the likelihood to only 5% of having further strokes or TIAs, it will not, of course, alter the chance of having a heart attack as a result of generalized arteriosclerosis. Neither will it have any effect on the symptoms of a patient who has had a previous completed stroke where brain cells are already dead before operation. It will not cure the paralysis of a previous stroke, it only *prevents* future trouble.

F When the carotid artery just below the skull is totally closed, it is sometimes possible to bypass this obstruction by connecting a blood vessel from the scalp into one of the arteries within the brain. This operation (extra cranial-intra cranial bypass) has not been performed long enough to predict what the long-term results will be in avoiding subsequent attacks, but the early data suggests that this operation will also prevent TIAs in this group of patients not previously able to be helped by operation.

G Like water flowing over rocks in a stream, blood flowing through a narrowed artery becomes turbulent. This produces a rushing sound (*bruit*—which means noise in French), just like the murmur of a fast-flowing brook. Such a sound can frequently be heard in a narrowed carotid artery before the patient has any symptoms (asymptomatic *bruit*). The first symptom of disease will be a sudden permanent paralysis (complete stroke) in 15% of patients with an asymptomatic *bruit*. A transient attack will be the first symptom in another 25%. On this basis, many vascular surgeons advise studies of blood flow and operation on persons who have a *bruit* (murmur) over the carotid artery, even though there are at that time no neurologic signs resulting from it.

H A completed stroke leaves the patient with permanent nerve loss (usually paralysis), due to death of some brain cells. This is in contrast to temporary nerve damage following a TIA. No operation can restore function to these dead cells or reverse paralysis. Operation performed after a stroke has occurred is intended only to prevent future attacks. There is a 25% probability of a TIA and another 25% chance of a further completed stroke if no operation is done to prevent it. Such an operation to prevent future attacks is usually delayed for six weeks after the stroke.

2. *High Blood Pressure*

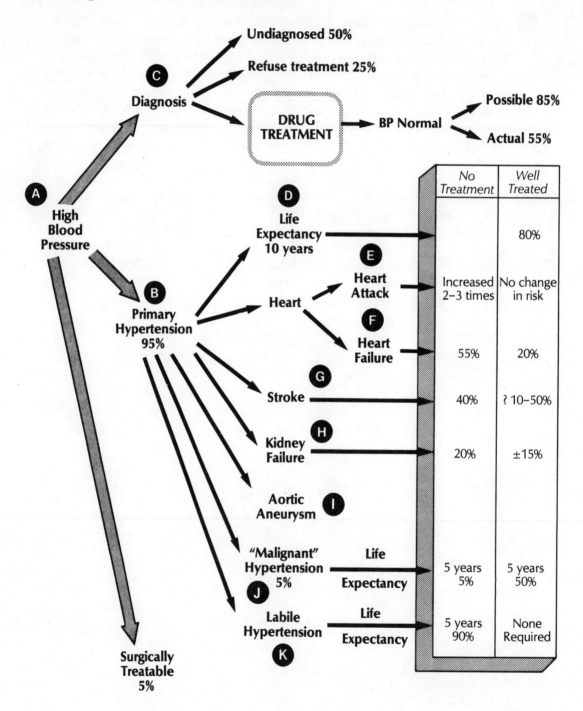

Undiagnosed 50%

Refuse treatment 25%

C Diagnosis

DRUG TREATMENT → BP Normal

Possible 85%

Actual 55%

A High Blood Pressure

C Diagnosis

D Life Expectancy 10 years

E Heart Attack

B Primary Hypertension 95%

Heart

F Heart Failure

G Stroke

H Kidney Failure

Aortic Aneurysm **I**

"Malignant" Hypertension 5%

Life Expectancy

J

Labile Hypertension

Life Expectancy

K

Surgically Treatable 5%

	No Treatment	Well Treated
Life Expectancy 10 years		80%
Heart Attack	Increased 2–3 times	No change in risk
Heart Failure	55%	20%
Stroke	40%	? 10–50%
Kidney Failure	20%	±15%
"Malignant" Hypertension Life Expectancy	5 years 5%	5 years 50%
Labile Hypertension Life Expectancy	5 years 90%	None Required

A There are twenty-three million people with high blood pressure (hypertension) in the United States. Normal pressure is 120/80 millimeters of mercury (mm Hg). The number at the top is called the systolic blood pressure; the one below the line the diastolic pressure. Arterial hypertension is defined as blood pressures at the elbow of over:

- 130/90 mm Hg for men under 45
- 145/95 mm Hg for men over 45
- 160/95 mm Hg for women.

B The cause of hypertension in 95% of people is not really known, and for lack of a better name is called primary hypertension. The higher the pressure, the greater are the chances of complication. The risks are also greater in blacks, in men, in those who are overweight, and in those whose hypertension appeared in childhood.

C Because hypertension often causes no symptoms for the first ten to fifteen years, about 50% of those with high blood pressure are unaware that they have the problem until they begin to have symptoms of heart disease, kidney failure, or a stroke. Of those who know they are hypertensive, as many as 50% will foolishly ignore the fact and refuse treatment, simply because at the moment, they are without symptoms. To do so is to invite disaster, for the ravages of unchecked high blood pressure slowly build up day by day, like an ignored loan at absurdly high interest rates. Unfortunately, the ignored hypertensive loan can never be repaid—only foreclosed. Of those who are treated, about 85% can, if they take their medicine meticulously, return their pressure to near normal.

D Untreated, the mortality rate (chance of dying in any one year) is two to three times that of a person with normal blood pressure. Proper treatment cuts the risk in half. The overall probability of a hypertensive person living ten years after the diagnosis is made is about 30%. If properly treated, the chances are increased to 80%. This is a 65% improvement in the likelihood of surviving and emphasizes the importance of treatment, even while there are no symptoms. The mortality rate is directly proportional to the severity of the hypertension.

Systolic Pressure	Mortality Compared to Normotensive Person	Diastolic Pressure	Mortality Compared to Normotensive Person
Below 127mm Hg	0.8%	68–82mm Hg	0.9%
128–137mm Hg	1.8%	83–87mm Hg	1.20%
158–167mm Hg	2.4%	93–97mm Hg	1.88%
		98–102mm Hg	2.34%

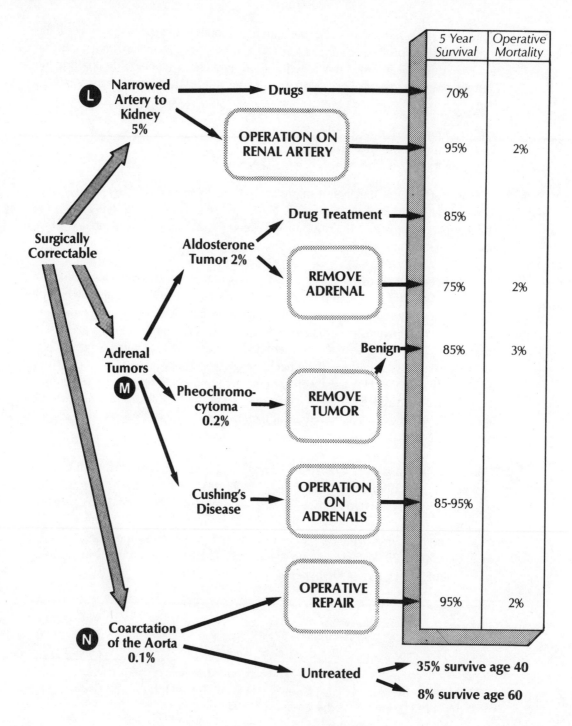

	5 Year Survival	Operative Mortality
Narrowed Artery to Kidney 5% → Drugs	70%	
OPERATION ON RENAL ARTERY	95%	2%
Aldosterone Tumor 2% → Drug Treatment	85%	
REMOVE ADRENAL	75%	2%
Benign	85%	3%
Cushing's Disease → OPERATION ON ADRENALS	85-95%	
Coarctation of the Aorta 0.1% → OPERATIVE REPAIR	95%	2%

Surgically Correctable

Adrenal Tumors

Pheochromo-cytoma 0.2% → REMOVE TUMOR

Untreated → 35% survive age 40

8% survive age 60

For example, a person with a systolic pressure of 160 mm Hg. has a 2.4% greater chance of dying in a given year than a normotensive cohort. The overall five-year survival of those with untreated mild hypertension is 65%; moderate hypertension, 40%; and severe hypertension, only 5%. About a third of hypertensives die of a heart attack, another third of heart failure, and the remainder, of stroke and kidney failure. Even after a person with hypertension develops one of the complications of the disease, treatment improves the chance of survival about three times, so it is well worth starting treatment if the person survives a stroke or heart attack.

E Hypertension increases the risk of coronary artery disease two to three times. About half of the hypertensive patients die of a heart attack, the risk being proportional to the degree of hypertension. Hypertensive patients suffering a heart attack have a five times greater risk of dying from the attack than do those with normal pressures. Once recovered from the attack, controlling the blood pressure with drugs does *not* decrease the chance of another heart attack in hypertensive patients.

F Just as a water pump wears out pumping against a high head of pressure and resistance, so does the heart fail when it has to work against high blood pressure in the arteries. Hypertensives have a five to six times greater likelihood of developing heart failure than do people with normal blood pressure. Good drug treatment will decrease this risk to slightly above normal by decreasing the work load of the heart.

Heart failure occurs in at least half of hypertensive patients during the last five years of their disease. Once such failure occurs, the probability of five-year survival is 50%.

G A person with hypertension has a ten times greater risk of blowing out a thin-walled artery in his brain and having a stroke than does a person with normal blood pressure. About 40% of all untreated hypertensives will develop such a stroke. As with heart attacks, the likelihood of stroke is proportional to the degree of hypertension. Drug treatment that will lower the blood pressure to near normal will decrease the likelihood of a stroke by about 75%. But once a stroke has occurred, even good drug treatment has a questionable effect on changing the risk of another stroke.

H The kidney not only plays an important role in causing high blood pressure, but itself is damaged by the hypertension. About 20% of untreated hypertensives have kidney failure—a risk that is decreased by good drug treatment.

I In an occasional hypertensive patient (about 5%) the big vessel leading from the heart (the aorta) will develop a swelling or blow-out in the chest due to hypertension. Untreated, very few such patients will survive. Treated with drugs and occasionally by later operation, about two-thirds of these patients can be saved.

J Patients with very high diastolic blood pressures (over 130 mm Hg diastolic) may develop an inflammation of their small blood vessels and are said to have "malignant hypertension." This has nothing to do with the malignancy of cancer or any other tumor, but describes the extremely bad course of this disease. Without treatment, only a few patients will even survive two years. At ten years, less than 3% of such patients are still alive. But with good treatment, survival at ten years is 50%.

K Some people have normal blood pressures most of the time, but occasionally are in the hypertensive range. On repeated examination, the blood pressure may be normal. This is called labile hypertension. Although no treatment is needed and survival is 90% in five years, such people have a much greater risk of ultimately developing sustained or constant hypertension than do others without labile hypertension.

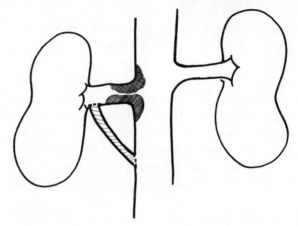

ARTERIAL GRAFT BY-PASSING A BLOCK IN ARTERY SUPPLYING
THE RIGHT KIDNEY

L A narrowed artery to a kidney starves it of its normal blood supply. Such obstruction is usually caused by arteriosclerosis. In response, the kidney releases a substance that raises blood pressure throughout the body as though it were trying to restore its accustomed blood supply. High blood pressure caused by disease of the arteries supplying the kidney is called renovascular hypertension. It is uncommon, and numerous tests must first be performed before operation is undertaken to improve blood flow to the kidney. Widening the narrowed artery leading to the kidney or bypassing the stricture has an 80% chance of reducing the hypertension within a few weeks. Occasionally, removing the kidney will cure hypertension if the other kidney is normal.

M The two tiny but powerful adrenal glands lie immediately above each kidney. Three kinds of adrenal tumors, each secreting a different hormone, will produce high blood pressure. Operations to remove these tumors can be expected to correct hypertension in 75–95% of patients, with a mortality of about 1–2%.

N An occasional child is born with a narrowing (or coarctation) of the large artery (aorta) near its emerging point from the heart. This is called coarctation of the aorta. If the constriction is not corrected it causes hypertension. Operation is performed through the chest, has a low mortality (2%), and will correct the hypertension in about 85% of children with coarctation. In adults where the hypertension has been present for some time, the response may not be quite so good.

3. Abdominal Aneurysm

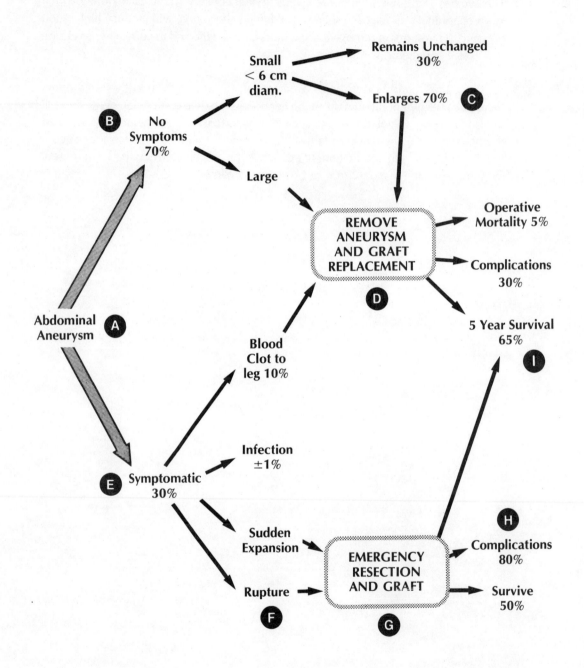

Small < 6 cm diam.

Remains Unchanged 30%

Enlarges 70% **C**

B No Symptoms 70%

Large

Abdominal Aneurysm **A**

E Symptomatic 30%

Blood Clot to leg 10%

REMOVE ANEURYSM AND GRAFT REPLACEMENT **D**

Operative Mortality 5%

Complications 30%

5 Year Survival 65% **I**

Infection ±1%

Sudden Expansion

Rupture **F**

EMERGENCY RESECTION AND GRAFT **G**

H Complications 80%

Survive 50%

A The big artery that carries blood from the heart to the abdomen and legs is located at the back of the abdominal cavity near the backbone and is called the aorta. With advancing age and arteriosclerosis (hardening of the arteries), the aorta may, like a balloon, enlarge and form a pulsating swelling. This is called an aneurysm.

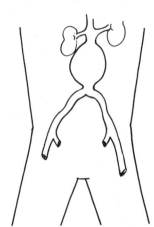

ABDOMINAL AORTIC
ANEURYSM

B Seventy percent of patients do not have any symptoms when the aneurysm is first discovered by a physician. When directly questioned, they may admit to mild abdominal discomfort, but little more . Aneurysms that are small (less than 6 centimeters in diameter) have a 30% chance of remaining that size and will not cause further trouble. Larger aneurysms, however, tend to enlarge rather quickly and break open like an over-inflated balloon. This is why aneurysms should be removed while they are still small and not causing symptoms.

C Aneurysms of over 6 centimeters in diameter, if not removed, have a 65% chance of rupture within two years. Half of the patients will have no symptoms from the aneurysm until it ruptures, by which time the chances of cure, even by an emergency operation, are only about 50%.

D When operated on electively (not as an emergency), 95% of patients can expect to survive the operation, which involves removing the aneurysm and replacing it with a soft, synthetic, cloth tube. Hospitalization is ordinarily ten days to three weeks. The low mortality (5%) of removing an aneurysm before its rupture contrasts with the 50% mortality if operation is performed after rupture. Aneurysms generally occur in the elderly, who have other associated diseases. About 30% of these patients will have some complication in the period after operation, including problems with the lungs (40%), heart failure (35%), acute heart attack 10%), and kidney failure (5%).

Abdominal Aneurysm

E The most common complaint of a person with an abdominal aortic aneurysm is vague awareness of a pulsating mass in the abdomen. About 1% of the time, a bit of debris from within the saccular aneurysm will be thrown off as an embolus and lodge in an artery in the leg or foot where it blocks blood supply. Small emobli cause pain and blue spots in the toes. Large ones, it not removed, may cause gangrene and require amputation.

F About 40% of aneurysms that overdistend and begin to leak blood (rupture) into the tissues around the back of the abdominal cavity cause death within a few hours. But with the remaining 60%, the original leak is small, causing pain in the back and some signs of blood loss, but they are not immediately lethal. Sixty percent of such patients will survive more than six hours, and about 40% will live twenty-four hours, while leaking blood from the aneurysm. When the embolus finally bursts, the patient's survival without operation is a matter of minutes. The important challenge for the patient and his physician is to recognize the condition before there is a massive fatal bleed.

G When the aneurysm begins to leak, the surgeon must operate immediately and replace the abdominal aorta with a cloth tube. The chances of survival are still about 50 to 60% even under these desperate conditions.

H After the operation, there is an 80% chance of some complication in the hospital period of elderly patients who have had to be operated upon under such unfavorable emergency conditions. This is greater than five times the risk of complication compared to an elective removal of an aortic aneurysm before it ruptures.

I After a patient has recovered from the operation, he has about the same life expectancy of anyone else of a similar age with an equivalent amount of arteriosclerosis. He is cured of his aneurysm.

4. Leg Claudication

A Claudication is pain or cramping in the leg, thigh, or buttocks, which follows walking or exercise and is relieved by rest. It is a signal from a muscle that its blood supply is inadequate and is usually caused by narrowing of the blood vessels (arteriosclerosis). If the arterial narrowing progresses, it can lead to gangrene and loss of the toes or part of the leg.

B Although claudication is a protest by muscles in the leg, it usually is a symptom of generalized arteriosclerosis, which affects blood vessels throughout the body. Forty percent of patients with claudication in the legs will still be alive after five years. Eighty-five percent of the deaths are from a heart attack or stroke, not as a complication of disease in their legs.

Average Survival for Patients Who Complain of Claudication	5 years	10 years
Expectancy for patients of the same age who do not claudicate	90%	—
Claudicators (overall)	73%	52%
• With associated coronary artery disease	55%	9%
• With associated stroke	61%	—
• With associated high blood pressure	69%	—
• With associated diabetes	—	17%
• With both associated diabetes and coronary artery disease	0%	

C In 80% of patients with claudication, the discomfort brought on by exercise will not progress appreciably. Stopping smoking, exercise, and weight reduction will all improve life expectancy. So much does smoking hasten the progress of the disease that many surgeons are in fact unwilling to operate on claudicators unless they promise to stop. With ideal non-operative care, 65% of claudicators will have increased exercise tolerance, and 80% will not require operation.

D But in at least 20% of patients, the symptoms of pain will get worse and tolerance to exercise decrease due to progressive narrowing of the vessels.

E Even with increasing symptoms, 45% of patients will refuse amputation and choose to live with these disabling symptoms.

F Of all those who claudicate, 6 to 7% will come to amputation because of gangrene of the toes, foot, or lower leg. This is most likely to occur in those who continue to smoke

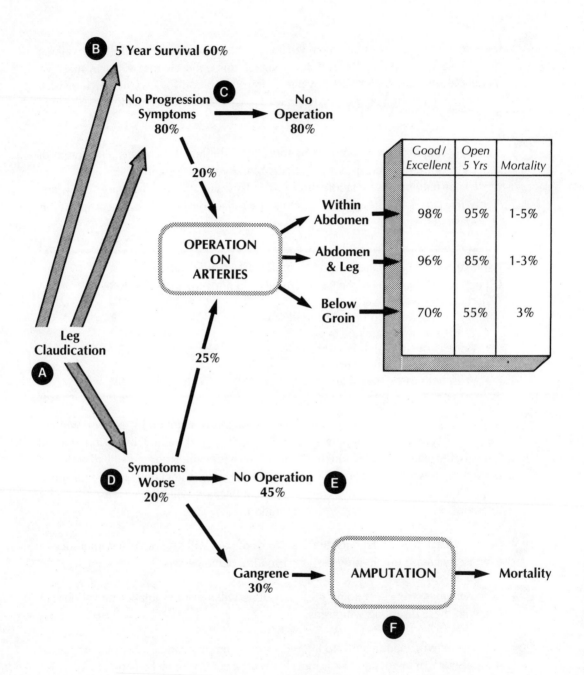

or have diabetes. In these patients, the leg usually must be taken off just below the knee (see "Amputation," page 143).

The exact operative technique chosen by the surgeon to increase blood flow to the calf depends on many factors, including the general condition of the patient, and the extent of arteriosclerosis in other organs—such as the heart—and large arteries in the abdomen, but, mainly, it depends on the condition of the arteries in the leg and calf. Usually, it is necessary to determine the outline of these arteries by X-ray examination before operation. The following table illustrates the expected operative mortality and chances for improvement following several types of operations used to increase blood supply to the leg. Possible types of operations include placing a vein or plastic tube

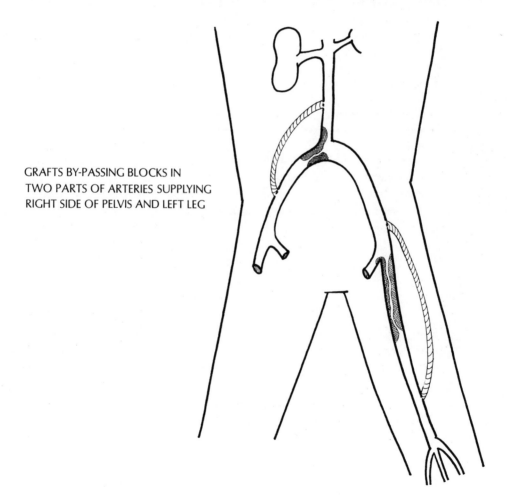

GRAFTS BY-PASSING BLOCKS IN
TWO PARTS OF ARTERIES SUPPLYING
RIGHT SIDE OF PELVIS AND LEFT LEG

bypass around the segment of blocked artery; opening the artery and removing the material that blocks it (endarterectomy); and a less commonly used procedure of cutting the sympathetic nerves that, in part, control the diameter of the artery. Benefit of such bypass operations depend on the graft remaining open (patent), so that this is a convenient measurement of benefit from the operation. As shown in the table, the likelihood of prolonged benefit is decreased when it is necessary to attach a graft at or below the knee.

Operation	Operative Mortality (%)	Improvement (%)	5-Year Patency (%)
Aorto-iliac endarterectomy	1	98	95
Aorto-femoral graft	1–3	96	85
Axillo-femoral graft	2–8	75	30–76
Femoro-femoral graft	5–15	70	50–80
Profundoplasty	4	60	75
Femoro-popliteal graft	0–5	80	74
Femoro-tibial graft	3	68	54
Lumbar sympathectomy	2–6	50–60	

These terms refer to the site at which the graft is connected to the patient's blood vessels. The aorta is high within the abdomen; the iliac in the lower abdomen. The femoral artery is in the leg, the popliteal artery behind the knee, and the tibial artery in the lower leg. The axillary artery is around the shoulder. Profundoplasty is performed in the upper part of the leg.

5. Amputation

A Amputation of the leg because of poor blood supply is usually caused by advanced arteriosclerosis. The arteries in the abdomen and leg become so clogged with obstructing material that sufficient blood cannot reach the foot and calf to keep the tissues alive. The need for amputation under these circumstances is a strong signal of generalized arteriosclerosis, which usually also involves the arteries of the heart, brain, and kidneys. The future of an elderly patient with generalized arterial disease following amputation is obviously very different than that of the young person who has an amputation after injury. The young have almost limitless ability to adapt to the loss of a leg.

B Elderly people may often live many productive years after amputation. Although the average survival is twenty-one months, this figure includes many who die of heart disease or a stroke a few days or weeks after operation. Expected survival at five years is 30%. These figures represent the attrition of generalized arteriosclerosis, not the result of the amputation.

C Arteriosclerotic narrowing of blood vessels usually affects both legs more or less equally. If one leg has such poor blood supply that gangrene is threatened and it has to be amputated, the chances are that blood supply to the other leg is also decreased. There is a 15% probability that the opposite leg will have to be amputated during the original hospitalization and a 50% chance of amputation on the other side within one year. This sobering fact dampens enthusiasm for buying an expensive, artificial leg ($1,500–$3,000), which can only be useful if the patient has a good leg on the other side. It is wiser to wait and see if the other leg will be strong enough to support the heavy burden of walking on an artificial limb without crutches.

D Sixty percent of the leg amputations for arteriosclerosis are performed above the knee (AK), where the wound almost always heals. Hospitalization is about seven to twenty-one days. A month after operation, the patient and his physician can decide whether it is desirable to order an artificial leg. An above-the-knee (AK) amputation sacrifices the knee joint, but in fact, this is often not as important as one would imagine in rehabilitating the elderly. Regardless of the site of amputation, only a third of the people amputated for arteriosclerosis ever order an artificial limb. Of those who do, only about 60% will ever use it for walking, with or without crutches. If a patient is to use crutches, saving the knee is of importance only for appearance.

The family of an elderly patient requiring amputation for arteriosclerosis must realize that the operation is performed to save life. They must not have undue hopes that the patient will soon walk without crutches on an artificial leg, since only about 20% ever will.

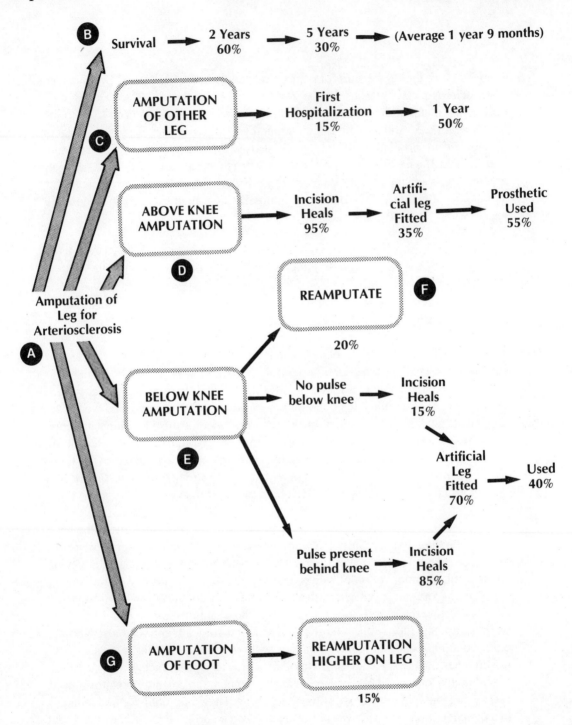

Survival → 2 Years 60% → 5 Years 30% → (Average 1 year 9 months)

B

AMPUTATION OF OTHER LEG → First Hospitalization 15% → 1 Year 50%

C

ABOVE KNEE AMPUTATION → Incision Heals 95% → Artificial leg Fitted 35% → Prosthetic Used 55%

D

REAMPUTATE **F** 20%

BELOW KNEE AMPUTATION

E

Amputation of Leg for Arteriosclerosis

A

No pulse below knee → Incision Heals 15%

Artificial Leg Fitted 70% → Used 40%

Pulse present behind knee → Incision Heals 85%

AMPUTATION OF FOOT → **REAMPUTATION HIGHER ON LEG**

G 15%

144

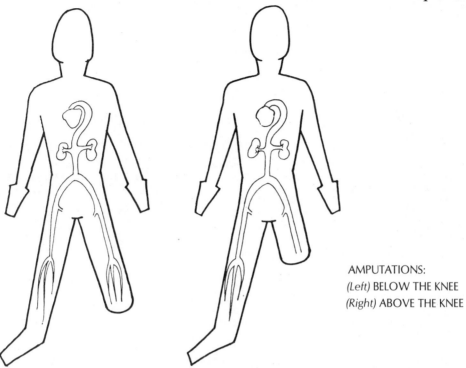

AMPUTATIONS:
(Left) BELOW THE KNEE
(Right) ABOVE THE KNEE

E Saving the knee by a below-the-knee (BK) amputation is desirable if the amputation stump will heal. There is an 85% chance of such healing if a pulse can be felt behind the knee before operation. If none can, the chances of healing are reduced to 15%. A number of more sophisticated tests of blood flow and blood pressure in the leg can more precisely predict the chances for a BK amputation wound to heal. If the BK stump heals, 70% of such amputees can walk on a temporary artificial pylon within two weeks after operation. A permanent prosthetic leg can be fitted eight weeks later, but, only about 40% of those amputated below the knee for arteriosclerosis ever use the artificial leg. They prefer to walk with crutches, which require much less effort.

F In about 20% of amputations below the knee, there is insufficient blood reaching the operative site to allow the wound to heal. This necessitates reoperation, removing the leg above the knee.

G In an occasional patient, where only the toes may be gangrenous, amputation can be performed across the middle of the foot. Hospitalization is prolonged (four to six weeks) while determining whether the wound will heal, but the excellent result, if the amputation site will heal, is worth the time. The chances are about 85% that patients selected for such transmetatarsal amputations will heal the wound in the foot. If not, reamputation higher in the leg (BK or AK) is necessary.

6. Varicose Veins

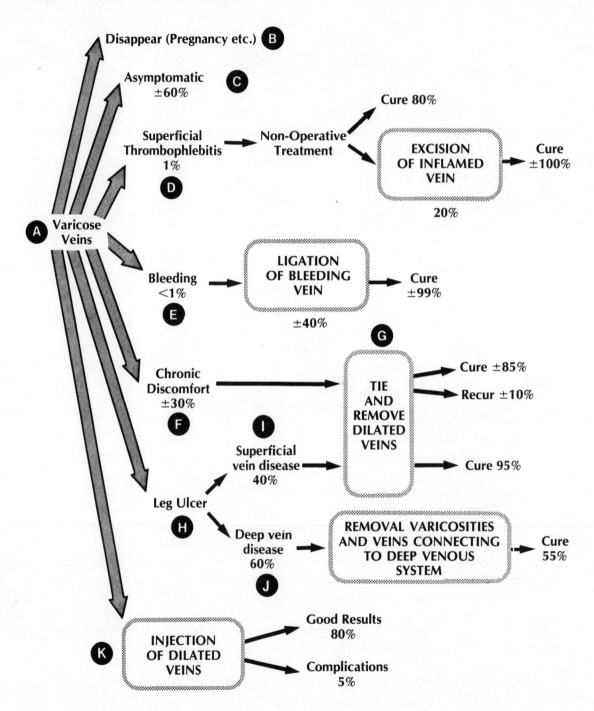

Disappear (Pregnancy etc.) **B**

Asymptomatic
±60% **C**

Superficial
Thrombophlebitis
1%
D

→ Non-Operative
Treatment

Cure 80%

**EXCISION
OF INFLAMED
VEIN** → Cure
±100%

20%

A Varicose
Veins

Bleeding
<1%
E

→ **LIGATION
OF BLEEDING
VEIN** → Cure
±99%

±40%

G

Chronic
Discomfort
±30%
F

→ **TIE
AND
REMOVE
DILATED
VEINS**

Cure ±85%

Recur ±10%

I Superficial
vein disease
40% →

Cure 95%

Leg Ulcer
H

Deep vein
disease
60%
J

→ **REMOVAL VARICOSITIES
AND VEINS CONNECTING
TO DEEP VENOUS
SYSTEM** → Cure
55%

K **INJECTION
OF DILATED
VEINS**

Good Results
80%

Complications
5%

A Because man stands upright, the veins in the legs must support the weight of a long column of blood extending from the ankle to the heart. Sometimes, these thin-walled veins cannot withstand the constant increased pressure and they dilate. Veins located deep in the leg are surrounded by muscles which help buttress their walls, but those lying under the skin have no such protection and are the first to increase in size. These are called varicose veins. Both sets of veins have valves, which help support the long column of blood and reduce the pressure inside the veins on standing. Valves in the dilated varicosities can no longer function. This further increases pressure within the veins when the person stands. Blood flow from the lower leg becomes sluggish, resulting in swelling of the calf, discomfort after prolonged standing, poor blood supply to the skin of the ankle, and frequently a skin ulcer in the lower leg.

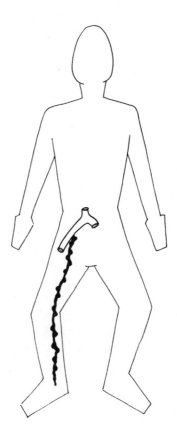

VARICOSE VEINS SHOWING
CONNECTION WITH LARGE VEIN
DEEP IN THE GROIN

Varicose Veins

B Varicose veins will seldom disappear without treatment. An exception are the varicosities that develop during pregnancy. After delivery, the veins will usually return to normal.

C Uncomplicated, dilated veins directly under the skin (superficial varicose veins) usually need no treatment, except for the sake of appearances.

D Occasionally, the long vein running down the middle side of the thigh just under the skin (saphenous vein) becomes inflamed, red, sore, and tender. This is called superficial thrombophlebitis. This differs from the more serious inflammatory involvement of the deep veins of the leg (see "Postoperative Thrombophlebitis," page 150). Almost complete relief can be obtained in 80% of superficial thrombophlebitis when treated with drugs such as steroids, which decrease the body's response to inflammation. In the 20% of patients who do not respond, the involved (saphenous vein) must be removed or tied at the groin. This operation promptly cures over 95% of such patients.

E Very rarely (0.2% of the time), a dilated varicose vein will burst through the skin and cause a frightening, but not really very serious, blood loss. This may require emergency operation to stop the bleeding. This complication is more feared by patients than is warranted. It seldom occurs, and when it does, is rarely dangerous.

F The most common symptom from varicose veins is a vague sense of tiredness and swelling in the calf after prolonged standing. This is due to slow flow of blood from the leg in the dilated veins. If the symptoms and swelling cannot be controlled with special fitted stockings or by other means, operation is required.

G Operation for varicose veins involves cutting the saphenous vein at the groin to disconnect it from the rest of the venous circulation. In addition, the rest of the varicosities that run down the thigh and leg beneath the skin are usually removed or "stripped." This removes all connections between the dilated superficial varicosities from the deep veins surrounded by muscles in the central part of the leg. Although this operation may require more than two hours, it has an insignificant mortality (less than 0.1%). Hospitalization may be from one to seven days. If the symptoms of swelling and fatigue in the leg were due to varicosities, the probability of cure is about 85–95%. In about 10% of patients, there may be a recurrence of a varicosity after operation. If the recurrence is small, the vein can often be made to clot by injecting an irritating solution into it (see K below). Re-excision is required in less than 5% of cases.

H Everyone occasionally skins his ankle. Such wounds normally heal promptly, but when varicose veins produce a poor blood supply to the skin of the ankle, an ulcer may persist. When the usual non-operative forms of treatment have failed, the only chance for permanent healing is by removing all the skin around the ulcer and covering the resulting defect with a skin graft taken from another part of the body.

I In the 40% of cases where the ulcer is associated with disease only in the superficial veins lying just under the skin, this operation will provide a 95% chance of permanent healing.

J In the remaining 60% of cases, where the veins deep within the calf and thigh are also diseased (deep venous insufficiency), simply removing the superficial varicosities will not heal the persistent skin ulcer. This requires excising the superficial varicosities, plus removing all the small veins that connect the superficial varicosities with the veins deep in the leg. This operation is tedious, but provides a 55% chance of cure for a crippling, chronic disease.

K Short segments of varicose veins can be made to clot by injecting into them various types of irritating (or sclerosing) solutions. After injection, the veins form fibrous cords beneath the skin. This injection technique characteristically requires eight to twelve office visits during several weeks. The chance of complication from injecting this irritating material into the vein is 0.1%. It can be expected to permanently cure about 80% of patients selected for treatment. The shorter the diseased varicosity, the better the chance for cure. It is ideally suited for treatment of recurrence or persistence of a small varicosity after operation.

7. Postoperative Thrombophlebitis

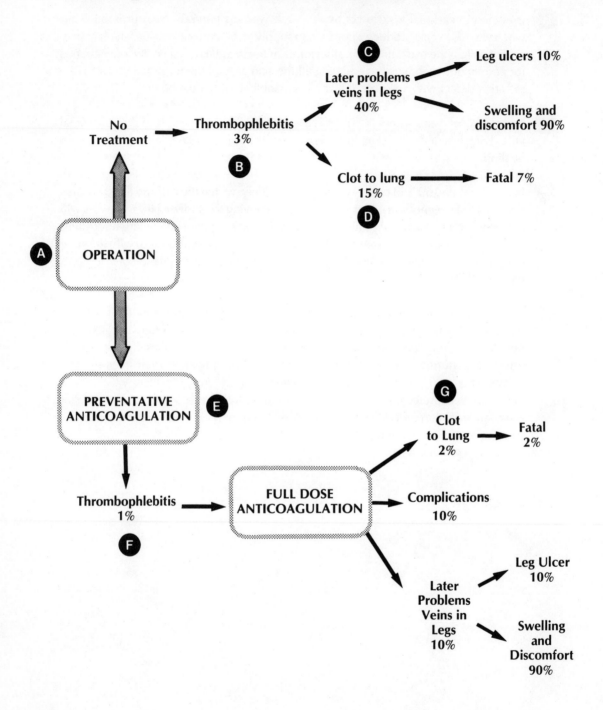

A Blood in the legs is ordinarily pumped back to the heart by the contraction and relaxation of the calf muscles. During an operation, blood in the legs stagnates. To complicate the situation, any operative wound increases the tendency of blood to clot. There is, therefore, a high probability that blood clots will form in the leg veins during and shortly after operations.

B The probability of such clot formation depends on many factors, such as the duration and type of operation, the age and weight of the patient, and the presence of heart disease. Some clots probably form in everyone's legs after a major operation. Special tests and X-rays of the veins will detect clots in 25% of patients after a major operation, but in only about 3% will there be any signs or symptoms of the clot.

C Normal veins contain a series of delicate one-way valves, which help support the long column of blood that lies between the ankle and the heart. Clots and inflammation within the leg veins (thrombophlebitis) will destroy these valves, so that the full weight of the column of blood presses on the leg veins. This will cause swelling and sometimes skin ulcers around the ankle (see "Varicose Veins," page 146). The chances are about 40% that a patient with thrombophlebitis after operation will have problems with the veins in his legs within four years. This might consist of varicose veins, swelling and discomfort after prolonged standing, or ulceration of the skin around the ankle. This usually results from involvement of the deep veins of the calf of the leg in the inflammatory process. This is called deep vein thrombosis, or deep venous insufficiency.

D If thrombophlebitis develops after operation, there is always a chance that a part of a clot that might form in the veins of the calf may break loose within the first two weeks and be swept up through the heart and lodge in lung. This is called a pulmonary embolus. Clinical signs are sudden severe pain in the chest and coughing up blood.

E In patients where the risk of thrombophlebitis is great, specific drugs may be given before or very soon after operation to interfere with clot formation. The most commonly used anticoagulant is heparin. In small doses ("mini-heparin"), this drug decreases the chance of clot formation in the legs. Excessive bleeding from the wound following mini-heparin treatment occurs about 1–2% of the time, but is usually of minor importance.

Postoperative Thrombophlebitis

F Despite the use of heparin to prevent clot formation in the legs, about 1–2% of patients may develop clinical evidence of thrombophlebitis following operation. This is about half as frequent as if mini-heparin were not used. As mentioned, special tests can detect blood clots in the legs of about 25% of patients not given mini-heparin, even when there is no other evidence of a clot. If mini-heparin is used, such small clots can be detected in only 5%.

G Once thrombophlebitis occurs following operation, the untreated patient has a 15% chance of having a pulmonary embolus. If, however, he is given a full dose of heparin, this reduces the probability to 2%. The likelihood of later deep-vein insufficiency is also reduced with heparin, from 40% without the drug to 10%, if it is started soon after the onset of thrombophlebitis. Although there is a 10% chance of some minor complications from heparin anticoagulation, the small risk is more than balanced by the decreased likelihood of the serious complications.

VII
Breast

1. *Breast Lump*

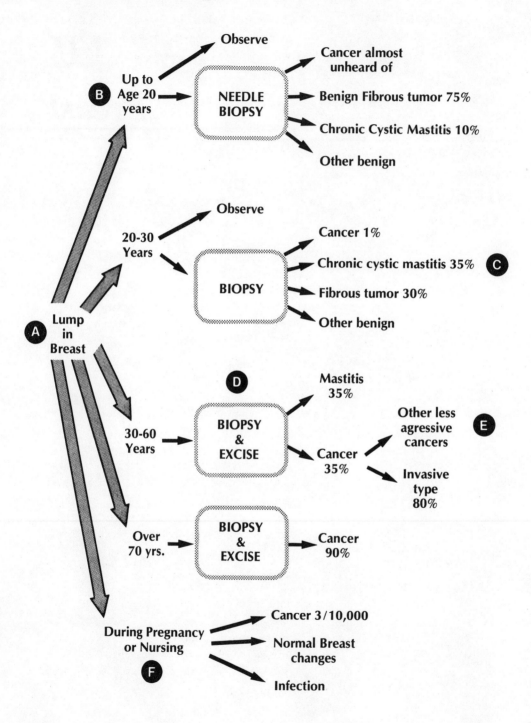

A Lump in Breast

B Up to Age 20 years
→ Observe
→ NEEDLE BIOPSY
- → Cancer almost unheard of
- → Benign Fibrous tumor 75%
- → Chronic Cystic Mastitis 10%
- → Other benign

20-30 Years
→ Observe
→ BIOPSY
- → Cancer 1%
- → Chronic cystic mastitis 35% **C**
- → Fibrous tumor 30%
- → Other benign

D 30-60 Years → BIOPSY & EXCISE
- → Mastitis 35%
- → Cancer 35%
  - → Other less agressive cancers **E**
  - → Invasive type 80%

Over 70 yrs. → BIOPSY & EXCISE → Cancer 90%

F During Pregnancy or Nursing
- → Cancer 3/10,000
- → Normal Breast changes
- → Infection

A The normal female breast changes in consistency during the monthly cycle, and a single firm area or lump is often difficult to differentiate from the multiple irregularities that often may normally be present. When a lump persists, it inevitably suggests the possibility that it might be cancer. Most, however, are not.

ABNORMAL LUMP IN LOWER PART
OF THE RIGHT BREAST

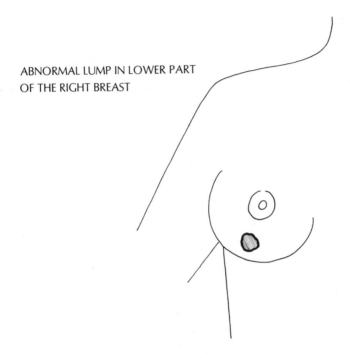

B Under twenty years of age, a lump in the breast usually indicates normal breast tissue. In teenagers with fully developed breasts, a persistent, solitary lump can be biopsied (often with a needle) and a piece of the tissue examined under the microscope. If absolutely necessary, the lump can be removed. Seventy-five percent of the time, it turns out to be a benign fibrous tissue (fibroadenoma), which is not cancer and will not turn into cancer.

C In the twenty to thirty-year-old age group, there is a remote chance that a persistent single breast lump will be cancer. A more likely diagnosis (35%) is chronic cystic mastitis, which is a variation in the normal changes that occur in the breast under the influence of a constantly changing, monthly, sex-hormone environment. A woman with chronic cystic mastitis is likely to continue to have lumpy breasts up to the time of menopause. It is not cancer, but such women must be particularly careful to discover new and persistent breast masses that might be cancer.

Breast Lump

D The high-risk cancer years are from thirty to sixty, during which time about one out of every twenty women will develop breast cancer. The average age at diagnosis is forty-eight. A persistent solitary breast lump in women in this age group has a 35% chance of being cancer.

Xeromammography, a special X-ray examination of the breast, may help decide whether a nodule warrants operative removal for microscopic examination for suspicion of cancer. Mammography is also used to detect very small cancers in the opposite breast when cancer has been found on one side.

E In addition to the common type of breast cancer (adenocarcinoma), which makes up eight out of ten cancers, there are a few far less active types of breast cancers, which have a better chance of cure.

F During pregnancy and lactation, lumps in the breast come and go and are seldom of importance. Very rarely (3 in 10,000 pregnancies), such a mass turns out to be cancer. The chances of cure are the same as in the non-pregnant woman with an equivalent type and grade of tumor. In nursing mothers breast lumps are often due to an abscess.

2. Breast Cancer

(A) Of all women found to have breast cancer, 40–60% are alive after ten years. Twenty to thirty percent have a normal life expectancy. In one-quarter of those cured, the tumor had spread to the lymph nodes under the arm when first treated.

(B) Two-thirds of women have some type of breast lump before menopause, but most, of course, are *not* cancer. Eighty percent of the lumps that are cancer are obviously malignant to the doctor when he first examines the patient.

(C) Breast cancer often travels or spreads to the lymph nodes under the arm (axilla) that drain fluid (lymph) from the breast. About 60% of breast tissue is in the upper-outer part of the breast, and this is where most cancers start. Cancers closer to the middle of the chest are more likely to drain into the lymph nodes within the chest under the breast bone (internal mammary lymph nodes). The chances of cure are slightly better for cancers in the outer part of the breast than those near the middle of the body, largely because the former are likely to spread to the lymph nodes under the arm where they can be more easily removed.

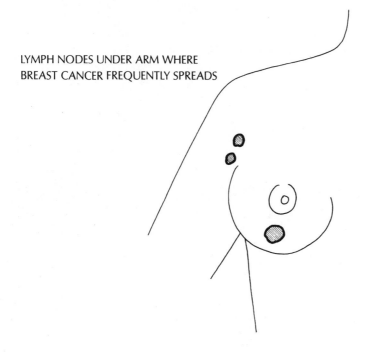

LYMPH NODES UNDER ARM WHERE
BREAST CANCER FREQUENTLY SPREADS

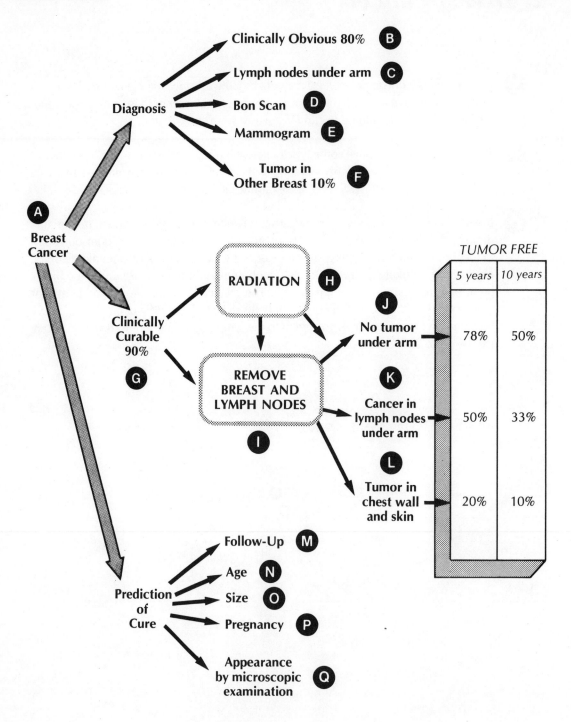

Chances are improved almost two times if there is no spread under the arm when the physician examines the axillae. If an experienced physician feels no suspicious nodes in the axillae, there is a 66% chance he will be correct and no tumor will be found. In 33% of cases, tiny deposits of tumor will be found in the tissue.

If a physician feels a mass, 66% of the time it will turn out to be a deposit of cancer. (The chances are about 33% that the enlarged node is *not* cancer.)

D A bone scan is a type of radioisotope (X-ray) examination that helps detect spread of tumor to bone. It is often performed on a patient with known or suspected breast cancer to determine whether the tumor has spread. If there is known tumor spread to bone, removing the breast tumor will not be curative, since some tumor will remain in the bone. But bone scan is grossly inaccurate in predicting spread of breast cancer to the bones. In only 33% of patients where the scan suggests tumor is cancer actually proven to be there. A "positive" bone scan, therefore, does not mean with certainty that the tumor has spread beyond resection for cure. Neither does a "negative" bone scan prove the reverse.

E A mammogram is a special X-ray picture taken to outline the soft tissue of the breast in order to detect small cancers that might not be detectable by ordinary physical examination. It also helps predict whether an easily palpable tumor felt in the breast is or is not cancer. The mammogram is about 90% accurate in predicting cancer. There is an 11% chance that a spot on the film that looks like cancer actually is not. Alternately, there is a 6% chance that a mass that looks like a benign (non-cancerous) tumor will turn out to be cancer.

F A woman who has a cancer in one breast has a ten times greater chance of developing cancer in the opposite breast than does a person without any breast cancer. In 10% of patients with breast cancer, there actually will be cancer on both sides when the original tumor is discovered. (Certain rare types of breast cancer are particularly likely to be present on both sides.) The tumor on the opposite side may be very small and difficult to detect. Mammograms often will help in finding such small tumors.

G Ninety percent of patients with breast cancer come to a physician while a breast cancer is still small enough so that there is a chance of cure. Only about 10% have distant spread—as, for example, in the lung or bones—and can only have tumor growth delayed, not totally cured.

H X-radiation kills cancer cells and is of great benefit in breast cancer, both in improving the chance of cure by operation and in prolonging comfortable survival in advanced breast cancer.

I Cure of breast cancer depends primarily on the operative removal of all the breast tissue on the side of the tumor along with the lymph nodes under the arm on that side. Details of the expectancy of this operation are described in "Mastectomy", page 166.

J An important factor in determining the chance of cure of breast cancer is whether there is spread of tumor to the axillary lymph nodes. If none is found, the overall survival for all types of breast cancer is 78% in five years and 50% ten years after operation.

K Even if cancer is found in the axillary lymph nodes, five-year survival is 50%, and ten-year survival 33%. If the cancer is located in the inner part of the breast (medial quadrants) and also in the lymph nodes under the arm, there is a 40% chance that it has also spread to the lymph nodes within the chest. Such tumor spread cannot be totally removed by operation and must be treated by radiation.

L Breast tumor that has spread into the chest wall or into the skin of the breast is considered in an advanced condition, and although the breast mass may often be removed by operation, treatment is mainly by X-ray or anti-cancer drugs and provides a 20% chance of five-year survival.

M Because a woman who has had a cancer develop in one breast is at a 10% risk of developing another cancer in the remaining breast after mastectomy (removal of one breast), it is very important that she and her physician remain alert to this possibility by frequent (six to twelve month) examinations of the remaining breast. The likelihood of such a new breast cancer is about 1% per year or about 10% in the ten years after mastectomy.

If no cancer has appeared by the end of 10 years after operation, the chances of cure are about 90%. There is a 7% chance that the cancer will recur in the operative incision.

N The age of the patient at the time the tumor is discovered does not appreciably affect the likelihood of cure. Those over thirty years of age have only a 20% better chance of cure than those who are younger.

O The smaller the tumor when removed, the less likely it is to have spread to the regional lymph nodes, and the more likely it is to be cured. This is why it is so important to detect breast cancer as soon as possible, while it is still small, localized, and more easily totally removed. More exact prediction of survival of varying size tumors is as follows:

Diameter of tumor	Probability of spread into axilla		Survival	
			5 years	10 years
2 cm	33%	Nodes +	45%	45%
		Nodes −	85%	
2–3 cm	50%	Nodes +	65%	40%
(1 inch)		Nodes −	83%	
4 cm	70%	Nodes +	35%	20%
		Nodes −	70%	

P Pregnancy does not in itself alter the chance of cure, except that the cancer may be overlooked in the usual changes that occur during pregnancy and only be discovered when the tumor is in an advanced stage. Breast feeding does not alter the likelihood of cancer very much one way or another. Breast cancer is slightly more frequent in women who have not had children.

Q The appearance of the cell under microscopic examination is important in predicting how fast the tumor will grow and, therefore, what the chances are for cure. When tumor cells resemble normal breast cells, they grow slowly and provide a better chance of cure. When, at the opposite extreme, they have lost almost all resemblance to their normal appearance, they are said to be undifferentiated, they grow rapidly, and the chance of cure is decreased. There are, in fact, several kinds of breast cancer called variously infiltrating adenocarcinoma, medullary carcinoma, and intraductile carcinoma, etc. Such diagnosis is made only after the pathologist looks at the tumor specimen under the microscope. Each has its own chances for probable cure.

3. *Advanced Breast Cancer*

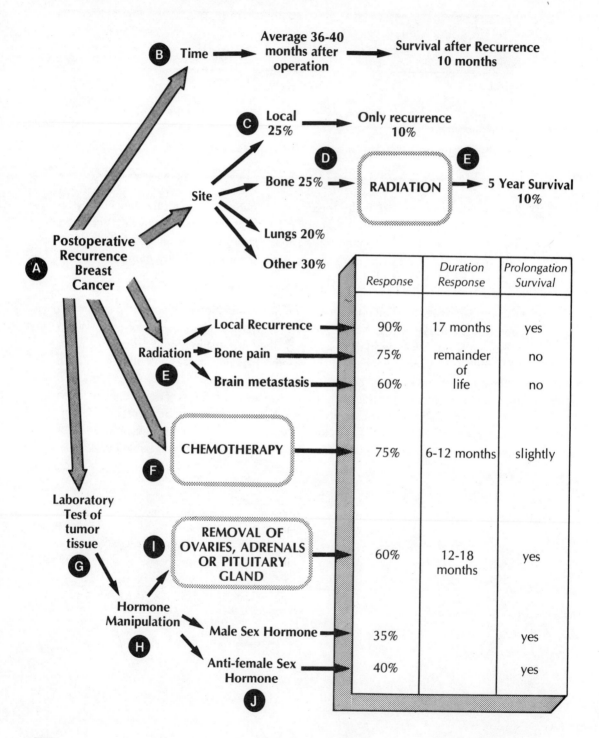

B Time → Average 36-40 months after operation → Survival after Recurrence 10 months

C Local 25% → Only recurrence 10%

D Bone 25% → **RADIATION** → **E** 5 Year Survival 10%

Site → Local 25%, Bone 25%, Lungs 20%, Other 30%

A Postoperative Recurrence Breast Cancer

Radiation → Local Recurrence, Bone pain, Brain metastasis **E**

CHEMOTHERAPY **F**

Laboratory Test of tumor tissue **G**

REMOVAL OF OVARIES, ADRENALS OR PITUITARY GLAND **I**

Hormone Manipulation **H** → Male Sex Hormone, Anti-female Sex Hormone **J**

	Response	Duration Response	Prolongation Survival
Local Recurrence	90%	17 months	yes
Bone pain	75%	remainder of life	no
Brain metastasis	60%		no
CHEMOTHERAPY	75%	6-12 months	slightly
REMOVAL OF OVARIES, ADRENALS OR PITUITARY GLAND	60%	12-18 months	yes
Male Sex Hormone	35%		yes
Anti-female Sex Hormone	40%		yes

A "Is it cured? Will the cancer come back? If so, where shall I look for recurrence?" These are the questions a woman asks after mastectomy for cancer. Then, "If it does come back, what may I expect?" The one in nine patients who has distant spread of breast cancer when first discovered and is not operated on for cure also wants to know "What can be done to make the rest of my life comfortable and last as long as possible?"

BREAST CANCER: COMMON SITES OF SPREAD

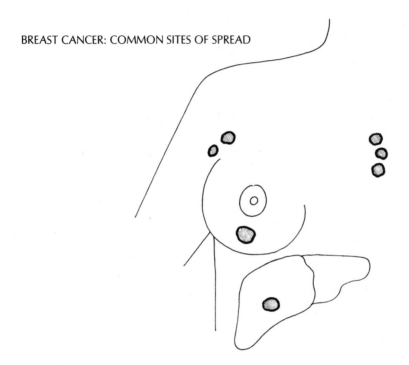

B The longer the time between the operation removing the cancer and the first reappearance of tumor, the better the chance of cure. The average time before such appearance is thirty-six to forty months after operation. Tumors that take longer to reappear are slower growing and can, in general, be expected to continue their relatively slow growth. Tumors that appear within a few weeks or months after mastectomy are fast growing. The average length of life after a breast tumor has recurred is ten months.

C One-quarter of recurrences appear at the site of the operation where the breast was removed. This often appears as a small nodule or firm ulcer in the scar. It is tempting to believe that this is the only bit of tumor remaining, but unfortunately, in only 10% of cases is this true. Usually, a local recurrence is a signal that there is more tumor elsewhere in the body. The local nodule can be removed to be certain that it is recurrence, but other means such as radiation or anti-cancer drugs are required to delay tumor growth.

D One-quarter of breast tumor recurrences are in bone, often the ribs or the bones of the spine. Often, the first symptom is pain. In others, there may be no symptoms, the recurrence being detected by routine X-ray examination or with a special study called a bone scan. (See "Breast Cancer," page 157). The repeated chest X-ray examination and bone scan are performed after operation to discover such metastases while they are still small and are more easily treated. Other relatively common sites of breast tumor recurrence are in the lungs, the brain, or the abdomen.

E X-radiation is more lethal to cancer cells than to surrounding normal tissue and, therefore, is used extensively to kill or contain tumor cells where the tumor is localized and radiation can be given in large amounts to a small target. Such, for example, occurs when there is recurrence in the chest wall or skin. The chances are nine out of ten that such localized tumor will shrink in size following radiation and that the tumor may be held in check for period up to one and one half years. Radiation has a 75% probability of relieving bone pain due to metastases. The likelihood of radiation providing relief of symptoms caused by metastases in the brain or lungs is somewhat less.

F Anti-cancer drugs are medicine that can either be taken by mouth or injected into a vein. These powerful chemicals may produce side effects, such as nausea or weakness, but these symptoms usually disappear when the dose of the drug is decreased. In contrast to X-ray, which is given only to a given site of tumor, these drugs spread throughout the body and affect tumor cells wherever they may be.

G Growth of normal breast tissue is obviously stimulated by female sex hormones; breasts wither after menopause when such hormones are in short supply. One way to predict whether a given breast cancer will respond to hormone manipulation is to determine by a special laboratory study whether female sex hormones will stick (bind) to the tumor cell surface. If cells of a tumor bind the female sex hormone (estrogen binding positive), the chances of its responding to hormone manipulation is about 60%. If the tumor does not bind estrogen (estrogen binding negative) the chance of response is only about 15%.

H The hormone environment of a breast cancer recurrence can be altered by removing the source of female sex hormones, giving male sex hormones which tend to counteract female hormones, or giving special anti-female sex hormone drugs.

I If the patient still has active ovaries (premenopause), removing them by operation will remove a major source of female sex hormones and can be anticipated to give six to nine months relief to 35% of patients with advanced breast cancer. Other glands, such as the adrenals, which lie over the kidneys, and the pituitary gland, which lies at the base of the brain, also control estrogen output and affect breast cancer growth. Removal of the adrenals or pituitary has a higher chance of complication than removing the ovaries, but can be expected to provide relief in about the same number of patients who have had help from removing the ovaries. The ovaries are often removed first, and if temporarily successful, the adrenal glands or pituitary gland can be removed later when symptoms recur.

J Life is prolonged about one year for the 35% of patients with advanced breast cancer who respond to hormone treatment, such as oophorectomy, adrenalectomy, or anti-female hormone drugs.

4. Mastectomy (Removal of Breast)

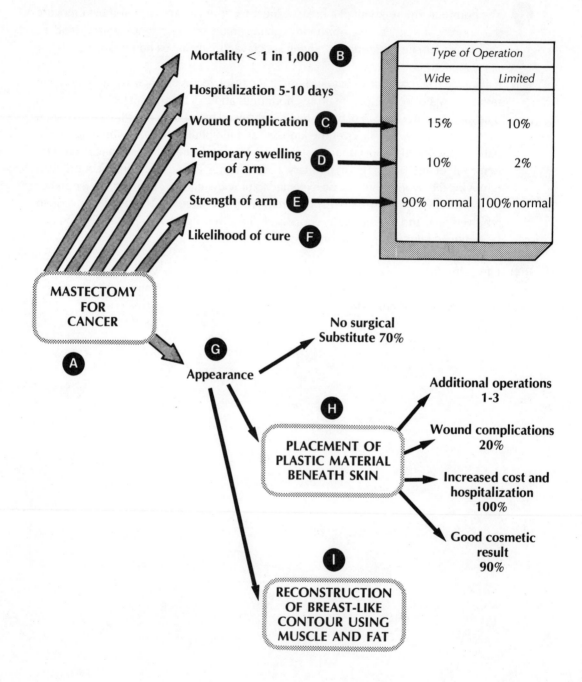

Mortality < 1 in 1,000 **B**

Hospitalization 5-10 days

Wound complication **C**

Temporary swelling of arm **D**

Strength of arm **E**

Likelihood of cure **F**

Type of Operation	
Wide	Limited
15%	10%
10%	2%
90% normal	100% normal

MASTECTOMY FOR CANCER

A

G
Appearance

No surgical Substitute 70%

H
PLACEMENT OF PLASTIC MATERIAL BENEATH SKIN

Additional operations 1-3

Wound complications 20%

Increased cost and hospitalization 100%

Good cosmetic result 90%

I
RECONSTRUCTION OF BREAST-LIKE CONTOUR USING MUSCLE AND FAT

A Mastectomy is the operative removal of part or all of the breast tissue. The operation is usually performed because of cancer. Breast tissue lies sandwiched between the skin and the firm sheet of underlying muscles on the chest wall. When only the breast tissue is removed, the operation is called a simple mastectomy. When, in an effort to get well around the tumor, some of the underlying muscles are also removed, the operation is called a radical mastectomy.

Cancers of the breast often spread to the lymph nodes under the arm (axillary lymph nodes). In operations for cancer, these lymph nodes are usually removed along with the breast tissue, both because they may contain tumor and to determine whether the tumor has spread to them beyond the confines of the breast. If such spread is found, treatment with drugs or X-ray after operation may be altered (see "Advanced Breast Cancer," page 162). There are many variations of the operation for removing the breast for cancer. They differ mainly in how extensively they remove both the muscles beneath the breast and the axillary lymph nodes. A modified radical mastectomy as frequently performed involves removing all the breast tissue and the lymph glands under the arm, but leaves the muscles under the breast tissue on the chest wall.

Much has been written with great emotion in the popular press about the virtues and differences between simple versus radical mastectomy. Their only difference is whether the muscles lying beneath the breast are removed along with the breast tissue. In the accompanying diagram, the two operations are referred to for simplicity sake as wide (radical) mastectomy or limited (simple) mastectomy.

B The chances of dying because of either operation are so remote as to approximate the risk of anesthesia alone (less than 0.1%). Mastectomy is almost always performed under general anesthesia. Hospitalization is five to ten days if all goes well, and the patient can return to normal activity within two weeks. With radical mastectomies, the time away from heavy work is prolonged a few more days.

C The incision usually heals and the stitches are removed from the wound within seven to ten days. In about 5% of cases, it may be necessary to remove so much skin over the tumor in order to get well around it that the remaining wound edges cannot easily be brought together. A skin graft, usually taken from the thigh, is used to cover such a wound. The graft becomes firmly attached in seven to ten days, and hospitalization may only be ten to fourteen days. Complications in wound healing can be expected in 10% of patients following simple mastectomy, 15% after radical or wide mastectomy, and about 20% if a skin graft is required to cover the defect over the tumor site. These occasional complications do not affect the chances of cure.

Mastectomy (Removal of Breast)

D Removing the lymph nodes under the arm is necessary because they may contain tumor. These nodes, however, normally are involved in draining fluid (lymph) from the hand and arm, so that after their removal there may be some temporary swelling of the arm. This occurs in about 10% of patients after wide (radical) removal of the breast and in about 2% of those following limited operation. Swelling usually subsides within a month after operation. Rarely, swelling persists, particularly if X-ray therapy is given to the area under the arm (axilla) or if there is tumor blocking lymph drainage.

E Even after wide (radical) mastectomy, where some of the muscles on the chest wall under the breast are removed, there is essentially no limitation of motion or strength of the arm or shoulder. Following radical or wide mastectomy, many women engage in every type of sports and lead perfectly normal lives.

F Mastectomy is performed to provide the best chance of cure from cancer. As with any operation, the ideal is to achieve this goal at the least cost in terms of deformity or disfigurement. There is much discussion (and a deluge of statistics) to support the benefits or drawbacks of limited versus wide resection (radical versus simple mastectomy) and variations of techniques in dealing with lymph nodes under the arm in breast cancer. The current trend is to remove all the breast tissue, save the muscles, and remove the axillary lymph nodes. There are conditions, however, when every surgeon thinks his patient is better served by changing this policy. The extent and type of tumor dictates the ultimate chance of cure far more than do details of operative technique.

G The breast contour is often important to a woman for many complex personal reasons. Whether the underlying muscles are removed (wide, or radical mastectomy) or not disturbed (simple, or limited mastectomy) does not actually alter the contour of the chest wall very much. Most of the contour similar to that of the opposite breast can be restored by a very simple insert in the bra immediately after operation. The patient can go home from the hospital with a normal appearance when dressed. This simple solution is permanently acceptable to about 70% of women following mastectomy.

H A few resent the insert and want something more permanent. One possible solution is the implantation of a plastic material, the shape and consistency of breast tissue, beneath the skin. This is usually done about six months after mastectomy. Its insertion has an early complication rate of about 20% and requires removal in about 10% of cases because of wound breakdown or discomfort.

I Another possibility is to restore breast contours using flaps of skin and fat brought into the area by another operation. This usually requires two to three operations in addition to mastectomy. Some women are eager to put up with the small additional risk and nuisance of at least one other operation. Others are not.

VIII
Abdomen

1. *Diaphragmatic Hernia*

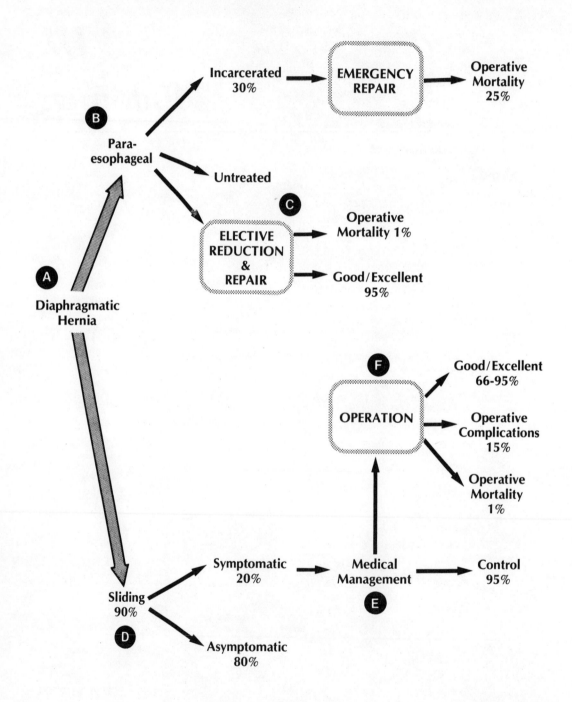

Incarcerated
30% → EMERGENCY REPAIR → Operative Mortality 25%

B Para-esophageal

Untreated

C ELECTIVE REDUCTION & REPAIR → Operative Mortality 1%

→ Good/Excellent 95%

A Diaphragmatic Hernia

F OPERATION → Good/Excellent 66-95%

→ Operative Complications 15%

→ Operative Mortality 1%

Symptomatic 20% → Medical Management → Control 95%

E

Sliding 90%

D

Asymptomatic 80%

A The point where the esophagus empties into the stomach is anchored beneath the diaphragm in the abdominal cavity. Sometimes, the normal attachments become loosened, and the stomach slides up into the chest through an enlargement of the normally small hole (hiatus) in the diaphragm. This is called a diaphragmatic or hiatus hernia. When this occurs, the valve mechanism that normally prevents food and stomach contents from backing up into the esophagus is destroyed, and the delicate esophageal lining is exposed to the erosive acid contents of the stomach juices. This causes inflammation and pain (esophagitis) and is the main reason for treating a diaphragmatic hernia.

B About 10% of all diaphragmatic hernias are called paraesophageal hernias. With this type, the junction of the esophagus and stomach remains in the abdomen, but the top part of the stomach works its way up through the diaphragm into the chest alongside

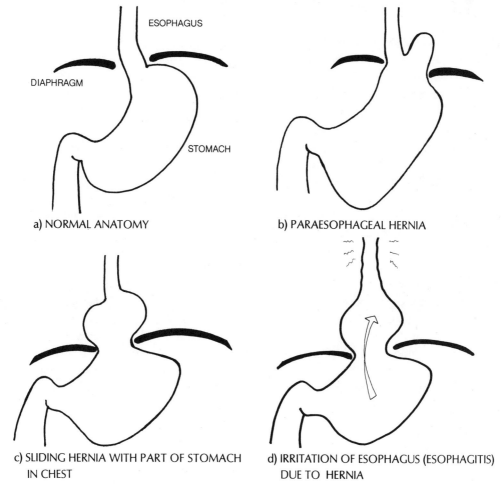

ESOPHAGUS

DIAPHRAGM

STOMACH

a) NORMAL ANATOMY

b) PARAESOPHAGEAL HERNIA

c) SLIDING HERNIA WITH PART OF STOMACH
   IN CHEST

d) IRRITATION OF ESOPHAGUS (ESOPHAGITIS)
   DUE TO HERNIA

the normally placed and fixed esophagus. The importance of this condition is the 30% probability that the stomach will become stuck (incarcerated) in the chest cavity, causing not only a block to the passage of food, but also interruption of its blood supply. Unless the hernia is reduced and the stomach returned to the abdominal cavity beneath the diaphragm, this will soon strangulate stomach tissue and cause death. Emergency operation reducing such a paraesophageal strangulated hernia has a 25% expected mortality.

C On the contrary, elective repair of a paraesophageal hernia before it becomes strangulated has about a 1% expected hospital mortality and about a 95% chance of cure. Elective repair is clearly preferable to waiting until the stomach has its blood supply cut off (strangulated).

D In the more common type of diaphragmatic hernia, the esophagus and stomach both slide into the chest. This is called a sliding diaphragmatic hernia, because the stomach and esophagus both slide back and forth into the chest. Radiologists find some degree of this defect in almost a third of all adults studied with special barium-swallow examination. The junction of the tubular esophagus with the stomach lies in the chest rather than where it belongs in the abdomen. In 80% of people with this slight deviation from normality, there are no symptoms. In the other 20%, however, the contents of the stomach reflux or regurgitate into the lower esophagus, causing irritation of the esophagus (esophagitis) and pain in the lower chest and back after eating a large meal. Lying down after eating makes the pain worse, as stomach contents back up and irritate the esophagus.

E Ninety-five percent of people with a diaphragmatic hernia and symptoms of esophagitis can manage quite well by avoiding large meals, use of antacids, sitting up after eating, and other methods short of operation.

F In 5% of patients, however, non-operative methods fail, resulting in persistent pain, bleeding, or narrowing (stricture) of the lower inflamed esophagus. Operative procedures to correct the hernia and prevent reflux or regurgitation can be performed either through the chest or through the abdomen. The various operations have in common the repair of the enlarged hole in the diaphragm, restoration of the stomach into the abdominal cavity beneath the diaphragm, and prevention of reflux of stomach contents into the esophagus. There is a 65–95% chance of a good to excellent result with these various operations, and about a 10% chance of hernia recurrence.

2. Stomach Cancer

A No one understands the reason, but stomach cancer is less common now in the United States than it was thirty years ago. It may be due to changes in our diet.

TUMOR AT LOWER END OF STOMACH

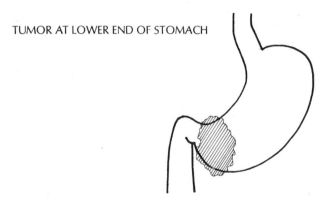

B Certain lesions in the stomach are likely to occur in people with stomach cancer. When such conditions are present, the patient and the physician must be particularly suspicious of the possible development of stomach cancer. Such lesions include:

- *Polyps in the stomach:* A polyp is a mushroomlike growth from the lining of the stomach. The larger its size, the greater the chances that it will be cancer. Polyps over 2 centimeters in diameter have a greater than 5% likelihood of being cancer. Often, several polyps protrude into the stomach.
- *Lack of stomach acid (achlorhydria):* Normal people secrete acid into the stomach. Fewer than 5% of people with stomach cancer have acid in the stomach secretions.
- *Pernicious Anemia:* This blood disease causes a decreased number of red blood cells (anemia) and is closely associated with lack of stomach acid (achlorhydria) and stomach cancer. The longer the patient has pernicious anemia, the greater his chances of developing stomach cancer. Ten percent of patients with pernicious anemia will develop a stomach cancer within ten to fifteen years.

C The only chance for curing a stomach cancer is by surgically removing the tumor together with a wide margin of surrounding stomach. Of a hundred patients with stomach cancer, forty will have such distant spread of tumors when first seen by a physician that operation is of no benefit. Of the remaining sixty who undergo operation, half will have tumors that have spread so extensively within the abdomen that total removal is impossible. In the other half, the tumor will still apparently be

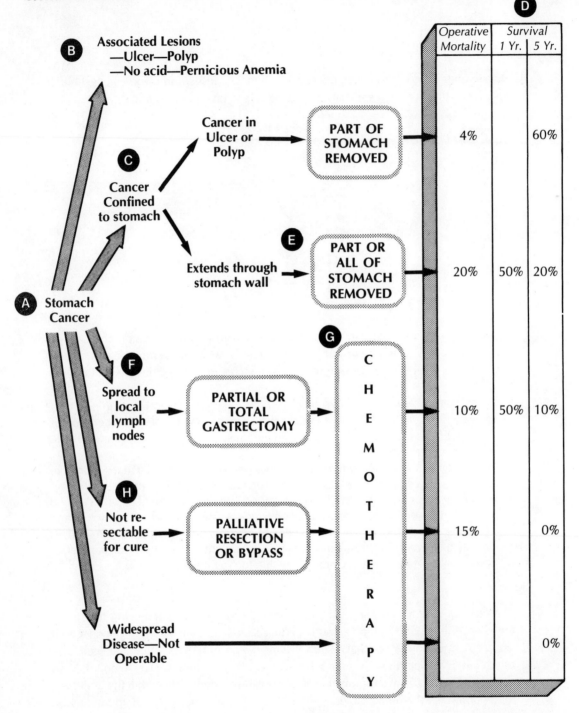

	Operative Mortality	Survival	
		1 Yr.	5 Yr.
PART OF STOMACH REMOVED	4%		60%
PART OR ALL OF STOMACH REMOVED	20%	50%	20%
PARTIAL OR TOTAL GASTRECTOMY	10%	50%	10%
PALLIATIVE RESECTION OR BYPASS	15%		0%
			0%

A Stomach Cancer

B Associated Lesions
—Ulcer—Polyp
—No acid—Pernicious Anemia

C Cancer Confined to stomach

Cancer in Ulcer or Polyp

Extends through stomach wall

E PART OR ALL OF STOMACH REMOVED

F Spread to local lymph nodes

G CHEMOTHERAPY

H Not re-sectable for cure

PALLIATIVE RESECTION OR BYPASS

Widespread Disease—Not Operable

confined to the stomach, where it can seemingly be removed totally. This represents 20% of all patients who are diagnosed as having stomach cancer.

D Of the original hundred patients diagnosed as having stomach cancer, 5–10% will be alive and apparently cured in five years, and half that number in ten years. Many of those cured will have had small cancers in an ulcer or polyp.

E When the cancer has penetrated through the stomach wall but still apparently has spread no further, the surgeon usually takes out the tumor and a large part of the surrounding stomach. Expected mortality is about 5% from this operation (partial gastrectomy). One-half of such patients will be alive in one year, and 20% in five years. Sometimes extensive stomach cancers require removing the entire stomach (total gastrectomy). The hospital mortality after this operation is about 20%. Patients, in fact, free of tumor, get along remarkably well without any stomach. They can eat almost normally, and although they seldom gain weight, they maintain their strength.

F None of the available anti-cancer drugs can cure stomach cancer. About 15% of such tumors will shrink in size for a few weeks or months after these drugs are given.

The average length of life after operation in which the tumor is unresectable for cure is less than a year.

G In about half of the patients who undergo abdominal operation for stomach cancer, the surgeon will find that he cannot remove all the tumor. If, however, the stomach tumor is obstructing passage of food, it is possible in 30% of cases to connect that part of the stomach uninvolved with tumor to the intestine, so that the patient can eat without vomiting. This will not cure the patient, but may make the remaining one to six months of life more comfortable.

H When the surgeon, at operation, finds tumor in the lymph nodes as well as in the stomach, there is a 10% chance of ultimate cure if the stomach and all the visible tumor in the involved lymph nodes are removed.

3. Gastric Ulcer

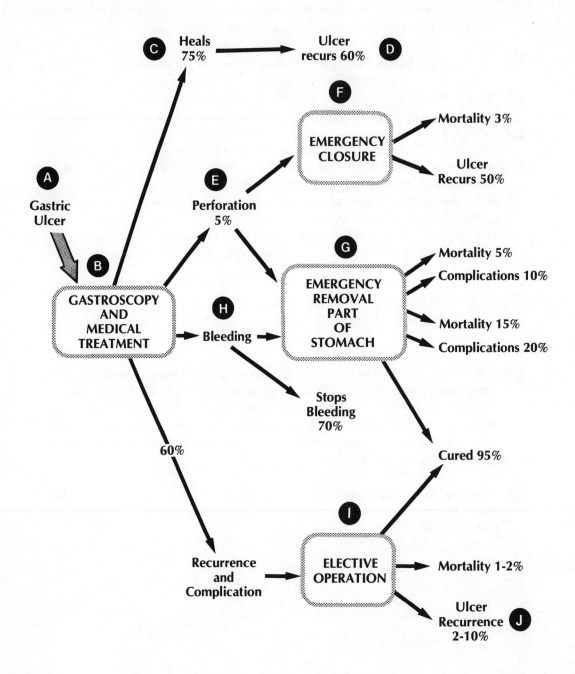

C Heals 75% → Ulcer recurs 60% **D**

F EMERGENCY CLOSURE → Mortality 3%
→ Ulcer Recurs 50%

A Gastric Ulcer

B GASTROSCOPY AND MEDICAL TREATMENT

E Perforation 5%

H Bleeding

G EMERGENCY REMOVAL PART OF STOMACH → Mortality 5%
→ Complications 10%
→ Mortality 15%
→ Complications 20%

Stops Bleeding 70%

Cured 95%

60%

Recurrence and Complication

I ELECTIVE OPERATION → Mortality 1-2%
→ Ulcer Recurrence 2-10% **J**

A A stomach (gastric) ulcer is a localized erosion or raw place in the tissue that lines the stomach. It differs from a duodenal ulcer, not only in its location but by the 5% possibility that it is associated with a stomach cancer. Almost never is there a cancer at the site of a duodenal ulcer. Gastric ulcers greater than 4 centimeters in diameter have a 75% likelihood of being cancer. Lack of acid in the stomach (achlorhydria) increases the likelihood of cancer three times in a person with a gastric ulcer.

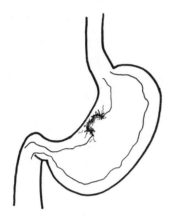 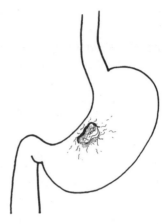

a) ULCER IN MIDDLE OF STOMACH   b) PERFORATION

B Once a gastric ulcer is suspected or diagnosed by X-ray studies, it usually is directly inspected by gastroscopy (see "Gastroscopy," page 180). This involves passing a flexible tube into the stomach through the mouth. Fitted with a lens system and a light at its tip, the gastroscope provides both a good look at the ulcer in the stomach and an opportunity to remove a small piece of the ulcer (biopsy) for study under the microscope. Such a biopsy is 95% accurate in proving the presence of cancer in the edge of an ulcer.

C If there is no evidence of cancer, medical treatment is usually tried for three to six weeks. If the ulcer decreases to half its original size with medical treatment for three weeks, it has a 95% chance of being benign (no cancer). Three-quarters of all benign ulcers will be totally healed within six weeks. If there is cancer associated with the ulcer, it may decrease in size but will never *totally* disappear.

D Even if a benign gastric ulcer heals, there is a 60% chance that the ulcer will recur within a few years and a 10% likelihood that the ulcer will cause so much trouble within two years that an operation will be needed for its cure. Most gastric ulcers go away quite promptly, but most come back and cause more trouble at a later date.

E About 5% of the time, a gastric ulcer will erode (perforate) through the entire stomach wall, spilling the acid stomach contents into the abdominal cavity. This dramatic and painful event requires an emergency operation.

F Eighty percent of the time, the surgeon will merely close the hole in the stomach. This relatively short operation has a 5% chance of mortality and a 10% chance of complications after the operation, but in the years thereafter, at least half of such patients will have recurrence of the ulcer. Simple closure of the perforation is the safest procedure, but doesn't usually cure the patient of his ulcer.

G In about 20% of patients with perforated gastric ulcers, the surgeon will decide to remove the perforation along with some of the stomach (partial gastrectomy) in order to not only take care of the immediate problem of perforation but also to give the patient a 90–95% chance of being cured of the ulcer by the operation. This is a bigger operation than a simple closure, with 10% chance of mortality and a complication rate of 15% when done as such an emergency. As usual, a price must be paid in order to provide a better chance of cure.

Ninety-five percent of perforated ulcers are benign. When perforation occurs through a cancer, the chances of cure are less than 5%.

H Many patients with a gastric ulcer will lose a little blood from the raw surface of the ulcer, but only about one in twenty will bleed so much that they require transfusion. Such bleeding from an ulcer in the stomach usually makes itself known by the patient vomiting up large amounts of bright red blood. About 15% of those who vomit up blood do so from a gastric ulcer.

At least two-thirds of patients who bleed from a stomach ulcer will stop bleeding without operation, If, despite all treatment, bleeding does not stop, an emergency operation is necessary. This usually requires removing part of the stomach (partial gastrectomy), and when done as an emergency, has a high (15% or more) expected mortality rate and a 20% chance of some complication in the early days after operation. Other types of operation are less risky, but are less likely to stop bleeding or to cure the ulcer.

I Pain, persistence of the ulcer complications such as bleeding, and suspicion of cancer will finally cause about 10% of all people who have a gastric ulcer to undergo operation for its cure. Operation at a convenient time (not as an emergency) is called an elective operation. The usual procedure is to remove a part of the stomach (partial gastrectomy). It cures about 95% of patients of their ulcer and when done electively has about a 2% chance of mortality—far less than when the operation is performed as an emergency.

(J) The chance of ulcer recurrence is only about 2% if partial gastrectomy is performed. If a lesser operation (vagotomy and pyloroplasty) is performed because of its lesser risks, the chance of recurrence is 10%.

4. Gastroscopy

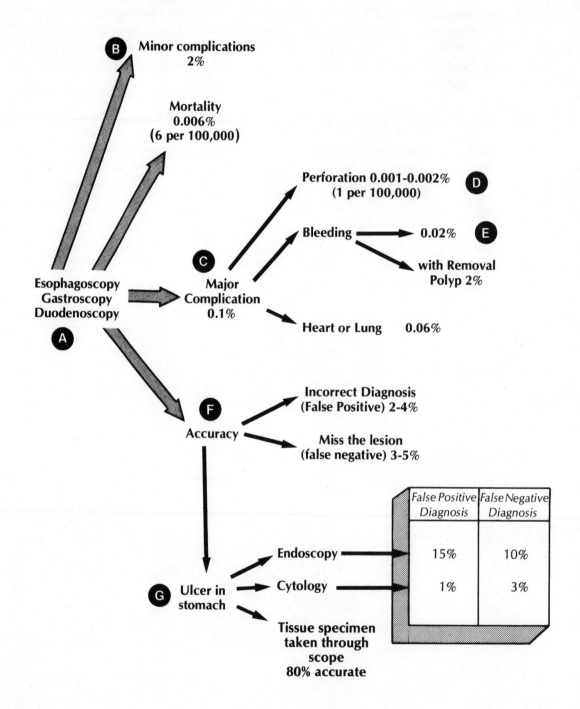

B Minor complications
2%

Mortality
0.006%
(6 per 100,000)

Perforation 0.001-0.002% D
(1 per 100,000)

Bleeding ➝ 0.02% E

with Removal
Polyp 2%

Esophagoscopy
Gastroscopy
Duodenoscopy

A

C Major
Complication
0.1%

Heart or Lung   0.06%

Incorrect Diagnosis
(False Positive) 2-4%

Miss the lesion
(false negative) 3-5%

F

Accuracy

	False Positive Diagnosis	False Negative Diagnosis
Endoscopy	15%	10%
Cytology	1%	3%

G Ulcer in
stomach

Tissue specimen
taken through
scope
80% accurate

A In the past, only a rigid lighted tube passed through the mouth was available to look into the stomach. This was extremely uncomfortable for the patient, roughly equivalent to sword swallowing. Lacking such a gastroscope, diagnosis of disease within the stomach was relatively inaccurate, relying on the shadow X-ray outline of swallowed barium in the stomach.

The recent development of a flexible gastroscope has changed all this. About 1 centimeter in diameter, this flexible tube, with a light at its tip, is swallowed by the awake patient, using only some sedative and a little local anesthetic applied to the back of the throat. The procedure is often done without the need for being admitted to

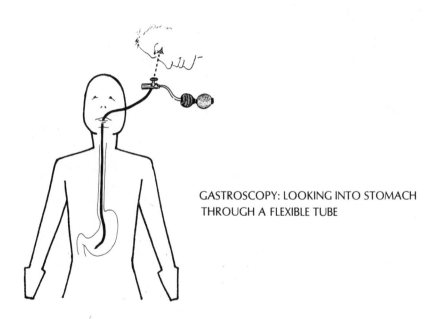

GASTROSCOPY: LOOKING INTO STOMACH
THROUGH A FLEXIBLE TUBE

the hospital and is completed in thirty minutes to an hour. The examining physician can direct the lighted scope toward any part of the stomach that he wishes to examine. If something suspicious is found, a small piece of the lesion can be removed with special forceps at the tip of the scope and the tissue examined under the microscope.

B Occasionally, there is damage to the teeth, gums, or back of the throat by the tube. Rarely, a patient is sensitive to one of the sedatives or local anesthetic agents used in the back of the mouth and throat.

C Major complications are so rare that the chance of their occurrence is less than 0.01%. The rare death occuring during gastroscopy results from bleeding or perforation of an already badly diseased stomach.

D In an occasional case, a hole is made in a friable area of the stomach already diseased and about to perforate before the examination. Over-distending the stomach with air passed down the tube can also perforate the stomach. When perforation occurs, the hole must be closed by immediate operation.

E The chance of significant bleeding resulting from gastroscopy is about 0.02%. The chance is greater if the patient is taking anticoagulant drugs. If a stomach polyp is removed through the gastroscope, there is 2% chance of significant bleeding. Such bleeding either will stop by itself, require electro-cautery (burning) of its base through the scope, or occasionally, an operation on the stomach must be performed to stop bleeding.

F Even when one can look directly into the stomach through the gastroscope, there is a possibility of overlooking a small, camouflaged or inconveniently located lesion. Sometimes in a stomach full of blood, a clot obscures the lesion. Accuracy improves with the experience of the endoscopist, but no one can guarantee a perfect record. The likelihood of overlooking a stomach lesion (false negative) is about 3–5%; of incorrectly diagnosing a lesion that is seen, 2–4% (false positive).

G The gastroscope is commonly used to determine whether a known stomach ulcer is cancer (see "Stomach Cancer," page 173). Sometimes, this is not easy. Even when a surgeon or pathologist has the stomach containing the ulcer in his hand after operation he can be wrong. Understandably, the endoscopist can do no better looking at the ulcer through a tube. The chances are about 15% that he will think a benign ulcer is cancer and about 10% that an ulcer containing cancer is thought to be benign. Examining cells under the microscope from washings taken through the gastroscope improves accuracy to 75–99%. Microscopic examination of a piece of a stomach tumor taken through the gastroscope is accurate in at least 80% of cases.

5. Duodenal Ulcer

A The stomach normally makes acid. Emotional tension or certain drugs make it produce more than a normal amount. But the lining of the stomach is designed to withstand acid and, like the inside of an enamel pot, doesn't erode or show signs of damage. However, the stomach empties into the duodenum, which, like an iron pipe, is *not* designed to withstand acid. When too much acid pours from the stomach into the relatively unprotected duodenum, its lining erodes and forms ulcers.

DUODENAL ULCER:

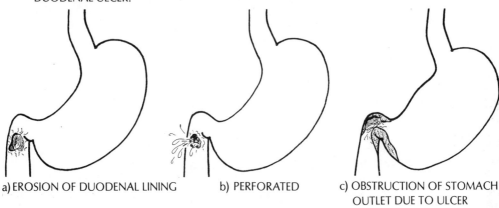

a) EROSION OF DUODENAL LINING   b) PERFORATED   c) OBSTRUCTION OF STOMACH OUTLET DUE TO ULCER

B Eighty-five percent of duodenal ulcers heal without complication. But a person who once has a duodenal ulcer has about a 50% chance of forming another one sometime in the future. About 15% of persons with a duodenal ulcer will ultimately require an operation for some complication of the disease. New drugs, called H-2 blockers, are of enormous benefit in stopping the acute symptoms of duodenal ulcer such as pain or bleeding, but do not permanently cure the disease.

C When all other means of managing the pain and discomfort of a duodenal ulcer have failed, as they do in about 15% of patients, operation is required. Such operations are designed to decrease the production of excessive stomach acid. This may be achieved by 1) removing the acid-producing portion of the stomach (partial gastrectomy), 2) removing that part of the stomach that stimulates acid production (antrectomy), and 3) cutting the nerve (vagus nerve) that stimulates acid production (vagotomy).

Choice of the proper operation for a given patient involves many factors such as age, general physical condition, chance of recurrence after operation, risk of the procedure, and chance of bad side effects resulting from the operation. The following table provides an idea of these risks with three operations commonly used to treat duodenal ulcer.

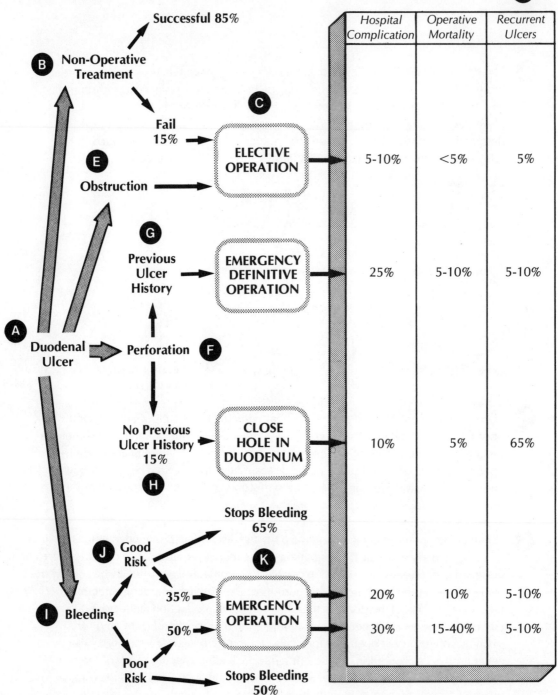

	Hospital Complication	Operative Mortality	Recurrent Ulcers
ELECTIVE OPERATION	5-10%	<5%	5%
EMERGENCY DEFINITIVE OPERATION	25%	5-10%	5-10%
CLOSE HOLE IN DUODENUM	10%	5%	65%
EMERGENCY OPERATION	20%	10%	5-10%
EMERGENCY OPERATION	30%	15-40%	5-10%

B Non-Operative Treatment → Successful 85%

Fail 15% →

E Obstruction →

C ELECTIVE OPERATION

G Previous Ulcer History →

EMERGENCY DEFINITIVE OPERATION

A Duodenal Ulcer → Perforation **F**

No Previous Ulcer History 15% →

CLOSE HOLE IN DUODENUM

H

Stops Bleeding 65%

J Good Risk

K

35% →

EMERGENCY OPERATION

50% →

I Bleeding

Poor Risk → Stops Bleeding 50%

D

	Operative mortality	Complication	Ulcer recurrence	Late complication
1. Cut vagus nerve plus an emptying procedure on the stomach (vagotomy)	5%	5–10%	15%	15%
2. Cut branches of the vagus nerve (selective vagotomy)	1%	1–2%	???	???
			Too new to be certain	
3. Remove part of the stomach and cut the vagus nerve (antrectomy and vagotomy)	5–10%	10%	5%	20%

D Following operation for duodenal ulcer, there is a 2–10% chance of producing what is called the post-gastrectomy, post-vagotomy, or dumping syndrome. These three names are all used for the unpleasant nausea, sweating, light-headedness, and diarrhea that may come on fifteen minutes to an hour after eating certain types of meals. The chance of having such symptoms differ from each operation. Unfortunately, the technique that provides the best chance for curing the ulcer (vagotomy and antrectomy) also has the highest probability of producing unpleasant side effects. The surgeon must choose which operation he judges the best for each patient on the basis of which has the least risk of death and complication and the best chance of cure of the ulcer. There is no universal simplistic answer.

E Each time an ulcer heals, it leaves a scar. After repeated attacks of ulceration, the accumulated scars narrow the duodenum to the point where the stomach cannot easily empty. Everything eaten is vomited. When this occurs, there is only a 10% chance that complete obstruction will even temporarily be relieved without operation. When obstruction continues, the obstructed area must either be removed or a short-circuit pathway created for food to bypass the obstructed duodenum. If the scarred area is only bypassed, the chance of future ulcer recurrence is at least 10–15%. The other possibility is to remove the obstructed portion of the duodenum and perform one of the operations designed to prevent future ulcer recurrence (vagotomy and antrectomy). This option has a 5–10% chance of mortality under these emergency conditions, but cures about 95% of the patients. The best compromise must be sought for each patient.

F Sometimes the ulcer erodes through the entire duodenal wall, spilling acid contents of the stomach into the abdominal cavity. This causes severe abdominal pain and is called a perforated duodenal ulcer. It requires immediate operation to prevent serious peritonitis.

G A perforated ulcer can be managed in either of two ways by merely closing the perforation or by closing the perforation and performing one of the definitive operations that will prevent further ulcer activity. The first type of operation is safer; the second option is more of an immediate risk, but provides a better chance for ultimate cure. Definitive operation prevents future ulceration in about 90% of patients. The mortality when performed as an emergency is 5–10%, and about one in four patients will have some sort of complication in the immediate period following this emergency operation. In general, the surgeon will choose to perform one of these definitive operations at the time of perforation if the patient has had a long previous history of ulcer problems.

H The other possibility for the surgeon is merely to close the ulcer. This operation has an expected mortality of less than 5%, but the chance of ulcer recurrence is 65%. One-third of patients with a perforated ulcer may do very well after simple closure of the ulcer. Another one-third will have various complications with recurrent ulcer. The final third will have so many complications with the ulcer that an operation will be necessary for its management. These stark possibilities must be understood by the patient as he recovers from the operative closure of his perforated ulcer. Simply closing the ulcer does not change the person's personality nor his future 66% chance of having future ulcer symptoms or complications.

I About 10% of patients with duodenal ulcer will bleed into the stomach, usually causing vomiting of blood or its passage in the stools. Severe bleeding requires admission to the hospital and blood transfusion. Once a person has a major bleed from a duodenal ulcer he has a 35% chance of rebleeding and a 40% likelihood of ultimately requiring an operation for his ulcer.

J Young good-risk patients can tolerate a good deal of blood loss, and only about 35% will have to undergo operation to stop the bleeding from the ulcer bed. Poor-risk and elderly patients, on the other hand, cannot tolerate as much bleeding, so about 50% must be operated upon to stop the bleeding. Anachronistically, old people with poor hearts and lungs have to be operated upon sooner than the young and healthy. The newer drugs for the treatment of ulcer (H-2 blockers) are of particular help in avoiding the need for risky emergency operations on patients for acute bleeding from duodenal ulcer.

K Emergency operation to stop bleeding from an ulcer has a high mortality rate that may approach 40% and a post-operative complication rate of 30% in very poor-risk or elderly patients. Emergency operation for bleeding ulcer is a life-saving procedure, but it is risky.

6. Diabetes Mellitus

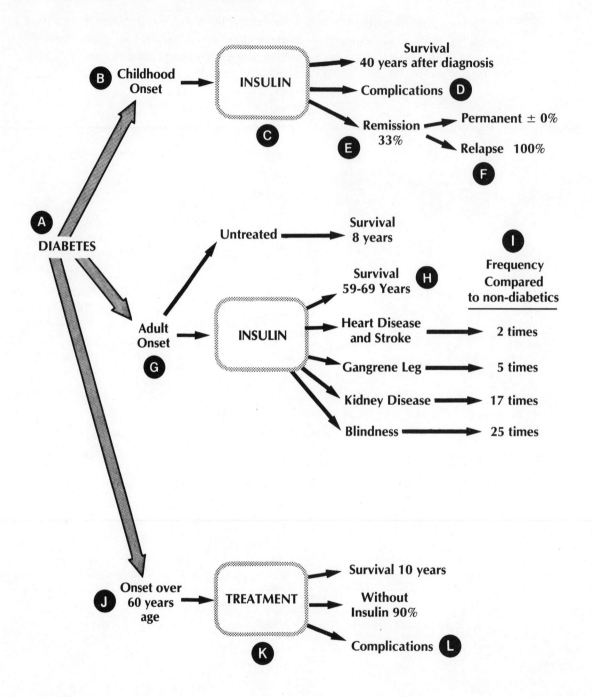

- **A** DIABETES
- **B** Childhood Onset
- **C** INSULIN
  - Survival 40 years after diagnosis
  - Complications **D**
  - Remission 33% **E**
    - Permanent ± 0%
    - Relapse 100% **F**
- **G** Adult Onset
  - Untreated → Survival 8 years
  - INSULIN
    - Survival 59-69 Years **H**
    - Heart Disease and Stroke → 2 times
    - Gangrene Leg → 5 times
    - Kidney Disease → 17 times
    - Blindness → 25 times
  - **I** Frequency Compared to non-diabetics
- **J** Onset over 60 years age
  - **K** TREATMENT
    - Survival 10 years
    - Without Insulin 90%
    - Complications **L**

A Diabetes is a generalized disease in which there is an abnormality in sugar metabolism. In 90% of cases this is due to a decreased production of insulin from special cells in the pancreas. Injections of this hormone bring the abnormally elevated blood sugar concentration toward normal and control many of the signs and symptoms of the disease, such as the early development of arteriosclerosis. At least 50% of diabetics have a family history of the disease. If one parent is a diabetic, there is about an 8–10% likelihood that a child will develop the disease. If both parents are diabetic, the likelihood is about 33%, with another 50% having occasional abnormalities in the level of sugar in the blood.

B Onset of diabetes before the age of twenty is usually abrupt, with sudden severe generalized signs of the disease, such as weakness and weight loss. This type of diabetes may even be due to a viral infection. Before the use of insulin, such children would live only a few months after diagnosis.

C With insulin, average survival is to about fifty-five years. Those with childhood onset often have very narrow limits for their tolerance for insulin and if not carefully controlled may either take too much insulin and go into insulin shock or take too little and have serious signs of diabetic coma (unconsciousness).

D Patients with childhood-onset diabetes have the same complications of the disease as do adults, except that high blood pressure is rare.

E About 33% of patients with childhood-onset diabetes will have a swift recovery from the initial attack and within a few weeks will have little evidence of the disease. Most will require little or no insulin.

F However, almost all of these children will, within a year, have some type of relapse of their disease. At first, there may be only an abnormality in one of the tests of blood sugar concentration. Gradually, however, they will develop full-blown diabetes.

G About 75% of diabetes starts in people between the ages of twenty to sixty. Survival, if untreated, is only about eight years, but diet, insulin, and oral antidiabetic drugs quickly provide improvement. Some type of treatment is required daily for the rest of the patient's life. Diabetes will not spontaneously disappear.

H The average life expectancy of a diabetic man is sixty years and of a woman, about seventy years. It is not certain whether close control of blood sugar levels with insulin appreciably increases life span, compared to those in whom there is less rigid control.

I Diabetics have an increased susceptibility to infection, to blindness, and to early onset of arteriosclerosis (hardening of the arteries). They are twice as prone to heart disease and stroke, five times more likely to develop gangrene of the leg due to poor blood supply, seventeen times as likely to have kidney failure, and twenty-five times more apt to have blindness. Causes of death in diabetes are: heart disease, 55%; stroke, 10%; renal failure, 8%; and infection, 6%. Cost of insulin is about $60 per year.

J About 30% of diabetes starts in people over sixty. In the elderly, the disease is usually mild. The normal value of blood sugar is higher in older persons than in the young.

K Only about 10% of patients with diabetes that starts after age sixty eventually require insulin. The vast majority may be controlled with diet and certain drugs taken by mouth. Patients with diabetes starting after age sixty have a life expectancy almost similar to non-diabetics, if they keep the diabetes under control with insulin or other means.

L Patients whose diabetes starts after the age of sixty are liable to the same complications as are ordinary adult-onset diabetics, except that blindness and kidney disease are less common.

7. General Anesthesia

A Most people are "put to sleep" during a major operation. Such a general anesthesia produces unconsciousness, blocks pain, and obtains muscle relaxation by a combination of drugs given into a vein or inhaled as a gas.

B Drugs given the night before operation and before the patient gets to the operating room are usually taken by mouth or administered by injection underneath the skin. They provide a reasonable night's sleep before operation and may involve an antibiotic to minimize the likelihood of infection after the operation. Drugs used in the operating room are usually given directly into a vein. Various salt and sugar solutions or blood are also often given intravenously during the operation.

C Every operation—no matter how minor—involves some loss of blood. Even operations such as hernia repair or dilation and curettage result in loss of 100–300 cc (cubic centimeters) of blood. During big operations, the loss may be ten times this amount. Adult man has a total of approximately 4,500 cc (4½ quarts) of blood in his body. He can lose about 500 cc without causing a problem, but when loss during operation is greater than this amount, even a healthy person may be better off having some of the loss replaced by a blood transfusion. The ordinary bottle of blood contains 500 cc.

Despite all precautions, blood from a blood bank has a chance of containing a virus that causes a certain type of liver disease called viral hepatitis. About 1% of patients receiving such virus-contaminated blood will contract viral hepatitis in the weeks after the transfusion. Two to ten percent will show changes in various sensitive tests of liver function that probably are due to the blood transfusion. This is difficult to prove for anesthesia, and the stress of operation may contribute to such chemical changes.

D Drugs used to produce general anesthesia not only make a person unconscious but also depress many other functions of the brain. Most decrease the rate and depth of breathing. Therefore, in 90% of the instances, respiration is assisted during operation by forcing air, oxygen, or anesthestic gases through a tube passed from the mouth into the airway (trachea) that leads to the lungs. The work of breathing during operation is often taken over by the anesthetist or by an artificial ventilator machine by his side. The endotracheal tube usually is removed soon after operation but sometimes is left in place for several days, if the patient needs help in breathing.

E In order to empty the stomach of its contents and avoid vomiting, a tube attached to suction is often passed through the nose into the stomach before or during operation. This may be kept in place for several days after operation. The likelihood of vomiting

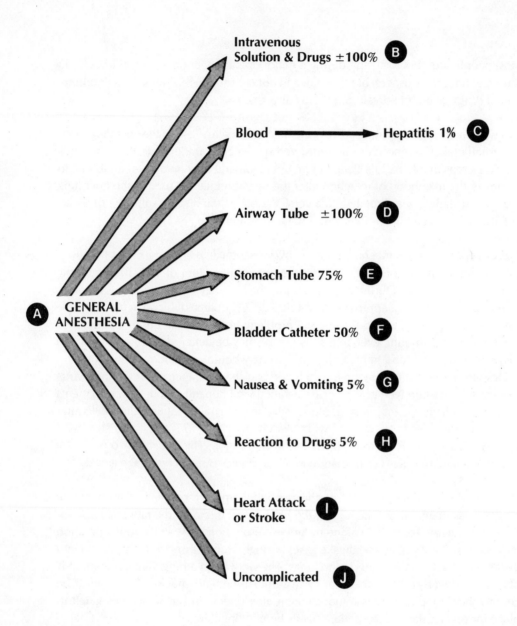

Intravenous
Solution & Drugs ±100% **B**

Blood ⟶ Hepatitis 1% **C**

Airway Tube ±100% **D**

Stomach Tube 75% **E**

Bladder Catheter 50% **F**

Nausea & Vomiting 5% **G**

Reaction to Drugs 5% **H**

Heart Attack
or Stroke **I**

Uncomplicated **J**

A GENERAL
ANESTHESIA

and inhaling irritating stomach contents during general anesthesia is about 0.02%. Usually, the amount aspirated is so small it is of little significance.

F Another tube (catheter) is often placed in the urinary bladder during anesthesia to drain off accumulated urine. It, too, may be left in place for some days after operation to be certain that urine is being made in proper quantities.

G Many people continue to hold an unjustified fear about the likelihood and severity of vomiting in the postoperative period. This dates back to the days when many irritating gases were used for general anesthesia. At the present time, about 5% of patients will experience some nausea and vomiting after operation, but this is usually so mild that it does not seriously bother a patient. If a nasogastric tube is left in the stomach, as described above, this essentially eliminates vomiting.

H There is always a possibility that a patient might be sensitive to one of the four to ten drugs that are administered by vein, by inhalation, or under the skin to a patient during a general anesthesia. Even when this is the case, the reaction usually is no more serious than a few hives on the skin or some other minor irritation. In less than 0.1% of cases is such a sensitivity reaction severe enough to interfere in any way with the operation or the clinical course following operation.

I Some of the drugs given during general anesthesia may affect the heart, causing irregularities in rhythm, rate, or its activity in pumping blood. Arrhythmias occur in over 50% of patients under general anesthesia; serious arrhythmias in about 20%. The anesthesiologist is trained to detect these abnormalities and to take appropriate action to correct them. Although the exact incidence depends on the age and prior condition of the patient, about 0.03% of patients who had no previously recognized heart disease will suffer a myocardial infarct (heart attack) during general anesthesia for a non-cardiac operation (see "Heart Attack," page 99).

J More than 99% of general anesthesias proceed without significant complication.

8. Pancreatic Cancer

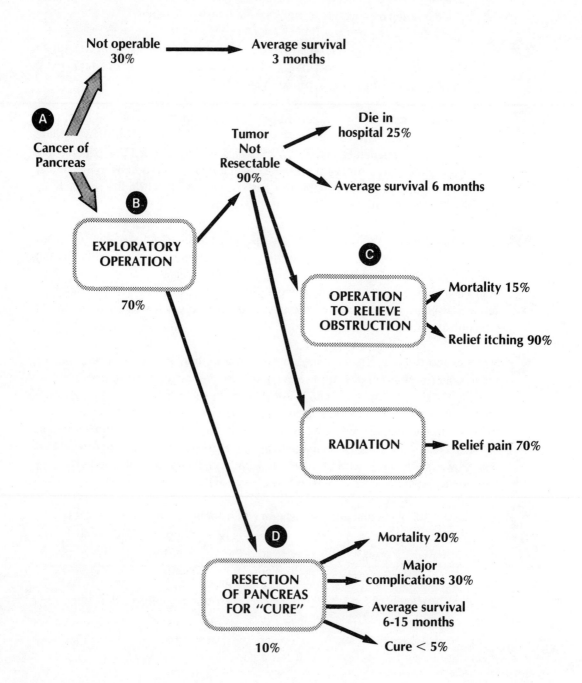

Not operable
30% → Average survival
3 months

A

Cancer of
Pancreas

B

EXPLORATORY
OPERATION

70%

Tumor
Not
Resectable
90%

Die in
hospital 25%

Average survival 6 months

C

OPERATION
TO RELIEVE
OBSTRUCTION

Mortality 15%

Relief itching 90%

RADIATION → Relief pain 70%

D

RESECTION
OF PANCREAS
FOR "CURE"

10%

Mortality 20%

Major
complications 30%

Average survival
6-15 months

Cure < 5%

A The pancreas lies across the upper abdomen in contact with many important organs. The right side of the pancreas encircles the common bile duct, a tube that drains bile from the liver into the intestine. When cancer develops in this part of the pancreas, it

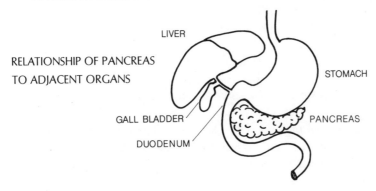

RELATIONSHIP OF PANCREAS
TO ADJACENT ORGANS

LIVER

STOMACH

GALL BLADDER

PANCREAS

DUODENUM

often blocks (obstructs) the common bile duct, causing bile to back up in the liver and resulting in a yellow color to the skin (jaundice). Although many other disease conditions cause jaundice, this is the hallmark of pancreatic cancer.

About 30% of such cancers have spread so widely when first discovered that operation cannot be of benefit. These patients survive an average of only three months. Drugs and radiation do not appreciably slow growth of pancreatic tumors.

B In the remaining 70% of patients in whom operation is thought to be of possible benefit, the chances are nine to one that the surgeon will, at operation on the abdomen, find that the tumor has spread so widely that it cannot all be removed. Average survival under these circumstances is about six months.

C When the bile duct is blocked by the pancreatic cancer, it often is possible to relieve the obstruction by diverting bile into the intestine around the tumor. This at least helps relieve the itching that plagues many patients with this type of jaundice. It also may prolong life a few more weeks.

D In 10% of patients with pancreatic cancer, the tumor appears only to involve the pancreas. But to remove tumors in the head of the pancreas, the surgeon must remove not only the pancreas, but parts of the stomach, duodenum, and common bile duct. This is a big operation, with a 20% chance of mortality and a 30% likelihood of some serious complication after operation. In some surgical centers, the chances are somewhat better. But regardless of the risk of operation, less than 5% of patients are ever cured of this type of cancer, and average survival, after what was thought to be curable operation, is only three to fifteen months.

Pancreatic Cancer

E Although cancer of the duodenum and nearby bile ducts is a different tumor than cancer of the pancreas, the two occur in almost the same location and usually cause similar symptoms of jaundice. Cancers arising in the duodenum and bile ducts have a slightly better chance for cure than those in the pancreas. About 85% of such patients are at least operable with a chance for cure.

F At such exploratory operation, 35% of bile duct or duodenal tumors cannot be removed, but at least relief of jaundice is often made possible by diverting bile into the intestine around the tumor. Average survival is four to nine months.

G In the remaining 65% of patients with bile duct or duodenal cancer, the tumor is resectable. Although the mortality of the operation is about 20% and the chances of major complication about 60%, almost a third of the patients who survive the operation are cured.

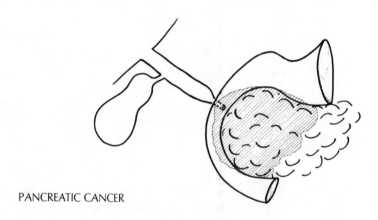

PANCREATIC CANCER

9. *Acute Pancreatitis*

A The pancreas is a long gland lying in the upper abdomen, over the backbone. In addition to insulin, the pancreas produces large volumes of very powerful digestive juices that are collected in a branching system of ducts that empty into the nearby intestinal tract. Anything that blocks the outflow of the pancreatic duct dams up these enzyme-rich juices, making them leak back into the gland, where they cause severe inflammation. Inflammation of the pancreas is called pancreatitis. The two most common causes of pancreatitis are a gallstone wedged in the outlet of the pancreatic duct where it empties into the intestine and alcohol, which stimulates the pancreas to feverish activity and gradually causes many points of obstruction of the pancreatic duct along its entire length. Pancreatitis often causes severe abdominal pain, which mimicks many other abdominal diseases and is often difficult to diagnose.

B Pancreatitis due to gallstones is usually only an incidental complication of acute gallbladder disease. Eighty percent of the severe attacks resolve as the gallbladder attack subsides. But the stone rarely passes into the intestine, and about 90% of those who had a severe attack of pancreatitis must have the stone removed by an operation at a later date in order to avoid recurrence. In about 20% of cases of severe gallstone-related pancreatitis, the acute attack will not subside and the patient continues to get worse. An emergency operation is then necessary to clear the obstructed pancreatic duct. If the stone is removed, the pancreatitis is cured, but frequently these patients are very sick for a few days after operation and have a 15% chance of complication. About 2% of patients will not survive.

C Most pancreatitis is associated with alcoholism, not gallstones. The acute attack of severe abdominal pain subsides in 9 out of 10 cases without the need for operation, but with each attack, the pancreas is further damaged and the patient usually ends up with chronic pancreatitis and a destroyed gland. Few if any of these patients stop drinking.

D There is swelling (edema) of the inflamed pancreas with every acute attack. In about 5% of cases, this is so severe that there is bleeding into the gland as the gland, in essence, begins to digest itself. This occurs uncommonly, but when it does occur, there is an 80% expected mortality unless an operation is performed. Operations involving removal of parts of the gland and various types of drainage may reduce the expected mortality from the acute attack to about 50%. The postoperative course is stormy in all the survivors, and about 80% will have evidence of pancreatic insufficiency because of the destruction of the gland. This may include diabetes.

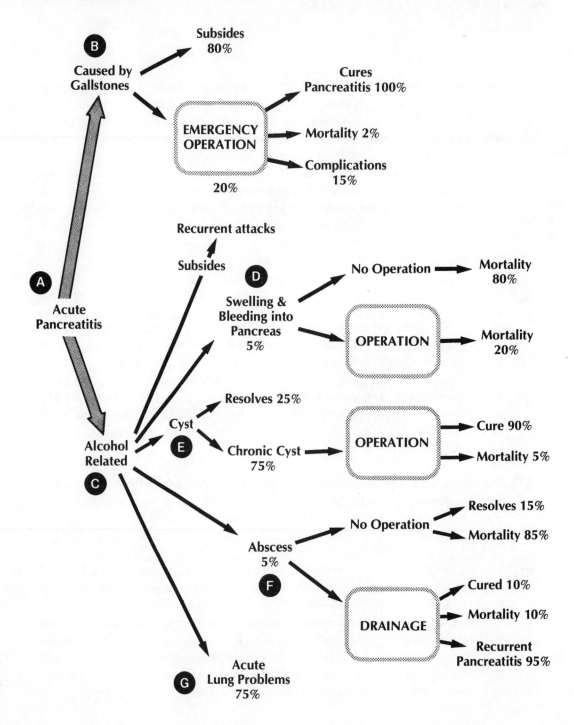

E There is swelling in the pancreas in all cases. In 40%, this can be felt as a mass in the abdomen. In about 10% of cases, special studies will show the formation of small fluid-filled cysts in the swollen gland. Most small cysts and 25% of larger ones (2 centimeters in diameter and over) will disappear. The remainder persist and end up as chronic thick-walled cysts arising from the pancreas.

F An infection (abscess) develops in the inflamed pancreas or in a cyst in about 5% of patients following an acute attack of pancreatitis. Treated without operation, the mortality of an established pancreatic abscess is very high (85%). Even with drainage, there is a 10% chance of mortality and a 50% chance of complications, which include prolonged drainage of pancreatic juice from the drain site.

G Problems with breathing accompany 75% of attacks of severe acute pancreatitis. Most clear as the attack subsides, but many patients require the use of a mechanical ventilator during the height of the attack.

10. Gallstones

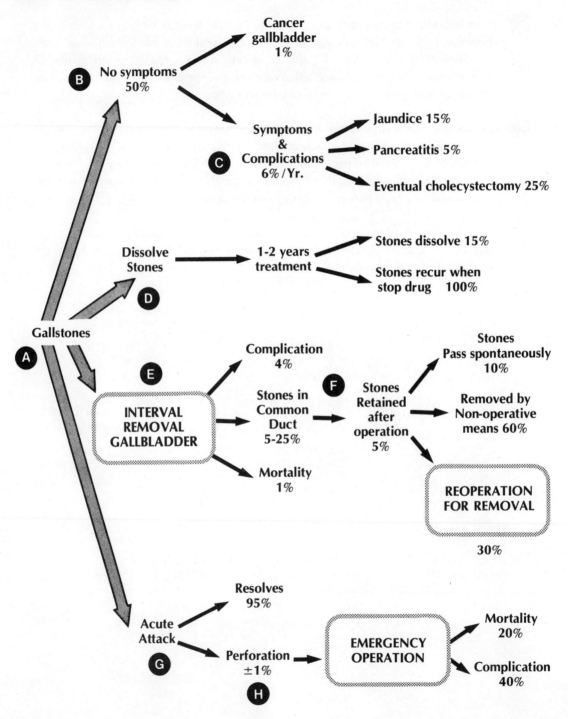

Cancer gallbladder 1%

B No symptoms 50%

C Symptoms & Complications 6% / Yr.
- Jaundice 15%
- Pancreatitis 5%
- Eventual cholecystectomy 25%

D Dissolve Stones → 1-2 years treatment
- Stones dissolve 15%
- Stones recur when stop drug 100%

A Gallstones

E INTERVAL REMOVAL GALLBLADDER
- Complication 4%
- Stones in Common Duct 5-25%
- Mortality 1%

F Stones Retained after operation 5%
- Stones Pass spontaneously 10%
- Removed by Non-operative means 60%
- REOPERATION FOR REMOVAL 30%

G Acute Attack
- Resolves 95%
- **H** Perforation ±1% → EMERGENCY OPERATION
  - Mortality 20%
  - Complication 40%

A Lying in the upper part of the right side of the abdomen just under the ribs, the gallbladder contains bile that is made in the liver. It drains into a small-diameter tube (the common bile duct), which empties into the intestine (duodenum). When the

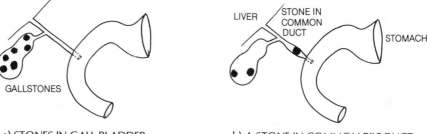

a) STONES IN GALL BLADDER   b) A STONE IN COMMON BILE DUCT

gallbladder becomes diseased, some of the material normally held in suspension in the bile precipitates out as stones in the gallbladder. Such stones may occlude the narrow end of the gallbladder where it empties into the common duct, causing attacks of acute pain under the ribs on the right side of the abdomen. Such a "gallbladder attack" is called acute cholecystitis.

Gallstones are more common in the elderly. Under forty years of age, 5% of the population have gallstones; thirty percent of those over sixty have gallstones.

Only about 20% of gallstones will show up on ordinary X-ray studies of the abdomen. Special X-ray studies and ultrasound examination are about 95% accurate in detecting gallstones.

B Half of the patients with gallstones are at first without symptoms. The question then arises, "Why take out the gallbladder if it is not causing trouble?" One argument involves the likelihood of gallstones causing cancer. This risk is less than 1%—too low to be a valid reason for taking out a stone-filled asymptomatic gallbladder.

C Much more important is the 6% likelihood per year of developing serious symptoms from the stones. This includes a 5–10% likelihood of ultimately developing serious inflammation of the pancreas (pancreatitis) due to the stones, and a 15–25% likelihood that stones will pass from the gallbladder into the common bile duct, where they are likely to cause jaundice (yellow skin) and liver damage.

About 25% of patients with "asymptomatic gallstones" will ultimately require an operation at a time when the operative risks may be greater.

D A drug taken by mouth for a year or two will dissolve the 10% of stones that are made of pure cholesterol. None of the other types of stones is affected. If the drug is stopped, stones will reappear. The drug obviously has very limited use.

E A quarter of a million cholecystectomies (operation to remove the gallbladder) are performed each year in the United States. Once the gallbladder has been removed, the patient is cured, if there are no complications. Hospitalization is four to fourteen days. The mortality rate is 0.05% for those under the age of fifty and about 2% for patients over the age of seventy years.

The postoperative complications are those that occur after any major abdominal operation. A unique complication involves possible injury to the common bile duct, which drains bile from the liver to the intestine and lies close to the gallbladder. Such an injury, which occurs about once in every five hundred cholecystectomies, usually requires reoperations for repair.

F The gallbladder empties into the common bile duct. Stones from the gallbladder that pass into this tube may obstruct bile flow into the intestine and cause jaundice. Stones in the common bile duct are more likely to damage the liver, make the person severely ill, and be more difficult to remove than if the stones are only in the gallbladder. The chances of having stones in the common bile duct as well as in the gallbladder increase with age. In those between thirty and forty years of age, the likelihood of common duct stone is 3%; in those over sixty, about 25%. In about 15–20% of patients, the surgeon must, at operation on the gallbladder, also open and explore the common bile duct for stones. When he does so, a tube is left in place in the duct and brought out through the skin for one to two weeks before it is removed. This prolongs hospitalization for several days.

Despite all precautions at the time of cholecystectomy, one or more stones are left in the common bile duct in about 5% of patients. About 10% of such stones will pass into the intestine spontaneously. In about another 60%, various maneuvers, short of operation, can be used to remove such common duct stones. Among such methods is removal of the stones through the drain tract left at operation or by use of an endoscope at the opening of the common bile duct into the duodenum. But after all these maneuvers have been tried, about 30% of retained stones in the common duct require another operation for removal.

G An acute attack of cholecystitis is painful and usually requires hospitalization for a few days, but 95% of the time it will subside without the need for operation. Predictably, after one attack, there will be others in the future.

H Less than 1% of the time, an acute gallbladder attack will result in perforation or rupture of the gallbladder, spilling the infected and irritative contents of the gallbladder into the peritoneal cavity. Even when operated upon promptly, this catastrophe has a 20% mortality rate and a 40% chance of serious complication. Sometimes, the gallbladder is only drained and not removed under this emergency situation. If not removed later, when the patient recovers, further attacks of gallbladder symptoms are virtually certain.

11. Jaundice in Adults

A   Jaundice is yellow discoloration of the skin and eyeballs. It is due to abnormal accumulations of bile that become deposited in the skin. Bile is made in the liver and drains through a small pencil-size common bile duct into the intestine. Anything that obstructs the bile drainage causes jaundice. It occurs as a part of many different diseases, some relatively trivial, others very serious.

B   Cancers of the pancreas, bile duct, gallbladder, and duodenum may each block bile drainage and produce jaundice. Although these tumors grow in slightly different ways, they are all, unfortunately, usually fatal, regardless of treatment. Fewer than 5% of patients with these tumors live five years (see "Pancreatic Cancer," page 174).

    There is a slightly better prospect for those with cancer of the duodenum than if the tumor is in the bile duct. Two-thirds are at least candidates for operation to see if anything can be done. Of those where the tumor is still contained within the site of origin in the duodenum, half are alive in five years. Bile duct tumors may grow slowly, and if jaundice is relieved by operation, the patient may live one to three years in relative comfort.

C   Middle-aged people who become jaundiced usually have gallstones (see "Gallstones," page 200). Stones form in the diseased gallbladder and then pass into the common duct, where they may block the flow of bile from the liver and cause jaundice.

    The likelihood of a patient with gallbladder disease having stones in the common duct increases with age. Between the ages of thirty to forty, the likelihood is 3%; after seventy years of age, 25%. The surgeon tries to remove all stones from the common bile duct at the time he removes the gallbladder (cholecystectomy).

D   But despite all precautions, in about 5% of patients operated on for gallstones, a stone will be left behind in the common duct, where it may block bile flow and cause jaundice.

E   If the stone is sufficiently small, it may pass into the duodenum without any treatment. After one to two weeks, this is unlikely. Fifteen percent of stones are made of a substance called cholesterol. They can be dissolved by many weeks of treatment with a solution dripped into a tube left in the common duct at the time of operation. Most retained stones are removed by various types of lighted tubes (endoscopes) passed into the drainage tract left at operation. Seventy to eighty-five percent of such retained stones can be removed by the endoscopist and radiologist without operation.

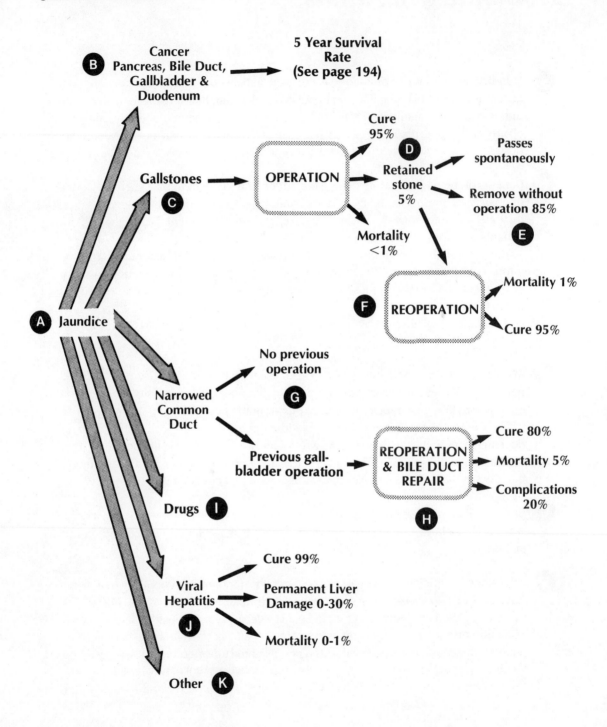

B Cancer Pancreas, Bile Duct, Gallbladder & Duodenum → **5 Year Survival Rate (See page 194)**

Gallstones **C** → **OPERATION**
- Cure 95%
- Retained stone 5% **D**
  - Passes spontaneously
  - Remove without operation 85% **E**
- Mortality <1%

Retained stone → **REOPERATION** **F**
- Mortality 1%
- Cure 95%

A Jaundice

Narrowed Common Duct
- No previous operation **G**
- Previous gall-bladder operation → **REOPERATION & BILE DUCT REPAIR** **H**
  - Cure 80%
  - Mortality 5%
  - Complications 20%

Drugs **I**

Viral Hepatitis **J**
- Cure 99%
- Permanent Liver Damage 0-30%
- Mortality 0-1%

Other **K**

F When these non-operative means fail, the stone can be removed with a second operation. The expected mortality is about 1%.

G A curious, low-grade tumor called sclerosing cholangitis can narrow the common duct and cause jaundice. The involved tissue can seldom all be removed at operation, but a tube passed through the tumor provides relief of jaundice for many months or even years.

H Most common duct strictures are due to a complication of previous operation on the gallbladder. Their repair is difficult, but good results can be anticipated in about 80% of patients. Mortality rate is 5–10%, and the chances of postoperative complication about 20%. Following repair, if any obstruction persists, there may be recurrent episodes of chills and fever.

I Many kinds of drugs can cause liver disease and produce jaundice. Usually, the jaundice will disappear when the drug is discontinued.

J Viral infections of the liver (viral hepatitis) produce jaundice by damaging the liver cells. There are at least three types of this disease; Type-A has a short interval between infection and the appearance of jaundice. Although these patients become very ill, the chance of dying of the disease is less than 0.5%, and almost all recover without any residual liver disease. In Type-B (serum) hepatitis, there is a long incubation period between exposure to the virus (often through a needle) and the appearance of jaundice. There is a 10% probability of permanent liver damage in this type of viral hepatitis. The expected mortality is about 1%. A third type of hepatitis, called Non-A Non-B, has a negligible mortality, but a 30% probability of leaving the liver permanently damaged. Infectious hepatitis may leave the patient weak and easily tired for many weeks before full recovery.

K Other rare causes of jaundice include diseases of the red blood cells, spleen, and specific inherited (congenital) biochemical abnormalities within the liver.

12. *Splenic Injury*

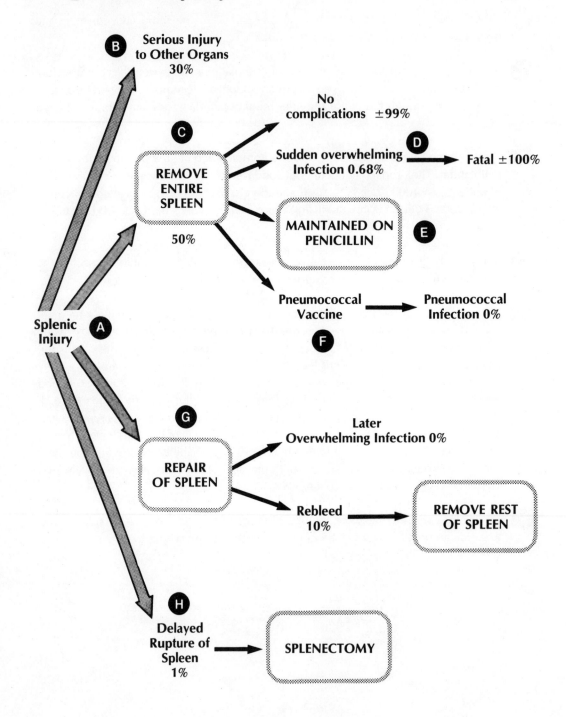

B Serious Injury to Other Organs 30%

C REMOVE ENTIRE SPLEEN 50%

No complications ±99%

Sudden overwhelming Infection 0.68% **D** → Fatal ±100%

E MAINTAINED ON PENICILLIN

Pneumococcal Vaccine **F** → Pneumococcal Infection 0%

A Splenic Injury

G REPAIR OF SPLEEN

Later Overwhelming Infection 0%

Rebleed 10% → REMOVE REST OF SPLEEN

H Delayed Rupture of Spleen 1% → SPLENECTOMY

A The spleen is a large bean- or kidney-shaped organ that lies on the left side of the abdominal cavity, up under the rib cage. It is loosely attached within the abdomen and is liable to injury in any severe blow to that area. When hit hard, its surrounding capsule often cracks in several places, like an egg shell. It has a rich blood supply and, when injured, often bleeds briskly into the abdominal cavity. Occasionally, the spleen is removed for reasons other than injury, such as part of other abdominal operations or as a part of the treatment of a disease of the blood or bone marrow.

B When the spleen is broken by a blow to the abdominal area, there is a 30% chance that the left kidney that lies just behind it will also be damaged and a lesser chance that the nearby liver or pancreas will be injured.

C For many years, the only accepted surgical treatment of an injured spleen was its entire removal. This is the quickest, simplest, and safest operation. Deaths following splenectomy are usually due to associated injury to the head or other parts of the body. But the spleen helps protect against certain infections, and when removed, the patient has an increased chance in the future of developing a sudden, severe, overwhelming infection caused by certain types of bacteria. Such risk is apparently greater in children than adults. For this reason, total splenectomy is only performed in those 25–50% of cases where the spleen is shattered beyond repair.

Current enthusiasm for saving the injured spleen must be considered in context. Overwhelming infections do occur after removing the spleen, but they are rare. Most patients, be they adults or children, never miss their spleens and have no complication from its total removal, which has been routinely performed for over fifty years.

D The chance of a child developing such an overwhelming infection after splenectomy is about 0.68%. This compares with a 0.05% chance in normal non-splenectomized children. Such an attack may occur years after the spleen was removed. Such sudden, frightening attacks of overwhelming infection are almost all fatal, running the course from onset to death within a few hours.

E Because of this remote chance of overwhelming infection, some physicians advise giving penicillin to children after splenectomy. There is no hard data to support this sensible but unproven policy.

Splenic Injury

F One-half of the overwhelming infections after splenectomy are due to a bacteria called pneumococcus. A pneumococcal vaccine exists that provides significant protection against infection by pneumococcus after splenectomy. Pneumococcal vaccine has no protective effect against other types of bacteria.

G If one-fifth of the spleen can be saved, its role in defending the patient against infection is maintained. The surgeon can preserve a part or all of the spleen in about half of the cases of splenic injury by stopping the bleeding with sutures, with the application of substances that form a clot over the torn area of the spleen, or even by taking out the part of the spleen that was injured and leaving the remainder. There is about a 10% chance that when the repaired spleen is left in place, it will start to bleed again within one to fourteen days and the rest of the spleen will have to be removed at a second operation.

H About 1% of the time, the damaged spleen will not bleed immediately after injury. A bruised area on its surface, however, may, after several days or even weeks, break down and suddenly bleed into the abdominal cavity. One-half of such episodes occur within a week after injury and another quarter during the second week. The remainder occur even later. Such delayed bleeding requires removing the entire spleen.

13. Small Bowel Obstruction

A The normal small bowel transports food and intestinal contents from the stomach to the colon (large bowel). Anything that obstructs this passage produces abdominal pain, vomiting, distention of the bowel, and swelling of the abdomen. If obstruction is

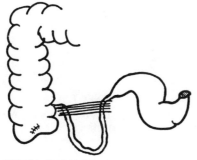

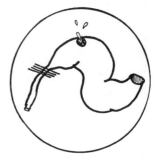

a) OBSTRUCTION OF SMALL BOWEL DUE TO ADHESION OR BAND FROM A PREVIOUS OPERATION

b) PERFORATION ABOVE THE SITE OF OBSTRUCTION

unrelieved, the blood supply to the swollen intestine may be cut off, leading to death of the bowel and, ultimately, to its rupture, peritonitis, and death of the patient. The chances for saving a person with small bowel obstruction depends mainly on how quickly the obstruction can be relieved before the blood supply is shut off and the bowel breaks open.

B Some inflammation and tissue reaction occurs around the site of every operation within the abdominal cavity. The reaction is particularly severe if there is an infection which forms bands of tissue or adhesions that run from one piece of intestine to another. Such adhesions may lie across and obstruct a segment of intestine. This causes 50% of small bowel obstructions.

C A tube passed through the nose into the stomach will remove the air and the secretions that accumulate behind the point of bowel obstruction and decrease the likelihood that the distended bowel will blow-out (perforate). In about 25% of patients, tube suction alone will relieve the obstruction, and the patient is cured of that episode. Three-quarters of these patients will have no further obstruction, but about one-quarter will have a subsequent episode.

D If obstruction of the small intestine is not quickly relieved, time soon runs out for the safe use of such naso-gastric tube suction. Suction does not relieve obstruction in 75% of cases, and in these patients, the shorter the delay in operation, the better are the

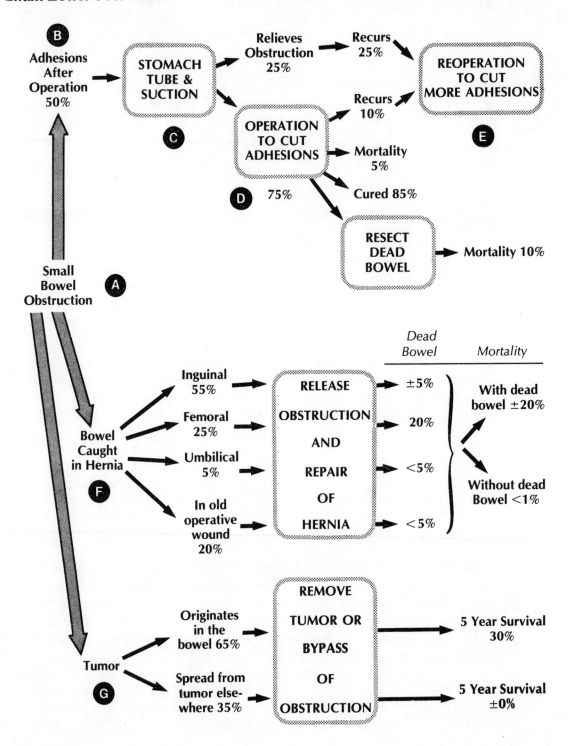

B

Adhesions
After
Operation
50%

**STOMACH
TUBE &
SUCTION**

C

Relieves
Obstruction
25%

Recurs
25%

**REOPERATION
TO CUT
MORE ADHESIONS**

E

**OPERATION
TO CUT
ADHESIONS**

D   75%

Recurs
10%

Mortality
5%

Cured 85%

**RESECT
DEAD
BOWEL**

Mortality 10%

Small
Bowel
Obstruction

A

Bowel
Caught
in Hernia

F

Inguinal
55%

Femoral
25%

Umbilical
5%

In old
operative
wound
20%

**RELEASE
OBSTRUCTION
AND
REPAIR
OF
HERNIA**

*Dead
Bowel*   *Mortality*

±5%

20%

<5%

<5%

With dead
bowel ±20%

Without dead
Bowel <1%

Tumor

G

Originates
in the
bowel 65%

Spread from
tumor else-
where 35%

**REMOVE
TUMOR OR
BYPASS
OF
OBSTRUCTION**

5 Year Survival
30%

5 Year Survival
±0%

chances that the blood supply to the distended obstructed bowel will still be intact and the bowel will not have to be removed.

If operation is undertaken within twenty-four hours after the obstruction begins, the expected mortality is less than 5%; if between twenty-four to forty-eight hours, 10%; and if operation is delayed beyond forty-eight hours, expected mortality is 15%. Death and complication is almost always due to the need to remove dead bowel.

E Operations to cut obstructing adhesions unfortunately stir up more reaction in the tissues and beget more adhesions. Having had an operation to cut adhesions, there is a 15% chance that obstruction will recur. If it does, and a fourth operation is necessary, the chances rise to 17%. After another such episode, a vicious circle is started, and the likelihood of still another operation rises to 40%.

F Intestine may slide from the abdominal cavity into a hernia sac. This in itself does not always cause obstruction. But if the bowel becomes caught (incarcerated) in the sac, it may become obstructed. This is particularly likely to occur in hernias where a small neck to the sac may trap bowel in the hernia. With a little inflammation at the constricted neck of the hernia, the bowel will be obstructed.

The most common type of hernia is an indirect inguinal type. This accounts for 55% of all obstruction due to hernia. A femoral hernia, though relatively rare, accounts for about 25% of all obstructions, because it has such a narrow neck to the sac. Wide-necked umbilical and postoperative wound (ventral) hernias, where bowel can easily slide in and out of the sac, rarely cause obstruction.

The size of the hernial opening also largely determines the chances of the trapped bowel having its blood supply shut off. The chances of finding dead bowel are 30% in obstructing femoral hernias compared to the 1–5% chance in obstructing umbilical hernias and about 10% in indirect inguinal hernias. As with obstruction due to adhesions, delay in operation on an incarcerated hernia increases the risk. If operation is undertaken within twelve hours of the onset of obstruction, the likelihood of finding dead bowel is about 10%; if between twelve–forty-eight hours, 30%; and if operation is delayed over forty-eight hours, about 50% will have dead bowel in the sac, which will have to be resected. Mortality varies between 10–40% if bowel must be resected.

G Cancers that start in the small bowel are rare, but in 35% of cases, obstruction is the first indication of such a tumor. There is a 30% chance of cure if such small bowel tumors are removed. If obstruction of the small intestine is due to tumor spread from another organ—as it is in about 35% of intestinal obstructions due to tumor—it is rarely possible to remove all the cancer. It is, however, frequently possible to divert or bypass the intestinal flow around the tumor and thereby relieve the symptoms of obstruction for the months of life that remain.

14. Appendicitis

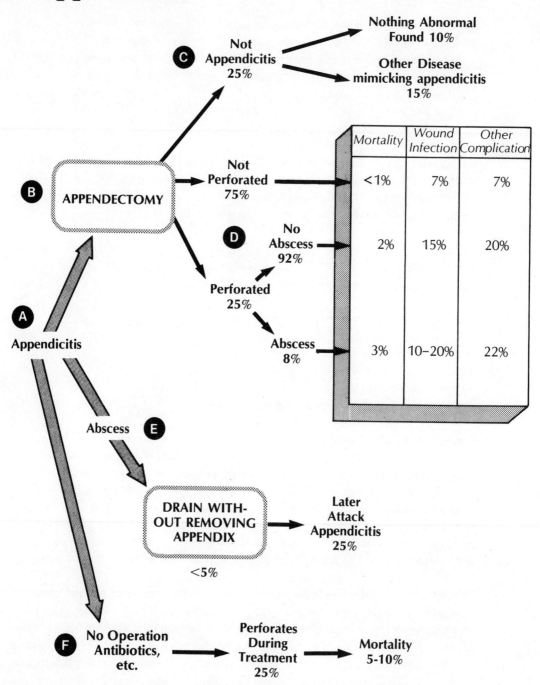

	Mortality	Wound Infection	Other Complication
Not Perforated 75%	<1%	7%	7%
No Abscess 92%	2%	15%	20%
Abscess 8%	3%	10–20%	22%

C Not Appendicitis 25%

Nothing Abnormal Found 10%

Other Disease mimicking appendicitis 15%

B APPENDECTOMY

A Appendicitis

Not Perforated 75%

D No Abscess 92%

Perforated 25%

Abscess 8%

Abscess **E**

DRAIN WITH-OUT REMOVING APPENDIX

<5%

Later Attack Appendicitis 25%

F No Operation Antibiotics, etc.

Perforates During Treatment 25%

Mortality 5-10%

A One of every fifteen persons will have acute appendicitis during his lifetime. It can occur at any age, but perforation is most common (up to 33% of the time) in children under five, due in part to difficulty and delay in diagnosis.

The appendix is a pencil-stub-sized tube of intestine that protrudes from the colon at

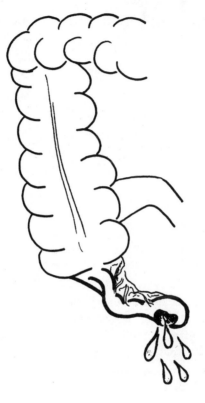

PERFORATION OF AN
INFLAMED APPENDIX

the point where it joins the small intestine. It lies on the right lower side of the abdomen. The appendix is of no value to body function, and nothing is lost after its removal.

Inflammation and infection of the appendix (appendicitis) is caused by a mechanical block to the small caliber tube. This causes pain and tenderness on the right side of the abdomen. If left untreated for twenty-four or more hours, the inflammation will progress and the appendiceal wall may break down (perforate), spilling its infected contents into the abdominal (peritoneal) cavity. This is peritonitis and is the cause of death in untreated appendicitis.

B Appendectomy means the surgical removal of the appendix. If there are no complications, the patient is usually in the hospital three to seven days after operation.

Appendicitis

(C) Appendicitis mimics many other diseases, so that the physician and surgeon are often not absolutely certain of the diagnosis before operation. The surgeon must play the odds in his decision to operate. He is wrong about 15–25% of the time, operating for what he thinks is appendicitis and finding none. But in most of these cases where the appendix is normal, he will find another disease that was producing the confusing signs and symptoms. In only about 10% of cases will no explanation for the symptoms mimicking appendicitis be found at operation. Why then does a surgeon take the chance of operation if he has a 15–25% chance of being wrong in his diagnosis and a 10% chance of finding no disease he can cure or benefit? The pertinent facts are:

- Since at least 7% of people will ultimately develop appendicitis, there is reason to remove the appendix to avoid future trouble.
- The risk in removing a normal or unruptured appendix is almost negligible whether measured by mortality (less than 1%) or complications after operation.
- If there is delay in operation and the appendix perforates, the risk of death and complication increases two to ten times. This is the most important fact to be considered.

The cost/benefit ratio to the patient clearly favors early operation if the responsible surgeon after careful study of the patient has a strong suspicion of appendicitis.

(D) The frequency of perforation at the time of operation depends mainly on how soon patients come to a physician after they develop signs of appendicitis. The longer they wait, the greater the chance of perforation—and subsequent complications. Infants and young children are particularly likely to perforate soon after the onset of symptoms. When, after perforation, there is pus in the abdominal cavity, the surgeon may leave the edges of the skin wound open for later closure. If there is an abscess, a wicklike tube (drain) may have to be left in the wound for a few days. The likelihood of wound infection (7–20%) depends mainly on whether the appendix has ruptured at the time of operation.

As with many abdominal operations, a tube passed through the nose into the stomach may have to be left in place for several days after operation until the intestines begin to function. During this time, nothing can be taken by mouth, and the patient must be fed by fluids given into the veins (intravenous fluids).

(E) About 1% of the time, when the appendix has ruptured, it is unwise to do more than drain the abscess, leaving the ruptured appendix in place. This results in a long hospital course. Draining the abscess does not remove the appendix, and 25% of such patients will suffer a subsequent attack of appendicitis. The appendix is, therefore, usually removed at some convenient time after the patient has recovered from the first operation when the area around the appendix was only drained.

F If for some obscure reason, appendicitis is treated by antibiotics and other medical means without operation, a quarter of the patients will go on to perforate the appendix while under treatment, and 5–10% will die unless operated upon. In the survivors, the complication rate is almost 100%. There is no support for the non-operative treatment of known appendicitis.

15. Ileostomy

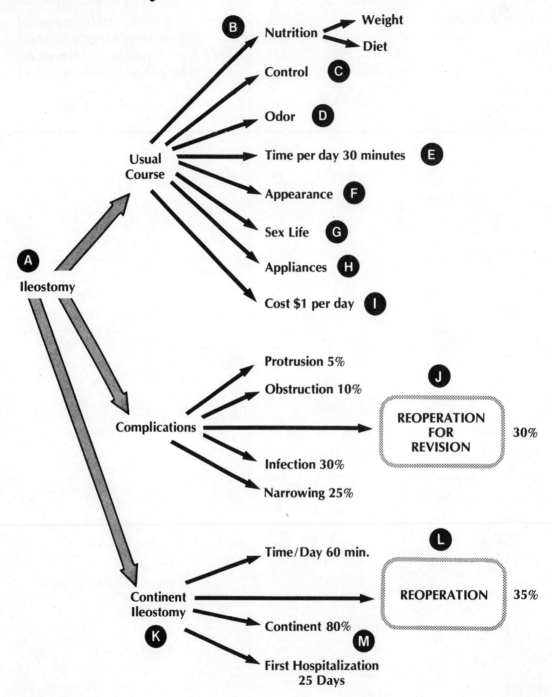

Nutrition → Weight, Diet **B**

Control **C**

Odor **D**

Time per day 30 minutes **E**

Appearance **F**

Sex Life **G**

Appliances **H**

Cost $1 per day **I**

Usual Course

A Ileostomy

Complications

Protrusion 5%

Obstruction 10%

Infection 30%

Narrowing 25%

J REOPERATION FOR REVISION 30%

Continent Ileostomy

K

Time/Day 60 min.

Continent 80% **M**

First Hospitalization 25 Days

L REOPERATION 35%

A When the rectum, anus, and entire large bowl (colon) must be removed, the end of the small bowel (ileum) must be brought out on to the abdominal wall as an ileostomy.

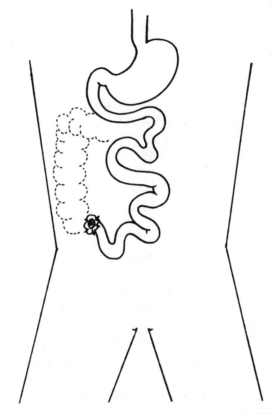

ILEOSTOMY: END OF SMALL BOWEL OPENING ONTO
ABDOMINAL WALL AFTER REMOVING THE COLON

Such an operation (total colectomy) requiring an ileostomy is often necessary for chronic ulcerative colitis and a few other disease conditions. There is no mechanism at the end of the ileum to control drainage of the liquid contents of the ileum, so it flows unchecked onto the abdominal wall.

B Because food is digested and absorbed in the small bowel, nutrition is not interfered with by an ileostomy, which leaves the small intestine intact. People with an ileostomy can eat normal diets and maintain normal weight, but as with anyone else, some foods are more likely to give them diarrhea. Patients with ileostomy soon learn to avoid such foods.

C Because there is no control to the discharge of watery bowel contents from an ileostomy, a plastic bag appliance is fitted over the opening of the bowel in the right side of the lower part of the abdomen.

D The appliance bag fits snugly over the ileostomy opening (stoma) so that there is no odor whatsoever resulting from an ileostomy.

E The patient carries out two procedures in the care of his ileostomy. The first is emptying the bag into a toilet when the bag becomes filled. This must be done about four times per day and requires about five minutes. The second procedure, performed about every two to three days, involves changing the ileostomy device that fits on the skin over the end of the ileostomy. This takes about forty minutes.

F The bag and appliance lie flat around the abdomen and are not noticeable when the patient is dressed. The entire device and bag is covered by a man's undershorts or a woman's panties.

G Simply bringing the end of the ileum out on the abdominal wall should not interfere with a normal capacity for sexual activity. Many patients, both men and women, with ileostomies have become parents. Other procedures often performed with ileostomy, such as abdominal perineal resection of the rectum, might interfere with sexual activity, but this is not due to the ileostomy.

H An adhesive paste is applied to the skin around the ileostomy opening. A lightweight plastic ring with a hole in its center fits closely around the protruding end of the ileostomy. A second ring, fitted with the bag, adheres closely to the first, so that no fluid or smell leaks out of the bag. The entire device is held in place with a small belt that encircles the waist. The bottom of the bag is occluded with a clamp, which can be quickly opened for drainage into a toilet bowl when convenient.

I The device itself costs about $200 and lasts about six months. Bags cost $1, and about three are used per week. The cost per year to a patient is about $500.

J Complications of the ileostomy itself are rare, if one excludes those caused by the underlying disease. The operation is often used in the treatment of ulcerative colitis or Crohn's disease (see pages 227 and 224). If there is disease in the remaining ileum, there may be complications, but this is a complicatioin of the disease, not of the ileostomy.

The ileostomy usually begins to function a day or two after its creation. The end of the bowel attaches firmly to the skin in about a week. Excess protrusion (prolapse) of the ileum through the opening (stoma) occurs in about 5% of patients and is usually easily reduced.

Uncommon (2–5%) complications include: the narrowing of the opening of the ileostomy, which requires dilation or, in 1% of cases, operative revision; and the obstruction of the intestine within the abdominal cavity around the ileostomy.

K Several techniques have been tried to create an ileostomy where drainage could be controlled. This is a so-called reservoir or continent ileostomy. The currently favored technique (Koch pouch) is successful in providing ileal continence (control) in about 80% of patients two to three months after the operation. The rate of complication after operation is 75%, and hospitalization averages four weeks, about twice as long as after a classic ileostomy.

L At least one extra operation for complications in the creation of such a pouch is needed in about 50% of the patients.

M If the patient is willing to risk the increased likelihood of complications, he can look forward to an 80% chance of controlling bowel movement through this type of ileostomy.

16. Colostomy

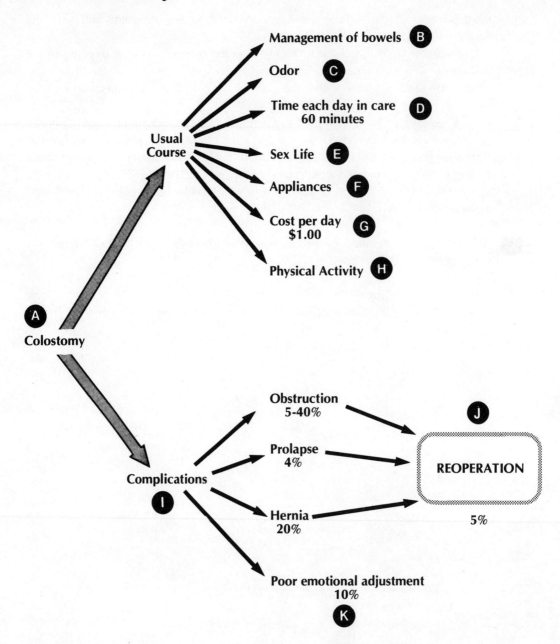

Management of bowels **B**

Odor **C**

Time each day in care
60 minutes **D**

Sex Life **E**

Appliances **F**

Cost per day
$1.00 **G**

Physical Activity **H**

Usual
Course

A
Colostomy

Obstruction
5-40%

Prolapse
4%

Hernia
20%

J

REOPERATION

5%

Complications

I

Poor emotional adjustment
10%

K

A It is occasionally necessary to bring the end of the large bowel (colon) out onto the skin of the abdominal wall, as either a temporary or permanent opening: this is a colostomy. It is usually performed because some part of the large intestine or rectum is

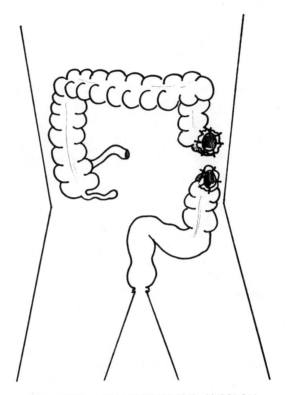

COLOSTOMY ON DESCENDING *(Left)* COLON

diseased and must be removed. The stool is discharged from the open end of the colostomy into a plastic collecting bag attached to the skin over a portion of the lower part of the abdomen. In its normal location between the buttock, a purse-stringlike muscle (the anal sphincter) controls bowel movements. Such control is lost when the bowel contents empty through a colostomy.

B For several weeks after operation, there is no control of the bowels, which discharge almost at random into the odor-proof plastic bag fitted over the end of the colostomy. The plastic pouch can be emptied several times daily and a new one applied every two to three days.

During the first few months after operation, patients soon find they can begin to manage discharge from the colostomy by altering their diet. Many people prefer irrigation of the colostomy every day or two, which helps prevent fecal discharge into the colostomy bag. Some patients do not bother with irrigation at all, simply emptying the pouch when it fills. Some people ultimately achieve such good control of the stool that they do not even wear a bag over the colostomy. Most people, however, wear some sort of small "security pouch" or covering over the colostomy opening.

C After the first few weeks, there is no greater odor of stool for a patient with a colostomy than there is for anyone else.

D Irrigation of the colostomy and arranging the appliance requires about one hour. Changing the pouch takes about fifteen minutes, which is not much longer than is needed for a person without a colostomy in going to the toilet.

E The colostomy itself does not interfere with the sex life of either a man or a woman. But the associated procedures, such as removal of the rectum or other pelvic organs, may cause impotence. Many men and women with colostomies enjoy an active sex life, and some have become parents.

F A disposable plastic drainage appliance fits over the end of the colostomy and is held in place with an adhesive that sticks to the skin. The average person with a colostomy uses one appliance bag per day.

G Total cost for the colostomy supplies depends on the type of appliance required and how often it is changed. It usually amounts to about $1.00 per day.

H Colostomy restricts activity very little. Many patients with colostomies are active housewives and office or manual workers. In general, people can continue their *normal* physical activity and life-style.

I Minor complications may be expected in about one of four patients with colostomies. Narrowing of the colostomy opening can in all but almost 5% of the instances be treated by dilatation with a finger inserted in a throwaway plastic glove. A hernial bulge in the muscles of the abdominal wall around the colostomy occurs in about 20% of patients with a colostomy, but seldom requires repair. Protrusion of the bowel through the colostomy opening (prolapse) is particularly likely to occur in infants. This might frighten the mother but is rarely of any danger. It can almost always be reduced by simple pressure over the protruding bowel.

J Reoperation and colostomy revision, because of one of the complications listed above, is necessary in about 5% of all patients with colostomy. Proper repair normally requires a major opening into the abdominal cavity and repair of the defect, but is curative 90% of the time.

K There is emotional as well as physical adjustment necessary for a patient with a colostomy. Society and rigid toilet training make much of odors, cleanliness, and continence, all of which bears on a patient's adjustment to alteration of bowel habits with a colostomy. All but 10% of patients come to accept colostomy without emotional trauma by the end of a year, particularly since it is so often associated with relief of pain, bleeding, or diarrhea from a severe underlying disease before operation. Many of the 10% who do have trouble with emotional adjustment had psychiatric problems before operation.

17. Crohn's Disease

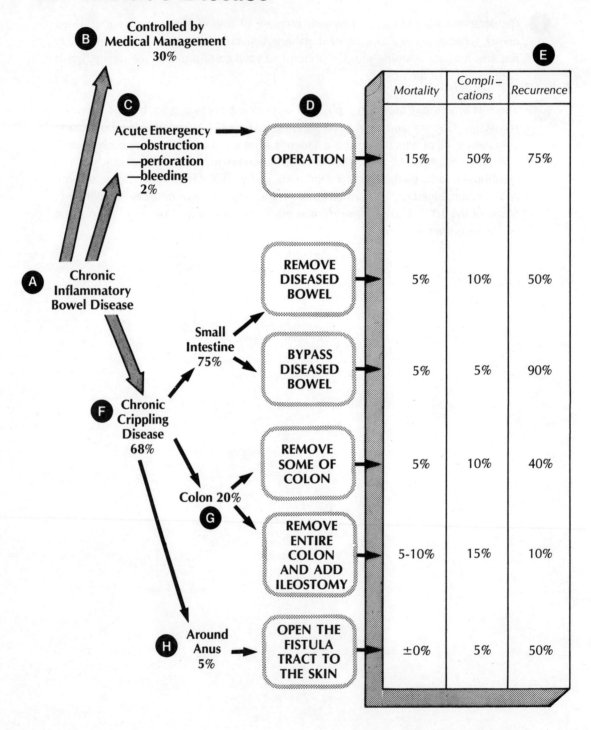

B Controlled by Medical Management 30%

C Acute Emergency
—obstruction
—perforation
—bleeding
2%

D OPERATION

A Chronic Inflammatory Bowel Disease

F Chronic Crippling Disease 68%

Small Intestine 75%

REMOVE DISEASED BOWEL

BYPASS DISEASED BOWEL

Colon 20%

G

REMOVE SOME OF COLON

REMOVE ENTIRE COLON AND ADD ILEOSTOMY

H Around Anus 5%

OPEN THE FISTULA TRACT TO THE SKIN

E

	Mortality	Compli-cations	Recurrence
OPERATION	15%	50%	75%
REMOVE DISEASED BOWEL	5%	10%	50%
BYPASS DISEASED BOWEL	5%	5%	90%
REMOVE SOME OF COLON	5%	10%	40%
REMOVE ENTIRE COLON AND ADD ILEOSTOMY	5-10%	15%	10%
OPEN THE FISTULA TRACT TO THE SKIN	±0%	5%	50%

A People with Crohn's disease characteristically suffer recurring attacks of abdominal pain, weight loss, and bloody diarrhea, which drag on for years. The symptoms are due to inflammation of the intestine. Patches of diseased bowel segments lie between relatively normal intestine. The disease usually affects the small intestine, but can also occur in the colon. After months and years of disease, the inflamed area may burrow a hole into an adjacent piece of bowel or out onto the skin, causing a fistula. Other complications are narrowing of the bowel and an increased likelihood of cancer of the bowel. The cause of Crohn's disease is unknown, and therefore there is no specific means of its treatment. The disease is also called regional ileitis or chronic granulomatous disease of the bowel.

B About 30% of patients with regional ileitis never require more than drugs and careful management of diet to control the symptoms of the disease. The longer the patient has the disease, the greater is the chance than an operation will be required. After seven years, about 40% of patients will require an operation for some complication of the disease.

C Acute emergencies are rare (2%) in Crohn's disease, but each requires immediate operation with an anticipated mortality ranging from 5–20% and a disturbing 40–80% expectance of serious postoperative complications. The more common reasons for emergency operations include:

- Perforation or rupture of the diseased bowel into the abdominal cavity causing peritonitis;
- Obstruction of the intestine by a narrowed, scarred segment of bowel;
- Bleeding from the bowel that will not stop by non-operative means;
- An abscess that requires drainage.

D Emergency drainage of an abscess resulting from a perforation has a low mortality (about 5%), but will result in a fistulous tract between the diseased bowel and the skin, which ultimately will require removal of the diseased piece of bowel.

If the bowel has perforated into the abdominal cavity, the blown-out segment must be removed. Sometimes, the bowel is brought out on to the abdominal wall as an ileostomy (see page 216), to keep the bowel contents away from the rest of the diseased segments of intestine.

When Crohn's disease causes acute obstruction, the surgeon tries to remove the narrowed diseased bowel, for this will give an 80% chance of avoiding further operation. Occasionally, a lesser operation must be chosen because of the patient's poor general condition, diverting the obstructed bowel contents, either as an ileostomy or into the colon.

When operation is for bleeding, the diseased bowel must be removed with an expected mortality of at least 15% and a 50% likelihood of complications after operation.

E Crohn's disease usually affects the entire small bowel in a patchy manner, and it is seldom possible for the surgeon to remove all of the diseased bowel. Even when the remaining intestine looks normal, recurrence of disease is to be expected.

F Crohn's disease is a chronic problem that usually causes symptoms for many years. Patients must learn to live with their illness. Operation is indicated when the symptoms become too unpleasant to bear or when a complication such as a fistula, abscess, or obstruction develops. Fistula from the diseased bowel, discharging stool onto the skin or into another piece of bowel, may close temporarily, but will always reopen unless the diseased area of bowel is removed by an operation. Similarly, once the intestine has become obstructed from scarring, it will never permanently remain open or return to normal. Even if an operation short-circuits or bypasses the narrowed area of the intestine and diverts intestinal contents from passing through the diseased bowel, the disease will continue and ultimately require operative removal.

G When Crohn's disease affects the large bowel (colon), it closely resembles the clinical course of chronic ulcerative colitis. Sometimes, the segment of diseased colon is so localized that only a part of the bowel needs to be removed, and the ends of the colon can be connected to each other. Mortality from this localized operation is only 5%, but there is a 30% likelihood that the disease will sooner or later show up in the rest of the colon. When the entire colon is involved and must be removed (total colectomy), an ileostomy is necessary (see page 216). If the small bowel is free of disease, this will function well, but if there is also disease in the small bowel, there is a 25–50% chance of needing a further operation on the ileostomy.

H Crohn's disease of the rectum often causes a fistulous tract from the bowel on to the skin near the anus. Ninety-five percent of such fistulae will close if they are opened widely by a relatively simple operation. But if the disease remains active in the colon, another fistula can be expected in half the cases. Rarely is it necessary to remove the rectum just to cure such a fistula.

18. Chronic Ulcerative Colitis (CUC)

A Chronic ulcerative colitis is an inflammatory disease of the large bowel that usually starts at the anus and progresses upward. Its characteristic clinical features are diarrhea, bloody stools, pain, fever, and weight loss. About half of all patients with chronic ulcerative colitis (CUC) will ultimately require operation.

B The first attack is often very severe. About 10% of patients will require an emergency or early operation to remove the colon (colectomy) as a result of this first attack. The other 90% will settle down to chronic disease and be maintained at least temporarily on medical treatment.

C CUC is particularly serious when it starts during childhood. Fifteen percent of such children will have a severe first attack, and half of these will require early emergency operation.

ULCERATION AND INFLAMMATION OF
LARGE BOWEL ABOVE THE ANUS

D The only totally curative operation for CUC is removal of the entire large bowel (total colectomy). This means removing the rectum and anus so that the bowel movements come out of an opening (ileostomy) on the abdominal wall, rather than from the anus (see "Ileostomy," page 216). After a few weeks, the patient cares for his own ileostomy, emptying the plastic bag two to three times per day. These patients usually can eat almost everything—far more than was possible when they had a colon diseased with CUC. Most are gainfully employed, married, and lead almost normal lives—merely having to devote a little more time to their bowel functions than normal

Chronic Ulcerative Colitis (CUC)

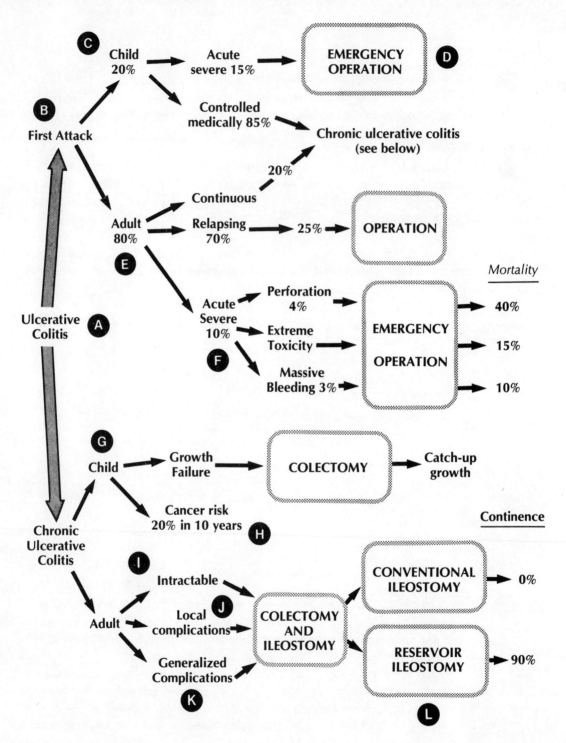

people. It is a price, but a relatively small one, to pay for being cured of CUC. Hospitalization is usually two to three weeks after total colectomy and ileostomy. The chances of complication in the early period following operation include:

- Wound infection: 10%
- Persistent drainage around the operative wound between the buttocks (perineal wound): 15%
- Reoperation on the ileostomy: 10%

E Adults with the first attack of CUC look forward to one of three possible courses. In 20%, the disease will retreat into a chronic continuous phase of constant diarrhea. Four out of five patients who fall into this group may ultimately need operation. A more common course (70%) will result in relatively disease-free periods, suddenly interrupted by acute episodes of diarrhea and pain.

F The 10% of adults whose disease progresses to catastrophic proportions may blow out (or perforate) the diseased colon, bleed massively by rectum, or develop a high fever, have a distended abdomen, and be very sick or toxic. This latter condition is called toxic megacolon. Such an acute complication requires an emergency operation. What the surgeon does depends on the condition of the patient. The only curative procedure is to remove *all* the colon and rectum, but the patient may be judged too sick to tolerate this big operation and a procedure involving a lesser compromise will be chosen. There is a high (60%) complication rate when these emergency operations are performed on such very sick patients.

A tempting operation occasionally urged by the patient or his family is to preserve the rectum and anus in the hope that it can some day be reconnected to the intestinal tract and the ileostomy closed. This is seldom wise for these reasons:

- If the rectum is left, three out of four patients will develop disease within the rectal stump, even if it is not connected to the rest of the intestinal tract.
- The added operation of connecting the ileum to the rectum (closing the ileostomy) has a 1–2% mortality.
- Cancer will develop in 2–3% of the patients where a rectal stump is left in place, even if it is not connected to the rest of the bowel.
- Assuming that the rectal stump is free of disease when cut off from the intestinal tract, it has at least a 75% chance of becoming diseased as soon as it once more has bowel contents flowing through it.

If subtotal colectomy is performed for bleeding, 5% will continue to bleed from the stump of rectum that is left in place and will soon require operative removal of the remaining rectum. In short, there is little chance of gain and a big chance of loss (cancer, new disease, bleeding, etc.) by leaving any rectum in patients with CUC.

Chronic Ulcerative Colitis (CUC)

G Children with CUC often are undersized but grow rapidly after removal of the entire diseased colon.

H The longer a patient has active CUC, the greater his chances are of developing cancer in the diseased bowel. The chances are about 20% per every ten years of disease. After thirty-five years of CUC, about half of patients will have developed cancer in the bowel. When it does develop, 20% of the time it is in more than one site and has a low chance of cure (40%, five-year cure), even if operated upon and resected. This is why it is advisable to resect the diseased colon *before* cancer develops, not wait for its almost certain occurrence.

I The sheer misery of constant diarrhea, pain, weight loss, and bleeding drives most patients with CUC to seek operation and a chance of cure, even though the price they pay is an ileostomy.

J Local complications of CUC that occur around the anus include:

	Incidence	Cure without removing the colon
Fissure (painful anal ulcers or sores)	10%	100%
Abscess	60%	85%
Fistula (opening from the rectum to the skin around the anus)	5%	50%
Fistulous tract from the rectum to the vagina (recto-vaginal fistula). This is the only local complication that requires colectomy.	35%	0%

K The patient debilitated and malnourished because of CUC may suffer a wide variety of generalized complications, such as liver disease (40%), arthritis, and eye complications.

L Many methods have been tried to make an ileostomy that will not constantly discharge its contents onto the abdominal wall. These are called reservoir, or continent, ileostomies. At best, there is an 90% probability of success in being able to control the ileostomy without a bag. But there is a 75% risk of complications, many of which require another operation. This is almost twice the complication rate of constructing a regular ileostomy that cannot be controlled and empties into a bag. It requires several months for most patients to learn how to manage a reservoir ileostomy (see page 216).

19. Diverticulitis

A The normal colon is a smooth, large-caliber tube with firm muscular walls. In older people, the muscular wall may weaken and tissue lining the bowel may protrude like a small hernia through the bowel wall. At first, these diverticula are small, but they usually enlarge to the size of small sacs (about 1 centimeter), which lie like a row of blisters on the outside surface of the colon. They usually first appear at the lower end of the colon not far above the anus, but later involve longer segments of the bowel. Infection may develop in these diverticular by-waters of the main fecal stream. This is diverticulitis.

DIVERTICULA ALONG THE ENTIRE
DESCENDING *(Left)* COLON

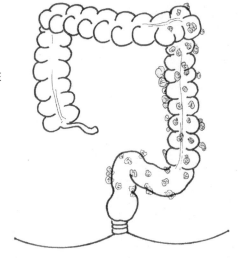

B Barium-enema X-ray examination of the colon demonstrates diverticula as a row of irregularities in the colon wall. The likelihood of finding diverticula in the colon increase with age:

- 10–20 years: 1%
- 20–30 years: 6%
- 30–40 years: 12%
- 40–50 years: 22%
- 50–60 years: 30%
- 60–70 years: 37%

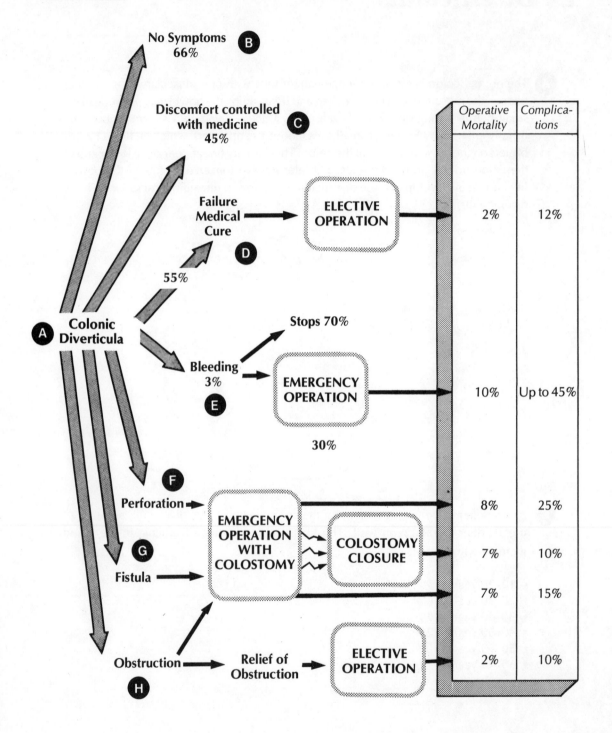

Sixty-six percent of such diverticula do not cause symptoms.

(C) Inflammation or infection of a colon diverticulum causes vague pain in the left lower part of the abdomen, similar to a "left-sided appendicitis." The first attack of diverticulitis is often mild and, in at least 45% of cases, will subside with proper medical treatment.

(D) Once a patient has an attack, he has a 25% likelihood of ultimately developing serious complications of the disease, including bowel obstruction, perforation, fistula formation, or bleeding. If there have been two attacks, the chances of such future trouble are 60%. If discomfort or pain persists, operation is necessary. Performed electively between attacks and not as an emergency, the part of the bowel containing the diverticula can usually be removed (colectomy) and the ends of the normal bowel joined together. Such an operation does not affect normal bowel habits.

(E) Bleeding occurs in 3–5% of patients with diverticula. In 70%, the bleeding stops spontaneously. If a patient bleeds once, he has a 22% chance of bleeding again. After two episodes of bleeding, the chances are 50% that he will again rebleed. If bleeding will not stop (30% of cases), emergency operation is necessary. Operation ideally consists of removing all the colon containing diverticula, including, of course, the area that is bleeding. The severed ends of the colon are then joined together. Occasionally, a temporary colostomy is necessary. The expected mortality rate for this emergency operation is 10%, and the chances of having postoperative complications 45%. Two percent of the time there may be rebleeding, even after all the colon that was thought to be involved is removed.

(F) A diverticulum may become so inflamed that it perforates or breaks open into the abdominal cavity, just as sometimes occurs in the appendix. Ninety-five percent of perforations from diverticulitis are localized, forming an abscess around the inflamed diverticulum. But a few cases (1–2%) break into the entire abdominal cavity and produce generalized peritonitis. The exact operation necessary for cure of this complicated problem depends on many factors, but carries a mortality of 6–8% and a complication rate of 10–25%. If a colostomy is performed, it often cannot be closed for three to four months, awaiting subsidence of the infection around the perforated diverticulum.

Diverticulitis

G One to two percent of the time, the diverticular infection penetrates into the urinary bladder or drains onto the skin, forming a fistula pouring bowel contents and gas into the urine or onto the abdominal wall. This usually requires at least two operations for cure: the first, a colostomy to divert bowel contents from the fistula, and the second, several months later, to remove the diverticulum and the tract and to close the colostomy. Occasionally colostomy closure requires a separate third operation.

H In 1–2% of cases, repeated infection around the inflamed diverticula produce obstruction to the passage of feces in the colon. This mimics the symptoms of cancer but rarely (2–3% of the time) do they coexist.

If the obstruction can be treated without emergency operation and the bowel put to rest, some of the infection subsides and the diseased area can be removed (colectomy) in a single operation with a mortality of 2%. But if a preliminary emergency colostomy is necessary for obstruction, operative mortality is 5%. As mentioned in G above, at least one and occasionally two more operations are then needed over two to four months to excise the colon containing the diverticula and then to close the colostomy and reconnect the remaining bowel. Each operation (colostomy, excision of the diverticula, and colostomy closure) carries at least a 3–5% mortality and a 5–10% complication risk. Many of these patients are old, and their associated heart and lung disease accounts for this high risk.

20. Cancer of the Colon

A The large bowel or colon is the lower end of the intestinal tract. It extends from the end of the small intestine in the right lower part of the abdomen around to the rectum. It is a frequent site of cancer in older people.

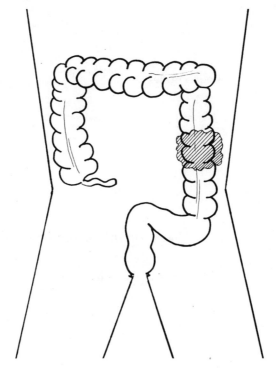

TUMOR IN DESCENDING COLON

B Colon cancer starts in the specialized tissue that lines the bowel. One of the most important indications for chance of cure is how far the tumor has grown when first discovered and treated. If it is still strictly localized in the colon where it started, the chances for total cure are 80%. If it has grown through all layers of the bowel wall, the likelihood of five-year survival is still 60%. But as the tumor spreads to local lymph nodes draining the area, the likelihood of cure drops to 40%, and to much less if it has spread to distant organs.

Cancer of the Colon

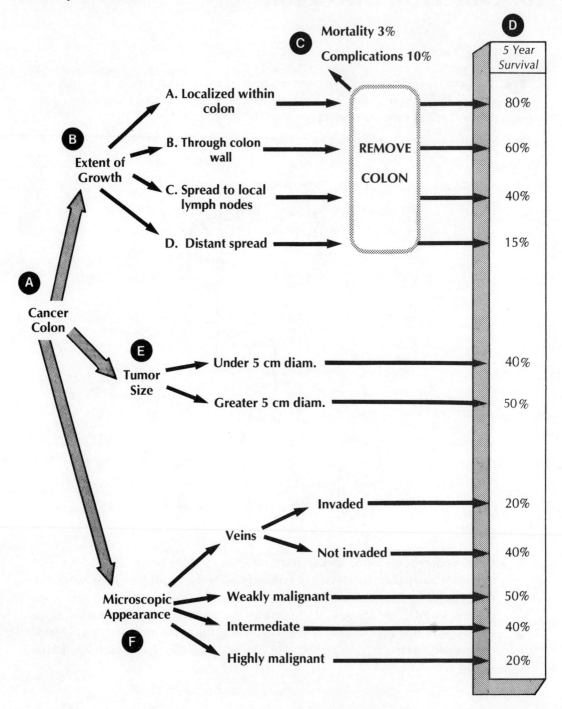

C The only chance for cure is by removing that part of the colon involved with the cancer. Fortunately, a person can do without almost all his large bowel without any particular difficulty—not even diarrhea. When the operation is performed electively (that is, not as an emergency), the bowel can be emptied and cleaned before operation and the procedure performed with a 3% chance of mortality and about a 10% likelihood of complication. Hospitalization is ten to twenty days. With most colon cancers, the bowel that remains after removing the tumor can be reconnected, and there is no need for a colostomy (see page 220).

D The chance of cure from colon cancer depends on many factors:

- How early it is detected and therefore how big the tumor might be when removed.
- How extensively it has spread.
- The appearance of the tumor cells when examined under the microscope.
- How it is treated by the surgeon.

A handy way to measure "curability" is by the likelihood of being free of tumor five years after discovery and treatment. Only an occasional case of tumor spread will turn up for the first time after five years.

E The sheer bulk of the tumor alone also helps to determine the likelihood of cure. Tumors under 5 centimeters in diameter have a 51% chance of cure; larger tumors, a 38% five-year survival.

F A third important indicator of curability is the appearance of the tumor when examined under the microscope. If tumor cells are found inside of veins, the chance of five-year survival is only 20%—half that if no such invasion is present.

The appearance of the tumor cells themselves also dictates the chance of cure after operation. Tumors with cells that are not too different than normal cells lining the colon are weakly malignant and have a 50% chance of cure five years after operation. Highly malignant-looking cells spread more quickly, and the chance of cure is decreased.

G Even when colon cancer has spread beyond the possibility of cure by operative removal, the patient's remaining months can often be made more comfortable by removing the tumor that involves the bowel. Such so-called palliative resection may relieve pain and stop diarrhea and blood loss into the bowel. An occasional person may even live five years with widespread disease. Operative mortality of removing such colon tumor in the presence of distant spread is about 5% and average survival two years in this selected group of patients.

Cancer of the Colon

H By the time a colon cancer perforates, spilling bowel contents into the abdominal cavity, it has usually been present for a long time and is in advanced state. Immediate operation with a colostomy and, if possible, removal of the tumor is necessary. The overall mortality of operation under these circumstances is about 20%, and the overall chances of cure about 25%. If at the time of perforation the tumor seems still to be localized to the bowel, the likelihood of cure is 40%. Perforation of a colon cancer is dangerous but does not inevitably mean incurability. The colostomy can be closed several weeks or months later, reestablishing normal bowel function.

Cancer of the colon is a common cause of large bowel obstruction and usually suggests a tumor of long-standing. Emergency operation is necessary to relieve the obstruction by a colostomy (see page 220). This has an expected operative mortality of 5–10%. If after several weeks or months the patient's general condition warrants it, the colon containing the tumor can be removed and the colostomy closed in a second operation. In about half of the patients so obstructed, the tumor will still apparently be limited to the tumor site. The chances of cure are only 5–10%, but the average survival is two years after the episode of obstruction.

Anti-cancer drugs do not increase the length of survival nor do they decrease the 30% likelihood of local recurrence of the tumor at the site of resection if given at the time of operative removal of a colon cancer.

Radiation can greatly relieve the pain of a local recurrence of colon cancer, be it in the bone, liver, or elsewhere.

21. Colonic Polyp

A A colonic polyp is a growth of the tissue that lines the inside of the colon. The polyp protrudes into the bowel. Frequently such polyps bleed. Their importance lies in the possibility that they may be or may become cancer.

B Colonic polyps in children are not and will never become cancer, but when they bleed, they usually must be removed, either through a lighted tube (sigmoidoscope) passed into the colon through the anus or by a formal abdominal operation. Removed by whatever means, they seldom recur.

C Members of certain families have an inherited tendency to form polyps throughout the entire colon (familial polyposis). Untreated, essentially all such patients with familial polyposis will die of colon cancer at an average age of forty-two years. By age thirty-six, two-thirds will have cancer, and in 50% there will be two or more polyps that have turned cancerous.

D One possible operation for familial polyposis is to remove the entire colon but to save the rectum, thus avoiding an ileostomy (see page 216). The appeal of having bowel movements through the rectum is real, but leaving the rectum invites its future involvement with cancer. Within five years, 5% of patients will have cancer in the rectal stump that has been preserved; in ten years, 13%; in fifteen years, 25%; and in twenty years, 42%. This risk is not worth taking.

E The only safe treatment is to remove *all* the colon, including the rectum and anus. This, of course, prevents any future colon cancer but requires an ileostomy. The mortality rate of total colectomy in this group of patients is about 1%.

F The common colon polyp in the adult is a so-called "adenomatous polyp." Ninety percent are within 25 centimeters of the anus and can be seen with a lighted tube (sigmoidoscope) passed into the rectum. When excised through a sigmoidoscope or a much longer colonoscope, the complication rate is 2%. When formal operation is required for removal of the polyp, the colon is opened through the abdomen, and the complication rate is 10–15%, largely consisting of infection. The overall likelihood of an adult adenomatous polyp being cancer is 5%. But the chances are related to the size of the polyp—those under 1 centimeter in diameter, 1%; between 1 and 2 centimeters, 10%; but in those over 2 centimeters in diameter, 45% are cancers.

Colonic Polyp

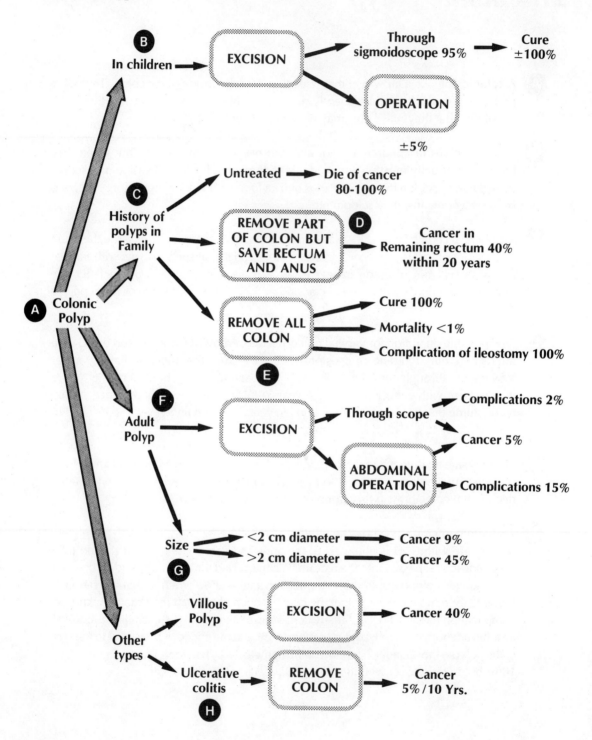

G A villus polyp is usually located just above the anus. It has a 40% chance of being cancer and, therefore, must be totally removed by performing an abdominal perineal resection. As detailed in the following section on rectal cancer, this means that the rectum and anus must be removed and a colostomy performed. The chances of cure are essentially certain if cancer has not yet appeared in such polyps and about 90%, even if there are cancerous changes in the tumor. As in other pre-malignant lesions, prevention is the best way to stop cancer.

H Polyps form in 2–3% of patients with chronic ulcerative colitis (see page 227). The longer the course of the disease, the greater the likelihood that such a patient will form a cancer in the polyps. Cancer develops at a rate of 5% for every ten years of disease.

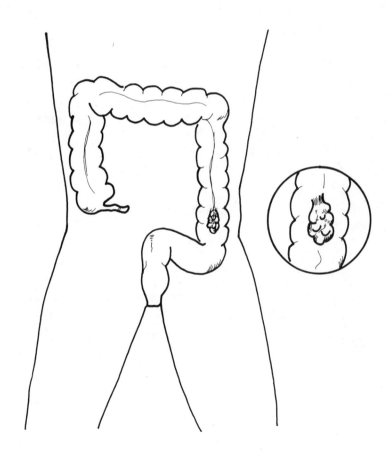

22. Rectal Cancer

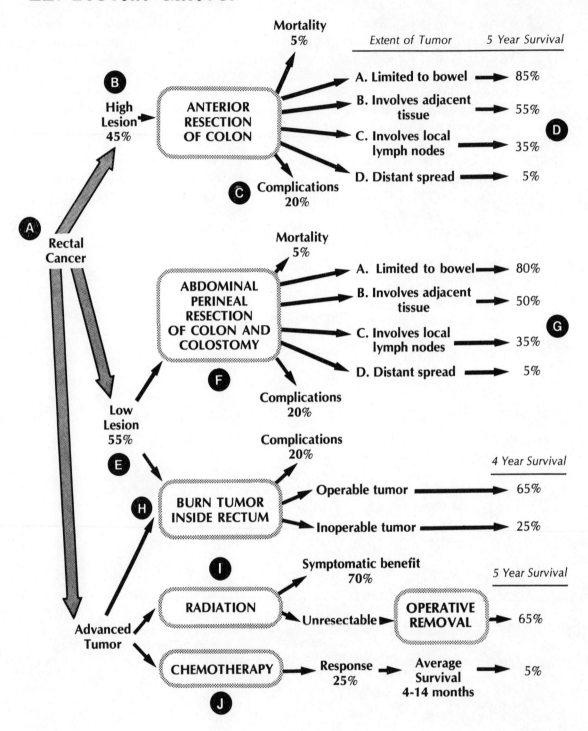

Mortality
5%

Extent of Tumor   5 Year Survival

B

**High
Lesion
45%**

**ANTERIOR
RESECTION
OF COLON**

A. Limited to bowel ➡ 85%

B. Involves adjacent
   tissue ➡ 55%

D

C. Involves local
   lymph nodes ➡ 35%

D. Distant spread ➡ 5%

C Complications
20%

A

**Rectal
Cancer**

Mortality
5%

**ABDOMINAL
PERINEAL
RESECTION
OF COLON AND
COLOSTOMY**

A. Limited to bowel ➡ 80%

B. Involves adjacent
   tissue ➡ 50%

G

C. Involves local
   lymph nodes ➡ 35%

D. Distant spread ➡ 5%

F

Complications
20%

**Low
Lesion
55%**

Complications
20%

4 Year Survival

E

H

**BURN TUMOR
INSIDE RECTUM**

Operable tumor ➡ 65%

Inoperable tumor ➡ 25%

I

Symptomatic benefit
70%

5 Year Survival

RADIATION

Unresectable ➡

**OPERATIVE
REMOVAL** ➡ 65%

**Advanced
Tumor**

CHEMOTHERAPY ➡ Response
25% ➡ **Average
Survival
4-14 months** ➡ 5%

J

A The rectum is that part of the large bowel (colon) lying just above the anus. It is the bottom of the intestinal tract. It functions to provide voluntary control of bowel movements. Although the rectum is only a small part of the large bowel, it is the site of about a third of all colon cancers. Cancer of the colon is seven times more frequent in men than in women.

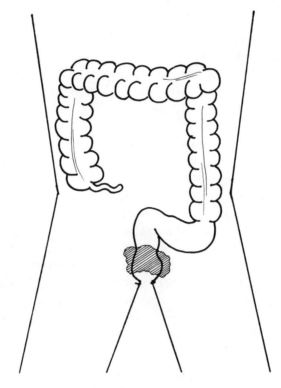

TUMOR IN RECTUM

B If the cancer is high enough above the skin of the anus, the tumor often can be removed with enough tumor-free rectum remaining so that the anus can be preserved. The two cut ends of the tumor-free colon can then be sewn together, and the patient can continue to have bowel movements through the anus in a normal fashion. This is called an anterior resection or anastomosis, because it is performed primarily anteriorly through an abdominal incision.

C The rate of complications following operation is high, because in addition to the usual problems connected with a big operation, it also includes the possibility of a leak and infection at the point where the two open ends of the bowel are joined together (anastomosed) deep in the pelvis.

D The chances for cure following removal of a rectal cancer depend mainly on the extent of the tumor at the time it is removed, just as in other colon cancers (see "Cancer of the Colon," page 235). If the tumor still is localized within the bowel, the chance of being alive five years after operation is 85%. As shown in the diagram, as the tumor spreads, the likelihood of cure by operation diminishes from 85% to 35% if it has spread to the lymph nodes draining that part of the colon containing the cancer. If there is distant spread of the tumor beyond the limits of possible removal at the time of operation, only an occasional patient ever survives five years.

E Cancers that lie 10 centimeters or less above the anus cannot ordinarily be totally removed and still leave a tumor-free margin of rectum above the anus. To remove all the tumor, it is necessary to remove the anus. This is called an abdomino-perineal resection, since it requires two incisions, one through the abdominal wall and the other around the anus in the perineum. After the rectum and anus are removed, it is necessary to bring the end of the remaining colon out through a small hole in the abdominal wall as a colostomy (see "Colostomy," page 220). Although at first the patient has difficulty controlling bowel movements through the colostomy, with time, the bowel movements can be brought under control. This may require giving oneself an enema through the colostomy every day and often some dietary restriction, but otherwise most of these patients lead normal lives and consider the colostomy a small price to pay for the good chance of cure.

F Two unique complications are apt to mar the immediate period following abdomino-perineal resection. The first (primarily in men) is difficulty in passing urine properly. This may require use of a catheter in the bladder for a week or more. The second is the possibility of intestinal obstruction either around the colostomy or deep in the pelvis where the tumor was removed.

G Chances for cure following abdomino-perineal resection for cancer are similar to those when the tumor is higher in the colon. If the tumor is localized to the rectum when removed, 85% of patients can anticipate cure; if tumor has spread locally, 50%; if local lymph nodes contain tumor, 30%; and if cancer has spread beyond the limits of removal by operation, the chances of cure are almost nil.

H The hot cautery has been used to burn the tumor that projects into the rectum. Normally, this requires four operative sessions of about one and a half hours each over six to nine months, under general or spinal anesthesia and is used only in an occasional case where the tumor cannot otherwise be excised. The value of this technique is debatable, but a four-year survival of 25% has been reported in tumors that were not otherwise thought to be removable by operation, and 65% survival where the tumor was considered resectable but cautery treatment was, for some reason, chosen instead of the usual treatment by operation.

I X-radiation therapy reliably controls pain from a local metastasis or spread of the cancer such as may occur in a bone. There is some evidence (though debatable) that an occasional cancer that seems to have spread locally, beyond the limits of operative excision for cure, can be shrunk by X-ray so that it *can* then be totally removed.

J About 15% of rectal cancers will have some response to anti-cancer drug therapy. Such drugs are never curative but may prolong life a few months and help control pain and other symptoms of advanced rectal cancer. Patients with advanced rectal cancer with distal spread only occasionally survive more than a year.

23. Hemorrhoids

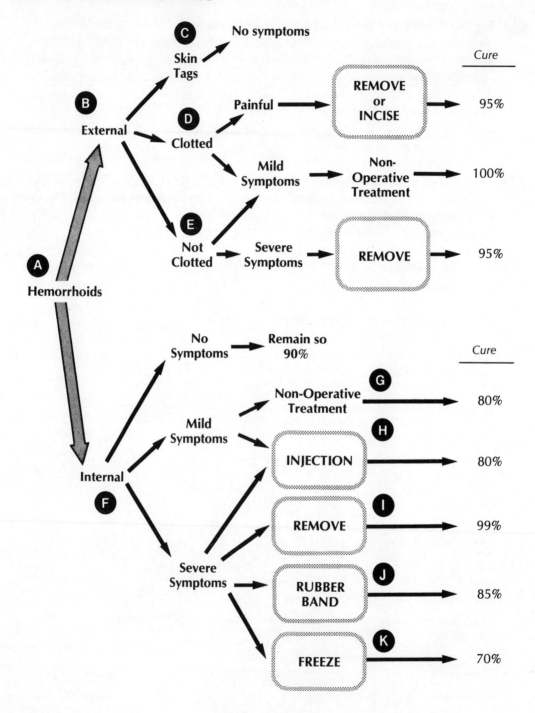

A Hemorrhoids are distended veins that arise from just inside the rectum and protrude through the anus. Their common name is "piles." Common symptoms of hemorrhoids are bleeding during bowel movement or discomfort or itching around the anus. Hemorrhoids can be seen by examining the anus or looking into the rectum with special lighted tubes or scopes.

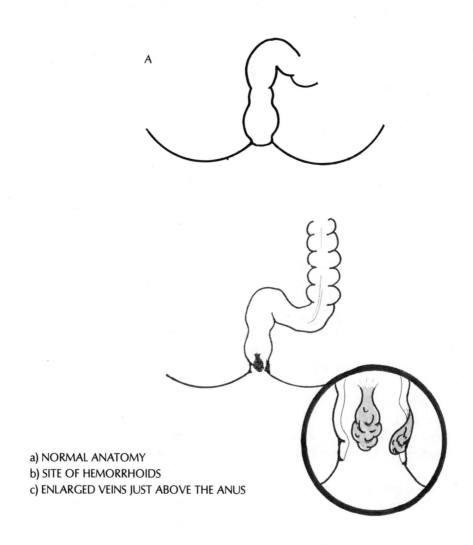

A

a) NORMAL ANATOMY
b) SITE OF HEMORRHOIDS
c) ENLARGED VEINS JUST ABOVE THE ANUS

Hemorrhoids

B External hemorrhoids protrude or stick out through the anus. Internal hemorrhoids arise from veins within the rectum and are not visible on the outside. They can only be seen with a scope put into the anus.

C Sometimes, small tags of skin around the anus represent old hemorrhoids that have filled with clot and become overgrown with skin. They seldom cause symptoms and only rarely need removal.

D Occasionally, the blood within an external hemorrhoid clots, forming a thrombosed hemorrhoid. This can be acutely painful. Relief is immediate by simply opening the vein with a scalpel and removing the clot. The procedure can be done under local anesthesia on an outpatient basis. If the pain is only mild, local treatment (cold or warm soaks, ointment, etc.) will give relief.

E Most hemorrhoids, like any veins, remain open and filled with blood. They may rupture and bleed, causing red blood on the stool or in the toilet bowl. Seldom is the amount of blood lost large enough to be significant, and it usually stops promptly without treatment. If bleeding recurs and the hemorrhoid is not cured by substances that soften the stool, the external hemorrhoids can be removed by an operation, with a 95% chance of cure. Because other more serious diseases such as cancer of the colon may also produce blood with bowel movements, any blood on the stool should be investigated by a physician and not be dismissed as being due to bleeding hemorrhoids.

F Hemorrhoidal veins that arise from above the anus are called internal hemorrhoids. They may remain within the rectum or protrude through the anus at the time of bowel movement. Most such hemorrhoids cause no symptoms and require no treatment.

G Non-operative treatment of mildly symptomatic hemorrhoids consists of diet and drugs that soften the stool and make it more bulky or application of local soothing ointments around the anus. Probability of success is about 80% and is greater with hemorrhoids that are only mildly symptomatic. In about 20%, symptoms will recur.

H Certain internal hemorrhoids can be made to disappear by injecting into them special drugs that cause the veins to clot. Although uncomfortable, this requires no anesthesia, is done on an office or outpatient basis, and does not require loss of time from work. But the hemorrhoids recur in about half of the cases and must later be removed by operation.

I Severe symptomatic, longstanding, or very large hemorrhoids usually require operative excision by one of many available techniques. This usually requires four to eight days hospitalization, one to three weeks off from work, a local, spinal, or general anesthesia, and an uncomfortable few days following operation. But it is a 99% effective way to cure hemorrhoids.

J Using a special applicator, a small rubber band can be slipped over the distended hemorrhoidal veins, choking off its base, resulting in clotting within the vein. The technique can only be used on internal hemorrhoids but there is an 85% likelihood of cure. The operation can be done using either local or no anesthesia at all. It is reasonably painful in about 10% of cases but can be done on an outpatient or office basis and often requires no loss of time from work. About 15% of internal hemorrhoids treated with the rubber-band technique will recur and require later operative treatment.

K Hemorrhoidal veins can be destroyed by freezing, using a special (cryo) probe that makes the vein clot. This cures about 70% of patients, but the resultant swelling around the site usually results in loss of two to three days of work. Sometimes, heat (cautery) is used instead of cold for destroying hemorrhoidal veins.

24. Pilonidal Sinus

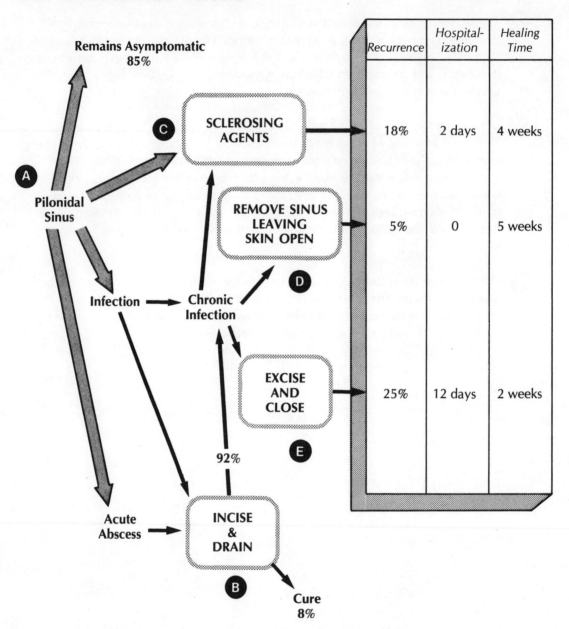

Remains Asymptomatic
85%

A Pilonidal Sinus

C SCLEROSING AGENTS

REMOVE SINUS LEAVING SKIN OPEN

D

Infection → Chronic Infection

EXCISE AND CLOSE

E

92%

Acute Abscess → INCISE & DRAIN

B

Cure 8%

	Recurrence	Hospital-ization	Healing Time
SCLEROSING AGENTS	18%	2 days	4 weeks
REMOVE SINUS LEAVING SKIN OPEN	5%	0	5 weeks
EXCISE AND CLOSE	25%	12 days	2 weeks

A At the lower end of the spinal column, about 5% of people have a dimple or skin depression, where the skin ended its folds over the spinal cord during fetal development before birth. This is a pilonidal cyst or pilonidal sinus, and in most people it causes no symptoms. However, occasionally this area becomes infected and causes pain and discomfort. It occurs four times as often in men and characteristically becomes infected in those with abundant hair growth in that area.

B When the pilonidal cyst forms an abscess, it becomes painful and must be drained of pus. But the chances are nine to one that the problem will recur after simply draining the infection. Permanent cure requires more extensive operative treatment.

C Occasionally, the sinus is treated by injecting it with a highly irritating (sclerosing) solution (phenol). This provides about an 18% chance of cure. It is painful and requires general anesthesia.

D Several techniques are used to remove the infected hair-containing tract by operation. The infected cyst can be totally removed and the skin left open, in which case the wound requires up to two months to heal. This is an uncomfortable but safe technique and is curative in about 95% of cases. If the cavity where the cyst was removed is very large, it may have to be packed open, requiring a week or more of hospitalization.

E An alternate operation involves sewing the skin closed after the infected tissue is removed. Seventy-five percent of the time the wound will heal, thus avoiding the uncomfortable problem of an open wound in this inconvenient part of the body. Hospitalization is about ten to twelve days. In the 25% where the wound breaks open after suture closure, the edges of the wound heal in slowly from the bottom over a period of several weeks.

25. Abdominal Operation

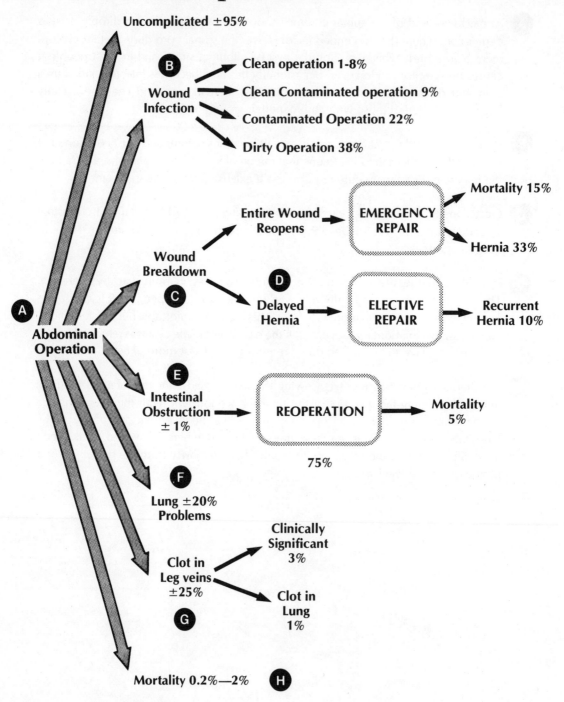

Uncomplicated ±95%

B Wound Infection
- Clean operation 1-8%
- Clean Contaminated operation 9%
- Contaminated Operation 22%
- Dirty Operation 38%

C Wound Breakdown
- Entire Wound Reopens → EMERGENCY REPAIR → Mortality 15% / Hernia 33%

D Delayed Hernia → ELECTIVE REPAIR → Recurrent Hernia 10%

A Abdominal Operation

E Intestinal Obstruction ±1% → REOPERATION → Mortality 5%
75%

F Lung ±20% Problems

G Clot in Leg veins ±25%
- Clinically Significant 3%
- Clot in Lung 1%

H Mortality 0.2%—2%

A This discussion relates to operations that are performed within the abdominal cavity. Such an operation is called a laparotomy (opening the abdominal cavity). The numbers cited as average in this chapter are only approximations, against which each patient's chances will have to be weighed. The probability of each complication and mortality is altered enormously by the type of operation performed and the general condition of the patient which must take into account his age, underlying disease in the heart, kidney, lungs, and brain and such factors as obesity and smoking history. About 95% of operations in the abdominal cavity will be uncomplicated.

B The likelihood of the operative wound becoming infected depends mainly on how heavily it is contaminated with bacteria at the time of laparotomy. Clean operations where the intestintal tract (bowel) is not entered, such as a hernia repair or operations on the arteries, have a 1–8% chance of wound infection. At the other extreme a frankly dirty operation within the abdominal cavity, such as one draining pus from a ruptured appendix, has a 38% likelihood of infection in the operative wound.

C In about one in 200 laparotomies (0.5%) the entire wound from the skin into the abdominal cavity will come apart. Such a wound dehiscence usually occurs between the fifth and tenth day after operation and is often associated with infection or chronic cough. It requires immediate reoperation and repair, with a 15% chance of mortality and a 33% likelihood that the repaired infected wound will itself not heal perfectly and will ultimately have a hernia defect beneath the intact skin.

D From 1% to 10% of all abdominal (laparotomy) incisions will break down beneath intact skin and form a hernia through the operative site. Seventy-five percent of such incisional herniae will develop within the first year. Infection, smoking, cough, obesity, and intestinal obstruction all increase the likelihood of such herniae.

If the hernia is repaired when it is small, the probability of cure is better than if it is allowed to reach a large size. Overall recurrence rate after repair of a ventral hernia is 10% (see "Hernia," page 282).

E During laparotomy, the bowel must be handled by the surgeon. This paralyzes normal bowel activity for a day or two. Infection will prolong such paralysis. In about 2.0% of abdominal procedures, the bowel either remains paralyzed beyond the expected 1–4 days or becomes blocked by a band (adhesion) caused by the inflammation and reaction around the operative site. Such paralysis of the intestine not due to adhesions can be managed by non-operative means. But when due to mechanical obstruction caused by adhesions it is necessary in 75% of cases to reoperate to cut these obstructing bands lying across the intestine (see "Small Bowel Obstruction," page 209).

F Complicated and delicate lung function studies will detect changes in anyone confined to bed for several days. X-ray studies will detect others. In only a fraction of those operated on and confined to bed will there be significant clinical changes in the lung. This may be caused and complicated by collapse of the lung, pulmonary embolus (see page 87), vomiting and aspiration, heart failure, obesity, pain, smoking history, and many other factors. After major operations a mechanical ventilating device is often used for a few days to help the patient breathe and prevent problems with breathing.

G Following operation and bed rest, blood in the veins of the leg and calf has an increased tendency to clot. When such blood clots form, the calf of the leg swells and becomes tender. This is called thrombophlebitis (page 150). Very small clots probably form in every patient's legs following laparotomy but in only about one in 100 is there any clinical evidence of thrombophlebitis. Of these few with symptoms about 20% will, if not treated, loosen a piece of the clot from the leg which will travel up the leg veins to the lung (pulmonary embolus). Drugs that interfere with clotting (anticoagulants) given before or shortly after operation decrease the probability of both thrombophlebitis and pulmonary embolus.

H Representative examples of expected mortality in several types of operations within the abdominal cavity include:

Remove appendix (Appendectomy) 0.2%
Remove gallbladder (Cholecystectomy) 1%
Operation on stomach (Gastrectomy) 1.5%
Remove part of colon (Colectomy) 2.1%

IX
Tumors & Skin

1. Major Burn

A A person with a deep extensive burn faces a long fight for life. During the first three to five days, he must be kept out of shock by receiving massive amounts of intravenous fluids to combat the water lost into the burned area. Once this hurdle is passed, he enters a long grueling race of attrition that is only won when the burn wound is permanently covered with good skin. Until this is achieved, his burn wounds will tend to become infected, and he will lose weight and strength unless extraordinary methods are used to supply large amounts of calories contained in intravenous solutions.

Chances for survival depend mainly on how much of the body surface area has been deeply burned. Serious burns destroy the full thickness of the skin (third-degree burn). The amount of the body surface involved is calculated by the "rule of nine," as shown below. One totally burned arm is 9% of the body surface; a totally burned leg is 18%; the skin on the front of the trunk 18%, and 18% on the back. The percent of the

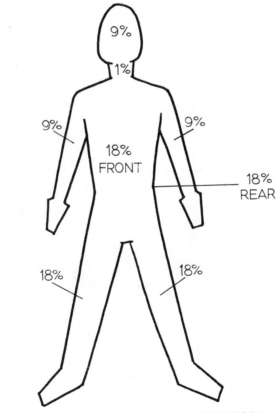

PER-CENT OF SKIN ON VARIOUS PARTS OF THE BODY

Major Burn

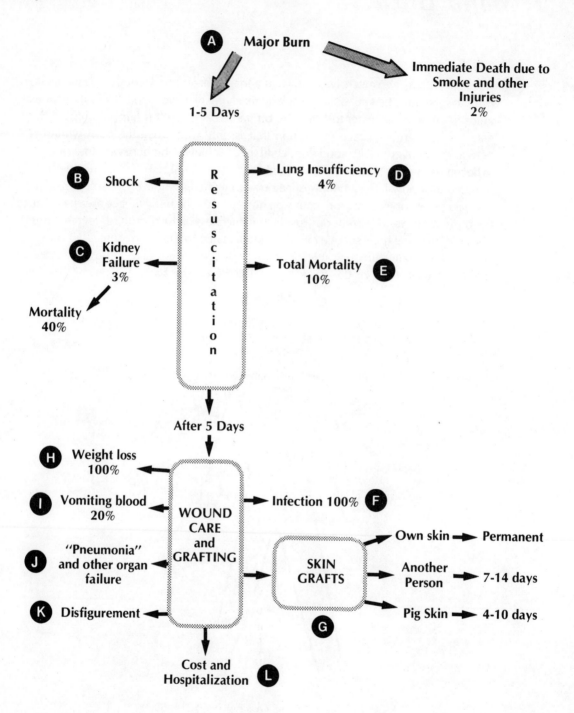

Major Burn

Immediate Death due to Smoke and other Injuries 2%

1-5 Days

A

B Shock

D Lung Insufficiency 4%

R e s u s c i t a t i o n

C Kidney Failure 3%

Mortality 40%

E Total Mortality 10%

After 5 Days

H Weight loss 100%

I Vomiting blood 20%

J "Pneumonia" and other organ failure

K Disfigurement

WOUND CARE and GRAFTING

F Infection 100%

SKIN GRAFTS

Own skin → Permanent

Another Person → 7-14 days

Pig Skin → 4-10 days

G

Cost and Hospitalization **L**

body surface burned is then calculated to determine the fluid needed to combat shock and the chances of survival.

Burns involving less than 20% of the body surface are considered minor as far as threat to life is concerned for ordinary adults. The very young or the very old withstand equivalent burns poorly. Burns involving the airway or lungs are usually less a matter of damage by heat than irritation of the lungs by inhaled smoke.

B A great deal of water and salt solution pours into the burned area and, if not replaced by intravenous infusion, results in severe or even lethal shock. Death from shock in the first one to three days is quite uncommon except with almost total body surface burns.

C Kidney damage with decreased or absent urine production occurs in about 3% of severely burned patients. If a patient develops such complete kidney shutdown, the chance of survival is 60%.

D Lung complications, manifested by difficulty in breathing, occur in the first few days after a burn in about 4% of severe burns and are usually related to the huge amounts of intravenous water and salt that have to be given to combat shock.

E Total mortality in the first day is about 10% and relates almost solely to the extent of the burn. The overall chance of survival of a patient with a severe burn as it correlates with the extent of the burn is as follows:

Surface Burn	Mortality
<20%	<10%
30%	30%
40%	45%
50%	60%
60%	80%

F After the fourth to fifth day, the burned patient is usually stable and the immediate threat past. The challenge then is to clean the burn wound and, as soon as possible, to cover the raw area with good skin. Not until it is so covered can there be protection against the ravages of infection. Antibiotics and other drugs put on the wound will delay bacterial growth but not until the skin covers the wound will the threat be over. This may require two to ten or more operations, depending on the size of the burn, to remove the thick, burned skin and to cover the area with skin grafts.

G Normal skin taken from an unburned area of the patients's body and placed on the burned area once it has been cleaned will grow and remain as a permanent skin cover. Skin grafts taken from another person will act as a temporary burn wound dressing but will last for only one to two weeks before the graft is gradually absorbed, leaving the wound raw once again. Skin from a pig will last as a covering for four to ten days before being rejected. Such temporary dressing, using skin from another person or an animal, may be helpful while the wounds are healing.

H A person with a burn wound consumes a huge amount of energy. The calories expended are equivalent to that of a marathon runner jogging all day and night. Unless an equivalent number of calories can be eaten or given intravenously, the patient loses a lot of weight and further delays his recovery. Seldom can all this food be tolerated by mouth, so special fluids high in calories must be given intravenously.

I Unless special precautions are taken, about 20% of patients with severe burns will develop stomach ulcers and 5–10% may vomit blood. These are called stress ulcers (see "Gastric Ulcer," page 176) and are often associated with burn-wound infection. Usually such stress ulcers can be managed with blood transfusions and do not require an operation to stop the bleeding. If operation cannot be avoided, the expected mortality is over 20%.

J Infection in the burn wound often affects many other organs at a distance from the burn including the lungs, liver, kidney, and heart. When these organs begin to fail because of the infection, the likelihood of survival is about 40%.

K A full-thickness burn inevitably will leave a scar. Surgeons can minimize the disfigurement and disability but cannot completely avoid it.

L A patient with a major burn is often in the hospital for four to eight weeks, undergoes two to ten or more operations, and receives four to twenty or more blood transfusions. The cost of this hospitalization alone often exceeds $20,000.

2. Malignant Melanoma

A   Everyone has a few freckles. But these have nothing whatever to do with malignant melanoma or cancer. They represent skin cells containing a brown pigment. An entirely different type of cell containing a black pigment called melanin may produce a cancerlike tumor called malignant melanoma. Every black spot on the skin is not, however, melanoma. Most people have a few such spots here and there.

    A typical melanoma starts as a black spot on the skin, and as it grows, it extends along the surface and burrows deep into the bottom layers of the skin. The tumor may then spread to the lymph nodes draining that area of the body. For example, the hand is drained by the lymph nodes under the arm (axilla), and the foot, from those in the groin. If unchecked, the melanoma will later spread throughout the body. The only certain way to diagnose malignant melanoma is by examining a piece of the tumor under the microscope.

B   The best chance for cure of melanoma is removal while the tumor is still localized to one area of the skin.

C   When the surgeon is suspicious that a black area of the skin is a melanoma, he will usually remove the black spot together with a wide margin of surrounding normal skin in order to be certain that he has removed all of the local tumor. This may seem to the patient like an excessively extensive operation for removal of such a simple skin lesion, but it has proven to be the safest procedure for treating this type of tumor. Sometimes the procedure leaves such a wide exposure that the edges of the remaining skin cannot be brought together and a skin graft must be used.

D   If when the surgical specimen is microscopically examined the melanoma is found to be limited to the superficial layers of the skin just beneath the surface, then nothing more need be done, and the chance of cure is 95–100%.

E   If, on the other hand, the melanoma is found to have burrowed deep into the skin, there is a 40% probability that the tumor has also spread to the local lymph nodes (axilla, groin, etc.), even though the physician cannot feel any evidence of such tumor when he examines the area. For this reason, the surgeon often removes the regional nodes under such circumstances, even though he can feel no evidence of tumor. If small deposits of tumor are found, the likelihood of cure is 40%. If no tumor is found, the chance of cure is 95–100%.

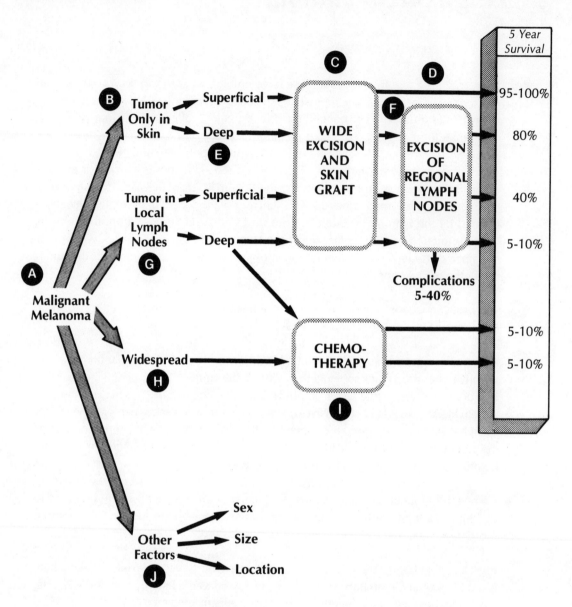

5 Year Survival

A Malignant Melanoma

B Tumor Only in Skin
Superficial
Deep E

G Tumor in Local Lymph Nodes
Superficial
Deep

C WIDE EXCISION AND SKIN GRAFT

D

F EXCISION OF REGIONAL LYMPH NODES

Complications 5-40%

H Widespread

I CHEMO-THERAPY

J Other Factors
Sex
Size
Location

95-100%

80%

40%

5-10%

5-10%

5-10%

F The operation to remove the lymph nodes draining the area of the tumor has a 1% operative mortality rate. The chances of complication after operation depend on the region in which the nodes must be removed. Removal of the nodes in the neck and under the arm requires hospitalization for about a week and leaves a scar, but otherwise, it is relatively free of complication. But removal of nodes in the groin has a complication rate of about 40%, largely because of continued leak of lymph from the wound and delay in wound healing.

G If the surgeon feels lymph nodes in the area draining the site of the melanoma that he suspects contain tumor, he has at least an 80% chance of being correct in his prediction. Under these circumstances, he usually removes all the nodes in that area at the time he removes the skin tumor. When the nodes contain tumor, the chances of cure are 40% if the original tumor was only in the superficial layer of the skin, and 5 to 10% if the melanoma has demonstrated its aggressiveness by burrowing deep into the skin.

H Melanomas can spread to any part of the body but are particularly likely to extend to the liver or lungs. They have an unpredictable course. Eighty percent of such metastases will appear within two years after removal of the original tumor, but others recur for as long as ten to fifteen years after the original tumor was removed. Even with widespread disease, 5 to 10% of patients will survive five years.

I A number of drugs are effective in decreasing the size of unremovable melanoma. The best drugs have about a 25% chance of decreasing the size of the tumor by one-half for at least a month.

Although there is great interest in trying to stop growth of melanomas by increasing the patient's immunologic resistance to the tumor, there is no evidence that such treatment as yet changes the progress of melanomas in humans.

J Other factors affect the chances of recurrence and survival after excision of a malignant melanoma:

Malignant Melanoma

- Men fare less well than women.
- Smaller (less than 3 centimeters in diameter) original tumors have a better chance of cure than big ones.
- Lesions on the leg, arm, and face have a better chance of cure than melanomas arising on the trunk or around the genital region.

3. Sarcoma

A Sarcomas are malignant tumors of the soft tissues, such as muscle, fat, and fibrous tissue. They are equivalent to cancers, which arise from different tissues.

Most soft tissue sarcomas usually are first noted as a non-tender swelling under the skin that gradually increases in size without any other symptoms. All such swellings are not sarcoma, however. Many factors affect the chances of cure of a sarcoma, including the cell type showing the tissue of origin, the size of the tumor when first treated, its location, degree of malignancy under microscopic examination, and the method of treatment.

B Sarcomas are, in general, classified by the type of tissue from which the tumor arose. Those from fat are called liposarcomas, those from fibrous tissue, fibrosarcoma, etc. Each type has its characteristic pattern of usual growth and probability of cure. Examination of the tumor under the microscope is necessary for final classification of sarcomas.

C The smaller the tumor when discovered, the more likely is the cure. Sarcomas less than 5 centimeters in diameter have, overall, a 65% probability of cure; those over 5 centimeters, a 40% likelihood of cure.

D The further away from the trunk of the body, the better the chances of cure. Sarcomas in the foot have a 75% cure rate; those in the thigh, 50%.

E The appearance of the tumor cells under the microscope are helpful in predicting the probability of cure. The more the tumor cells look like normal tissue cells, the better the chance of cure. Those of low-grade malignant appearance (e.g., they look similar to normal cells) have an overall 75% cure rate. Those of high-grade malignancy, a 17% chance of cure.

F As with most malignancies, treatment and the probability for cure depend upon being able to remove the tumor with a border of surrounding normal tissue to be certain that no tumor cells remain. Limited local excision of the tumor with a thin rim of surrounding tissue is a less disfiguring and crippling operation for sarcoma but implies a 40–90% chance of the tumor recurring at the original site.

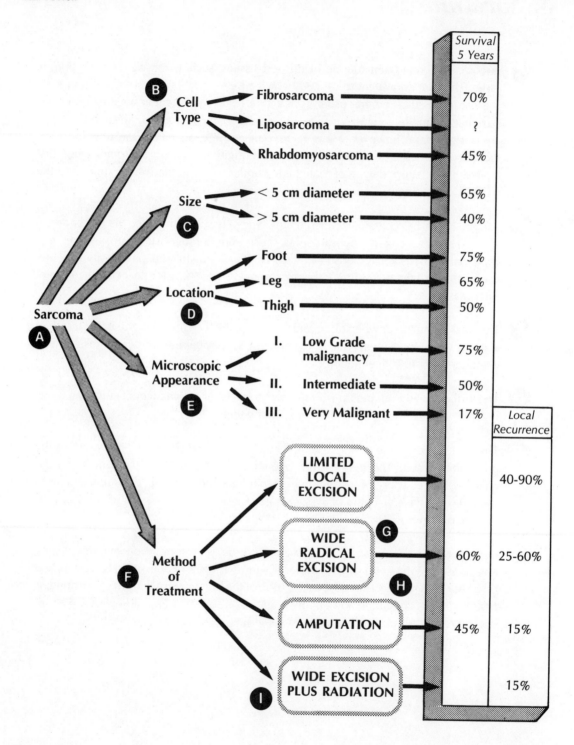

G Much wider excision, removing large muscle bundles around the tumor, decreases the likelihood of local recurrence to 25–50%, depending on the type of sarcoma involved. There is no additional benefit from removing local lymph nodes, which is effective in many cancers. Sarcomas spread differently than do cancer. If the lymph nodes in the area draining the sarcoma contain tumor, there is only a 20% chance of five-year cure, regardless of treatment.

H Applying radiation to the tumor bed after its operative removal decreases the likelihood of local recurrence of the tumor to 15%. Sensitivity to x-radiation differs between various cell types of sarcomas. Lymphosarcoma and liposarcoma are particularly sensitive. Fibrosarcomas are more resistant. Seventy percent of all recurrences after excision or X-ray therapy are at the site of the original tumor. When the tumor recurs locally, there is a two-thirds chance this is the only remaining sarcoma, so repeat wide excision is warranted. Even a second local recurrence can be cured in half the cases, with wide operative removal. Such strictly local recurrences have the same chance of cure as do the original lesion. Where the size, location, and microscopic appearance of the recurrent sarcoma require amputation of an arm or leg, 20% of cases will have a second recurrence at the amputation site.

Fifteen percent of patients will have distant spread of sarcoma when the tumor is first diagnosed and will not usually be helped by operative removal of the tumor. Survival after one year is 80%. With such wide, diffuse disease, radiation and anti-tumor drugs are used to delay tumor growth and control pain.

A single anti-tumor drug decreases the size of 15–20% of widespread sarcomas. The chance of response is increased to 50% if a combination of drugs is used.

I Radiation therapy is of great benefit to those with advanced sarcoma. It will decrease the size of about half such metastases and provide relief from pain to about 80%.

Occasionally after removing a sarcoma, a single metastatic deposit of tumor will appear in the lung on chest X-ray examination. If after three to six months no other tumor has appeared, it is worth exploring the chest and if only the one tumor nodule is found, removing it. The chances of cure is a heartening 25% under these unusual circumstances.

4. *Childhood Leukemia*

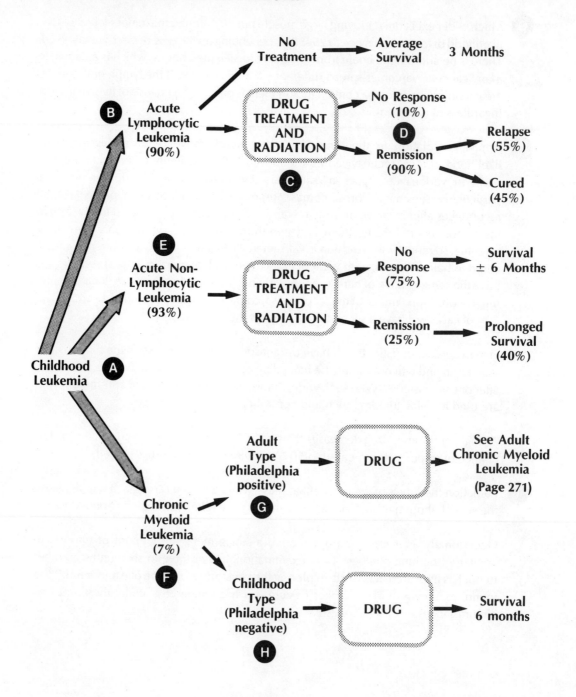

No Treatment → Average Survival 3 Months

B Acute Lymphocytic Leukemia (90%)

C DRUG TREATMENT AND RADIATION → No Response (10%)

→ **D** Remission (90%) → Relapse (55%)

→ Cured (45%)

E Acute Non-Lymphocytic Leukemia (93%)

DRUG TREATMENT AND RADIATION → No Response (75%) → Survival ± 6 Months

→ Remission (25%) → Prolonged Survival (40%)

A Childhood Leukemia

G Adult Type (Philadelphia positive) → DRUG → See Adult Chronic Myeloid Leukemia (Page 271)

F Chronic Myeloid Leukemia (7%)

H Childhood Type (Philadelphia negative) → DRUG → Survival 6 months

A Normally, there is delicate control of white blood-cell production in the bone marrow. But sometimes the body is flooded with abnormal forms of these cells. The condition is similar to a cancer of the bone marrow and is called leukemia.

B The type of the leukemia (lymphocytic, myeloid, etc.) is determined by examining the abnormal cells in the blood and in the bone marrow. Acute lymphocytic leukemia has an overgrowth of white blood cells known as lymphocytes. There is a sudden (acute) onset of symptoms, such as bleeding or infection. This accounts for 90% of the leukemia in children.

C Treatment is with several types of drugs, plus x-radiation to the brain and to the spinal cord. The drug treatment is continued for one to two years.

D In 90% of children, improvement will be seen within one to three weeks. This is called a remission. The other 10% of children do not respond to treatment and usually live less than six months. Of those who respond, about 55% will do well for about one to three years before having another attack (relapse). When retreated, about 50–75% will obtain another good temporary response. They are, however, seldom totally cured.

E An occasional child (about 3% of all leukemias in children) will have an acute onset of symptoms, but the cell will differ from those found in lymphocytic leukemia. This is called acute non-lymphocytic leukemia. Treatment is with drugs and radiation to the brain and spinal cord. About 75% of these children will not improve and live only about four to six weeks. The other 25% respond, and of these, about 40% will live for several years.

F In about 7% of leukemic children there will be gradual (chronic) onset of symptoms, with the cells found flooding the blood stream appearing normal but present in totally abnormal numbers. This is called chronic myeloid leukemia.

G Most of these children have a disease similar to one also found in adults. They have abnormal (Philadelphia) chromosomes. Treated with drugs, most of these children respond promptly, just as do adults (see "Adult Leukemia," page 270).

H The other children with chronic myeloid leukemia have a special childhood type of the disease (Philadelphia chromosome negative). Very few of these children will respond to any drug treatment.

5. *Adult Leukemia*

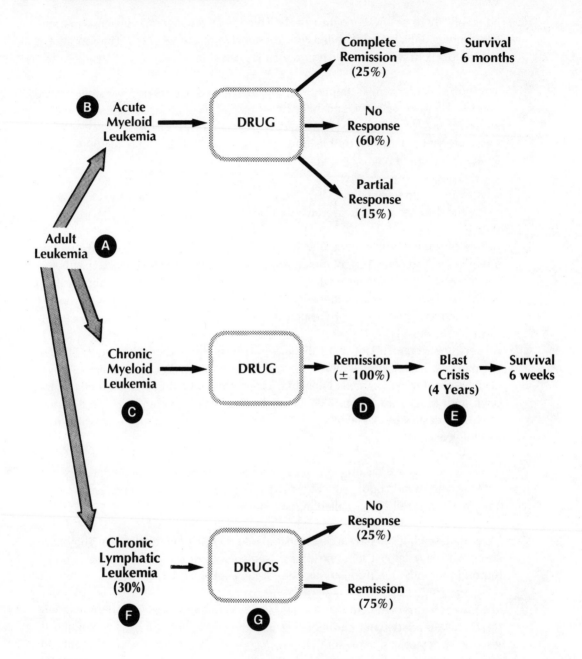

A Adults may develop leukemia, which, as in children, resembles a cancer or overgrowth of the white blood cells in the bone marrow. These cells are released into the blood in abnormally large numbers.

B Acute myeloid (or myelogenous) leukemia involves sudden onset of symptoms, such as bleeding, weakness from anemia, or infection. The bone marrow and blood stream is flooded with white blood cells that look like very immature forms of cells often found in normal people. Treatment with drugs only helps about 25% of such patients, who may live six to twelve months. There will be essentially no response in about 75% of such patients, who can expect to live but a few months. The chances of living two years with this disease are almost nil.

C Chronic myeloid leukemia has a gradual onset, the average age of which is thirty-five. The disease usually makes itself known by weakness and fullness in the left upper abdomen because of an enlarged spleen. Treatment is usually with a drug called Myleran, given by tablets once a day for many months. The average survival is about four years after the onset of symptoms.

D Almost all patients with chronic myeloid leukemia respond to initial treatment with Myleran. This treatment makes the patients feel better, reduces their blood cell counts and spleen size, but does not alter the expected length of life. Patients usually live normally during this time even though leukemic cells persist in the blood and bone marrow.

E After one to six years (average four years), these patients have a sudden change in the disease, which turns into acute leukemia. The expected course is then as described for acute leukemia.

F Thirty percent of the leukemia found in old people (average age about sixty years) is called chronic lymphatic leukemia. It is often found on a routine physical examination in a patient who has no symptoms. Average survival of such asymptomatic patients with this disease is five to six years.

G There may be no need to treat patients with chronic lymphatic leukemia. If symptoms develop, as they do in 75% of cases, then treatment is with a drug, Chlorambucil. About 75% of patients can be expected to respond. Of these, about 25% will never have other symptoms. It is simple enough to bring the white blood-cell count to normal, but this is not the disease, merely a sign of it. Average survival after treatment is about four years in these elderly people.

6. Hodgkin's Disease

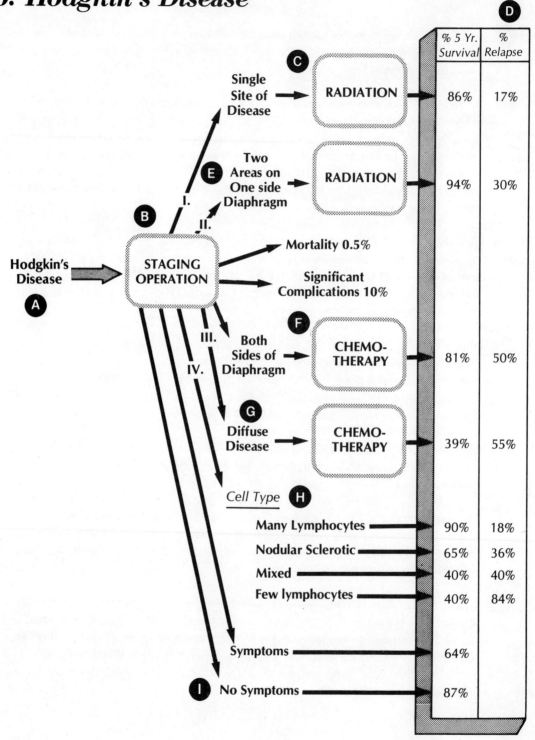

	% 5 Yr. Survival	% Relapse
Single Site of Disease → RADIATION	86%	17%
Two Areas on One side Diaphragm → RADIATION	94%	30%
Both Sides of Diaphragm → CHEMO-THERAPY	81%	50%
Diffuse Disease → CHEMO-THERAPY	39%	55%
Many Lymphocytes	90%	18%
Nodular Sclerotic	65%	36%
Mixed	40%	40%
Few lymphocytes	40%	84%
Symptoms	64%	
No Symptoms	87%	

Hodgkin's Disease

STAGING OPERATION

Mortality 0.5%

Significant Complications 10%

Cell Type

I. II. III. IV.

A Cells called lymphocytes are spread throughout almost every organ of the body. They are particularly concentrated in the spleen and lymph nodes. For unknown reasons, this lymphatic tissue sometimes forms a tumor which is called Hodgkin's disease. Sometimes, the tumor is strictly localized to one or a local group of lymph nodes. Other times, it appears almost simultaneously in many parts of the body, such as in the neck or in the spleen. Even when the tumor is localized, it may cause generalized symptoms, such as fever and fatigue.

B Because the tumor cells in localized Hodgkin's disease are very sensitive to X-ray, it is important to know as precisely as possible exactly where the tumor deposits of Hodgkin's disease are located so that the X-ray beam can be aimed directly at the tumor. Locating the disease is best achieved by a so-called "staging operation" in the abdomen. The spleen is removed and specimens taken from representative lymph nodes throughout the abdomen and from the liver. Each is examined under the microscope to determine whether it is involved with the tumor. Such a staging operation alters the clinical impression of the extent of the disease in 35% of cases and thereby changes the plan for treatment. Chances of dying from this operation are less than 0.5%, but there is some sort of complication after operation in about 10% of these people already ill with Hodgkin's disease. Hospitalization for the operation is usually about five to seven days.

C If the disease is localized to one area of the body such as the neck, X-ray therapy is given in large amounts to that area alone, and the chances of five-year survival are about 85%. Seventeen percent of patients so treated will have a return of tumor at the original site and can be given more radiation at that point, or the mass can be removed by an operation.

D A relapse is a recurrence. About 90% of recurrences of Hodgkin's Disease after treatment occur within three years, and 97% within five years. If no new tumor has reappeared after five years, the chances of it ever doing so are 3%. Recurrence should be expected in this disease, but fortunately there are so many effective methods of treatment that recurrence does not mean the disease is incurable.

E If after physical examination and a staging operation, two areas of the tumor are precisely located on one side of the diaphragm (that is, either within the abdomen or the chest), then radiation still can be directed only at these spots and the chances of five-year cure are 94%. The 30% who have a relapse can be retreated with X-ray, or the mass can be excised.

Hodgkin's Disease

F When tumor occurs in both the chest and the abdomen, that is on both sides of the diaphragm, it is too diffuse a target for x-radiation, so drugs are used that kill Hodgkin's disease cells throughout the body. Five-year survival can be expected in 81% of such cases. The chance of cure decreases when the number of tumor sites is great.

G When Hodgkin's disease is spread throughout the body, drug therapy is required. Even with such advanced disease, 39% of patients can anticipate a cure. In the 55% who relapse, a different drug may make the tumor disappear. Chemotherapy, like radiation, may make the patient feel miserable for a few days after it is given. Some of the possible unpleasant symptoms include nausea, vomiting, inflammation of the bladder, loss of hair, and diarrhea. Fortunately, these symptoms go away when the drug is stopped. A sense of well-being returns as the tumor recedes.

H As with most tumors, the appearance of the tumor cell under the microscope helps predict the chances of cure. Hodgkin's tumors with many lymphocytes, for example, have an exceedingly good chance of cure (90%); those with few lymphocytes, a 40% likelihood of five-year survival.

I Many patients with Hodgkin's disease have no symptoms of illness. They merely may have noted a mass in the neck, for example. Such patients have a better chance for cure than those who have symptoms of illness when the tumor was first diagnosed. Of all those whose only evidence of disease at first diagnosis is the tumor mass, 87% will be alive in five years, compared to a 69% chance of survival if the disease has made them ill.

X
Hernia

1. Neonatal Umbilical Hernia

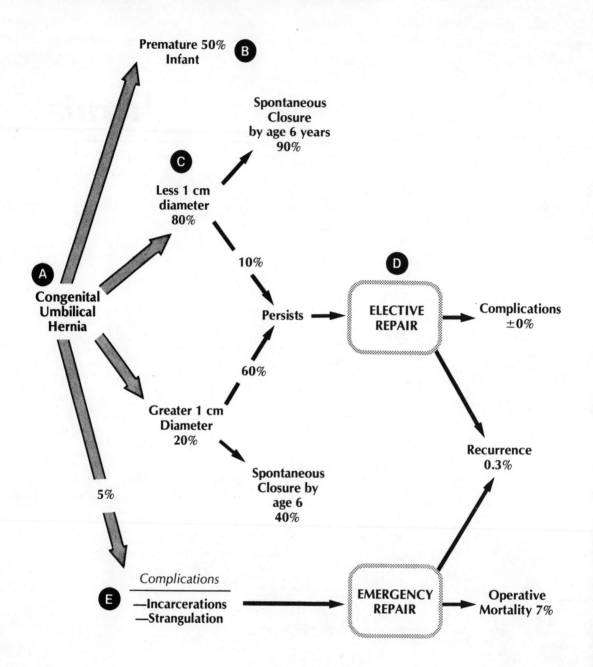

A The lifeline of the fetus before birth (the umbilical cord), which connects to the placenta of the mother, passes through a hole in the abdominal wall. At birth, the umbilical cord is tied, and its remnant is the umbilicus (belly button). Normally, the muscles surrounding the umbilicus shut like a gate over it. But in a few infants, a weakness exists at this point, providing a point where the abdominal lining can protrude as a sac through the umbilicus. This is an umbilical hernia. Half of all premature infants, born before their muscles are fully developed, will have a defect at the umbilicus at the time of birth. Most umbilical hernias, in contrast to hernias elsewhere, will close without any treatment.

B If birth weight is below 1500 grams, three out of four premature infants will have an umbilical hernia. Even in full-term black children, 25% have such a hernia at birth.

C Most umbilical hernias close spontaneously, regardless of treatment. Putting pressure over the defect with adhesive tape or a waistband does not help. The probability of spontaneous closure depends on the size of the defect and how long the hernia persists. By three months of age, the neck of the hernia is usually (80%) less than 1 centimeter in diameter, and of these, 90% will be closed by six years of age. The other 10% will persist into adulthood. Of the 20% of hernias greater than 1 centimeter in diameter at age three months, 40% will close spontaneously by age six. In the other 60%, the defect will persist. From these facts, many surgeons conclude that an umbilical hernia should be repaired if it persists after six years of age, or if the defect is greater than 1.5 centimeters in diameter at age two to four years.

D Elective repair of an umbilical hernia is an operation usually lasting about one-half to one hour and carries such a small mortality that it approaches that of only the anesthesia itself (less than 0.1%). Hospitalization usually is only one to three days. Sometimes, this operation can be performed without the need of being admitted to the hospital. The probability of recurrence is 0.3%.

E If for some reason the umbilical hernia is not repaired, there is about a 5% chance that a complication will develop. This may be an inability to replace the hernia contents into the abdomen (incarceration), intestinal obstruction (blocked bowel), or, rarely, an interruption of the blood supply to the bowel in the hernia sac (strangulation). Emergency repair of such complications has an operative mortality of 7%, compared to almost no chance of death if the operation is performed before any trouble develops.

2. Infant Groin Hernia

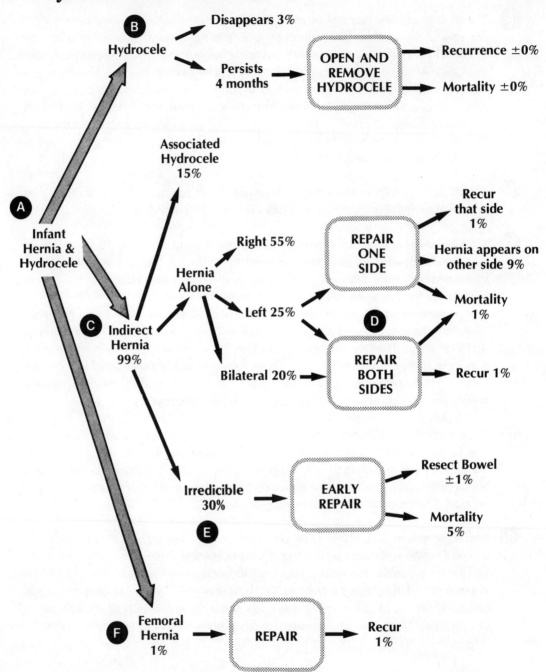

B Hydrocele → Disappears 3%

Hydrocele → Persists 4 months → **OPEN AND REMOVE HYDROCELE** → Recurrence ±0%

OPEN AND REMOVE HYDROCELE → Mortality ±0%

A Infant Hernia & Hydrocele

Associated Hydrocele 15%

C Indirect Hernia 99%

Hernia Alone → Right 55%

Left 25%

Bilateral 20%

REPAIR ONE SIDE → Recur that side 1%

REPAIR ONE SIDE → Hernia appears on other side 9%

Mortality 1%

D **REPAIR BOTH SIDES** → Recur 1%

Irredicible 30% → **EARLY REPAIR** → Resect Bowel ±1%

E **EARLY REPAIR** → Mortality 5%

F Femoral Hernia 1% → **REPAIR** → Recur 1%

A The abdominal wall is composed of firm overlapping layers of muscle and tough sheets of fascia. There are certain weak points where the muscles don't quite overlap, through which sacs of abdominal cavity lining may appear as an abdominal bulge or hernia. Intestine or other contents of the abdominal cavity can enter the hernia sac through the connecting neck of the hernia. Infants born before full term (premature) are particularly liable to have hernias. Sometimes the hernia sac is sealed off from the abdominal cavity and becomes filled with watery fluid. This is called a hydrocele and appears as a swelling in the scrotum.

B Ninety-three percent of hydroceles in premature infants have an associated hernia. Although 3% of hydroceles in newborns will disappear spontaneously, if they persist more than four months, they certainly will not go away and must be repaired. This is usually done under general anesthesia, either with a day of hospitalization or as an outpatient. The risk to the infant of recurrence is almost nil.

C Almost all groin hernias in newborns or infants are known as indirect hernias, and in 15%, there is an associated hydrocele. Fifty-five percent are on the right side and only 25% on the left, leaving 20% with hernias on *both* sides.

D It is often difficult to be certain that a small hernia does not exist on the side opposite from a clearly detected hernia sac. If only the known hernia is repaired, there is a 9% chance that a hernia will show up at a later date on the other side. Because of the doubled likelihood of hernia on the right, some surgeons repair *both* sides, even when they only can feel a hernia on the left. The chance of recurrence is about 1% after hernia repair in these infants.

E When the contents of the hernia sac cannot be pushed back into the abdominal cavity, the hernia is said to be incarcerated or irreducible. This occurs in about 30% of hernias in infants under four months of age. Because the intestine caught within the hernia sac might become obstructed or have its blood supply shut off, such incarcerated hernias should be repaired as soon as possible. There is only about a 1% likelihood that the bowel will be obstructed or dead in these infants, but when the bowel has to be resected, there is a 5% expected mortality rate. There is far more chance of benefit than of loss by early operation on an incarcerated hernia.

Infant Groin Hernia

 Hernia protrusion in the top part of the thigh (femoral hernia) is very rare in infants but should be repaired because of its tendency for incarceration. Rarely (about 2% of all incarcerated hernias in infants), the blood supply to the bowel in the hernia sac is cut off and the bowel becomes gangrenous and will break open if not repaired as an emergency. Such a strangulated hernia requiring bowel resection carries a mortality of up to 10%. It is far less common in infants than in adults, but when it occurs, it is a serious acute emergency. Mortality with an irreducible but not strangulated hernia is not more than 1%.

3. Adult Groin Hernia

A A hernia is an abnormal protrusion or bulge of the lining of the abdominal cavity through a weak place in the muscles of the abdominal wall. The hernia sac connects with the abdominal cavity through a narrow neck, which constricts the contents of the sac where it goes through the abdominal wall. Although there are several types of

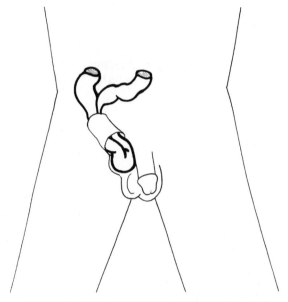

LOOP OF SMALL INTESTINE WITHIN HERNIA SAC

hernia, the ones commonly associated with the term are in the groin. It is a common condition, 90% of which occur in males. Repair is indicated for the discomfort they cause, because they tend to grow in size and because intestines may drop into the sac and become irreducible (incarcerated). Occasionally, the blood supply to the trapped bowel is shut off, resulting in gangrene. The latter is called a strangulated hernia.

B The most common type is called an indirect hernia, because it starts in the groin and travels obliquely (indirectly) down toward the scrotum. This is the kind of hernia found in infants and associated with hydrocele (see "Infant Groin Hernia," page 278). Forty-five percent of groin hernias in adults are of this type. The hernia occurs on the right side alone 55% of the time, on the left, 25% of the time, and on both sides, 20%. Twenty-five percent of adults with a left-sided hernia will ultimately develop a hernia on the right. On this basis, some surgeons faced with a hernia on the left advocate exploring the right side as well to prevent a future hernia on that side.

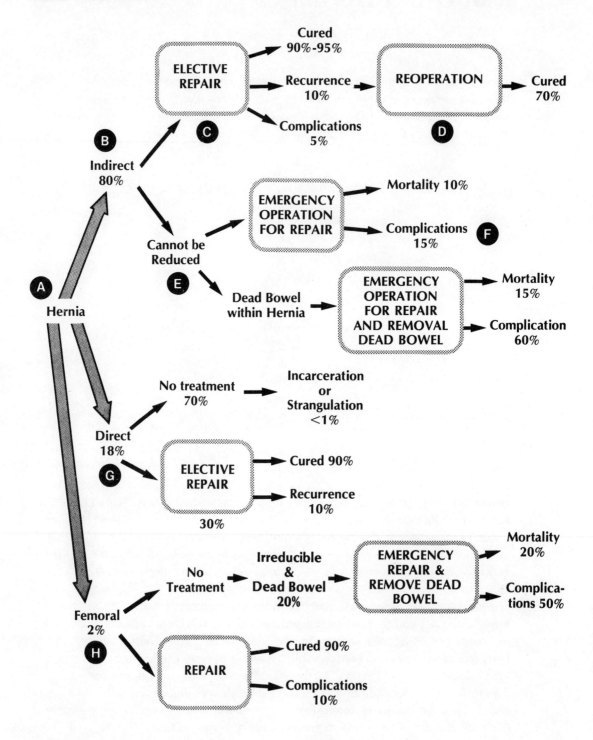

C Various types of operations are used to cure a groin hernia, but all involve removing the sac, closing its connection to the abdominal cavity, and closing the muscles and tendons around the weakened area from which the hernia arose. General, spinal, or local anesthesia can be used, and hospitalization is usually for two to seven days.

Complications with elective repair are about 5%, compared to a 50% or more expectancy if the operation is delayed and then has to be done as an emergency. This is why elective repair while the hernia is still small is so important.

D The repair will not hold and the hernia will recur 5–10% of the time. A chance of recurrence is less in young men where such hernias often occur. Sixty-five percent of such recurrences appear within five years following operation. Factors that increase the likelihood of recurrence include technical problems at the time of repair, very weakened tissues, or conditions such as chronic cough or constipation, which consistantly put a strain on the area of repair by increasing the pressure within the abdomen. Following a second repair for a recurrence, there is an even greater (up to 30%) chance of the hernia once again breaking down.

E When the contents of the hernia sac cannot be pushed back into the abdominal cavity, this is called an incarcerated hernia. In itself, this is not dangerous, but it is in this type of hernia where the blood supply to the bowel may quickly become shut off and produce gangrene and perforation of the confined intestine. This is called a strangulated hernia, and if not promptly relieved is 100% fatal, since infection spreads throughout the abdominal cavity (peritonitis).

F Emergency operation for strangulated hernia (dead bowel) has a very high mortality rate (15%) and an awesome rate of complication (60%). In the elderly, where it often occurs, the chances of disaster are even worse. This is why an irreducible (incarcerated) hernia should be promptly repaired before it becomes strangulated and bursts.

G Direct hernias cause a bulge in the groin and usually appear in elderly men. They only rarely become irreducible or cause gangrene of the bowel (strangulation), but they are often uncomfortable and, for that reason, only require repair. Anesthesia, hospitalization, and cure rate is about the same as for indirect hernia, but complication rate in the elderly is higher than in young people, where most indirect hernias are found.

Adult Groin Hernia

H The bulge of a femoral hernia occurs in the upper thigh a little lower down than the point where the far more common indirect hernias are felt. This is the most common groin hernia in women. Because the opening of the hernia sac is usually narrow, an untreated femoral hernia has a 20% chance of having bowel contents trapped within the hernia and with it the further dangerous complication of strangulation. Even if small, a femoral hernia should therefore be promptly repaired, for if one waits until the hernia strangulates, the operative mortality done as an emergency is 15–25%. In contrast, elective femoral hernia repair has an almost negligible mortality.

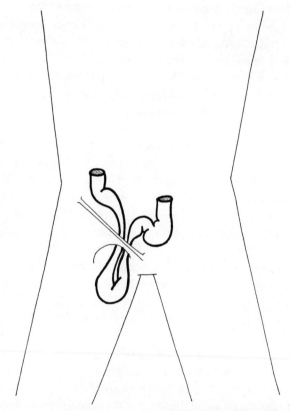

LOOP OF SMALL INTESTINE IN FEMORAL HERNIA SAC

XI
Gynecology

1. Uterine Fibroid

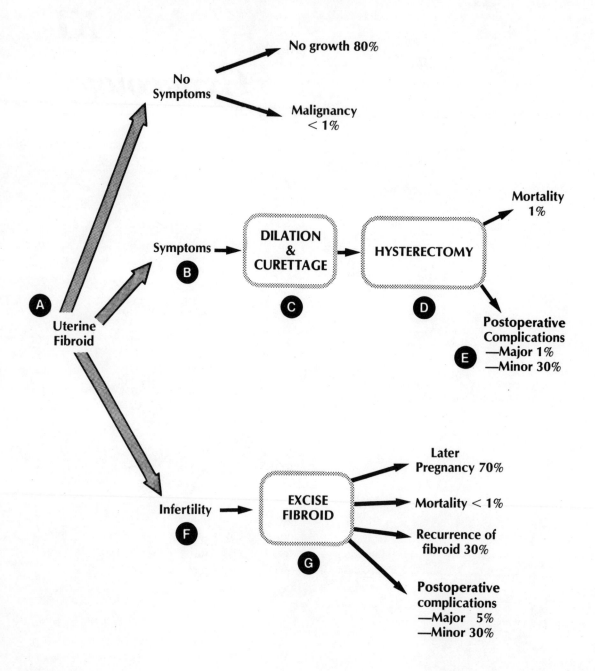

No Symptoms

- No growth 80%
- Malignancy < 1%

A Uterine Fibroid

Symptoms **B** → **DILATION & CURETTAGE** **C** → **HYSTERECTOMY** **D**

- Mortality 1%
- Postoperative Complications
  —Major 1%
  —Minor 30% **E**

Infertility **F** → **EXCISE FIBROID** **G**

- Later Pregnancy 70%
- Mortality < 1%
- Recurrence of fibroid 30%
- Postoperative complications
  —Major 5%
  —Minor 30%

A In about 25% of all women, a firm scarlike tumor grows on the womb (uterus). Because it is made of fibrous tissue, it is called a fibroid. It is not cancer, and in only the rarest of instances (less than 1%) will it ever become cancer. For unknown reasons, this condition is about six times more likely to occur in a black woman than in a caucasian.

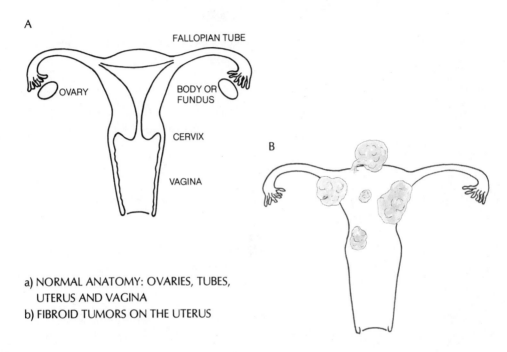

a) NORMAL ANATOMY: OVARIES, TUBES,
   UTERUS AND VAGINA
b) FIBROID TUMORS ON THE UTERUS

B Common symptoms are lower abdominal discomfort, a sense of pressure or pelvic pain, or abnormal vaginal bleeding. Sometimes a fibroid may grow to a large size without causing any symptoms. Large fibroids or ones that grow quickly are usually removed.

C Fibroids are common and often cause abnormal vaginal bleeding, but so do cancers of the uterus, and the two very different conditions can be confused. The best way to exclude cancer is by dilation and curettage (D&C), a relatively minor operation in which the contents of the uterus are scraped out and microscopically examined. If bleeding is due to fibroids, no cancer tissue will be found.

D Except in unusual circumstances (infertility, pregnancy, etc.), a fibroid that becomes symptomatic is best treated by removing the entire uterus (hysterectomy). Since most hysterectomies for fibroids are performed near the time when the ovaries stop functioning (menopause), and since there is always a chance (about 1% in women over forty years of age) that cancer of the ovary may later develop, both of the ovaries are usually removed along with the uterus. This is called a bilateral oophorectomy and hysterectomy. If the ovaries are not removed at that time, about 5% of patients will require another future operation for some disease of the ovary.

E Major complications requiring reoperation following hysterectomy are rare, but postoperative fever usually caused by infection in the urinary tract may occur in up to a third of cases.

F About a third of patients with multiple fibroids are unable to become pregnant, primarily because these benign growths interfere with the process of conception and the normal growth and delivery of the fetus.

G Excision of one or more fibroids, while leaving the rest of the uterus intact (myomectomy), is occasionally indicated when all other causes of infertility have been excluded. Probability of success decreases with age. Subsequent fertility following myomectomy is almost certain if the patient is below twenty-five years of age, is 29% for those between thirty-six and forty years of age, and is almost never successful in those over forty. Even those who become pregnant after myomectomy, however, have a 40% chance of losing the pregnancy (spontaneous abortion).

H Complications following myomectomy are about the same as those following hysterectomy: 5% major and 30% minor.

2. Endometriosis

(A) The tissue lining the uterus is called the endometrium. It grows and then sloughs off as a part a woman's monthly (menstrual) cycle. When some of this tissue grows outside of the uterus, the endometrial implants are called endometriosis. This is *not* cancer.

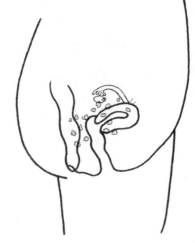

IMPLANTS OF UTERINE
(ENDOMETRIAL) TISSUE IN
THE PELVIS

(B) Although 15% of women have some endometriosis, only one in five will have symptoms from this abnormally located uterine tissue.

(C) Endometrial implants can be found anywhere in the pelvis. They cause pelvic pain in about 80%, painful menstrual periods (dysmenorrhea) in 90%, or pain during sexual intercourse (dyspareunia) in about 45% of women.

(D) To relieve the unpleasant symptoms of endometriosis but still to allow childbearing, a wide variety of operations have been tried. These include removing a part of the ovaries, cutting adhesions around the implants, cutting the nerves to the uterus, burning or removing the implant in the pelvis, suspending the uterus, etc. Although far from specific, these operations all seem to benefit about 80% of such patients, for reasons that are difficult to explain.

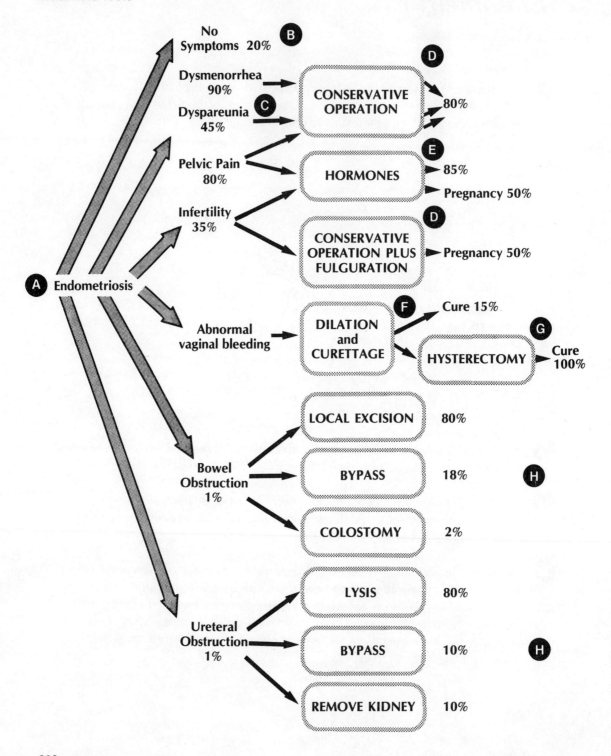

E Various combinations of two types of female sex hormones (progestins and estrogens), either alone or in combination, relieve pain in about 85% of patients. Another drug, derived from a male sex hormone, shrinks the endometrial tissue, stops menstruation, and provides pain relief in 90% of these patients.

Infertility correlates with the severity of the disease. Possibility of becoming pregnant is 75% for mild disease, 50% for moderate disease, and 33% for severe endometriosis.

F Both uterine cancer and endometriosis cause abnormal vaginal bleeding, and the two must be differentiated by a dilation and curettage (D&C) and by looking at the pelvic area through a lighted tube (laparascope). Occasionally (15% of the time) D&C will stop the symptoms, presumably by removing abnormally placed endometrial tissue in the wall of the uterus.

G If, despite treatment, symptoms are unbearable or the woman has completed having children, it may be wise to remove the uterus and ovaries (hysterectomy and oophorectomy) and maintain the patient on a female sex hormone. Operative mortality is less than 1%. In about 3% of patients, any endometrial tissue left in the peritoneal cavity after taking out the uterus and ovaries may be reactivated by sex hormone replacement therapy, and pain occurs.

H In the less than 1% of instances where endometrial tissue obstructs the bowel or urinary tract, various types of operations may have to be performed to relieve the block. These include surgical removal of the tissue (80%), bypassing the bowel contents or urine around the block, or in the case of bowel obstruction, even a colostomy, an operation in which bowel contents are diverted onto the abdominal wall. Rarely, one kidney may have to be removed when endometriosis has blocked urine excretion and has destroyed the kidney. The symptoms of endometriosis range from the mere unpleasant to life-threatening urine or bowel obstruction.

3. Cancer Cervix

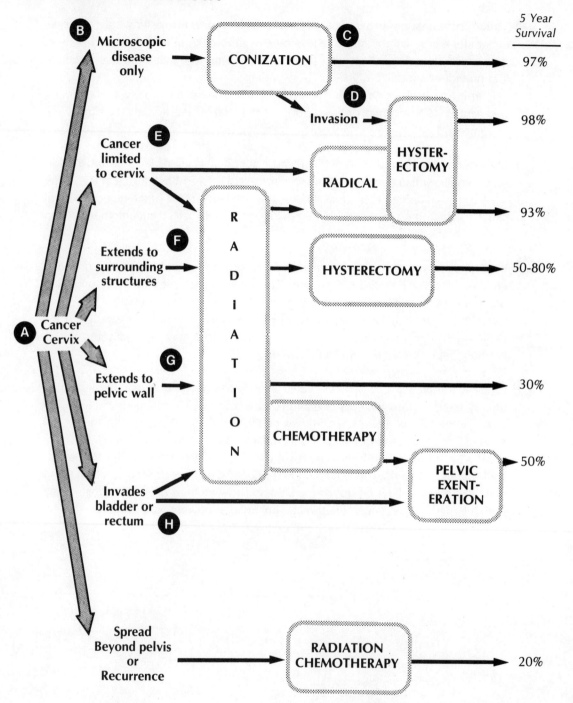

5 Year
Survival

B Microscopic disease only → **CONIZATION** **C** → 97%

→ Invasion → **D** **HYSTERECTOMY** → 98%

E Cancer limited to cervix → **RADICAL** **HYSTERECTOMY** → 93%

F Extends to surrounding structures → **RADIATION** → **HYSTERECTOMY** → 50-80%

A Cancer Cervix

G Extends to pelvic wall → 30%

CHEMOTHERAPY → **PELVIC EXENTERATION** → 50%

Invades bladder or rectum **H**

Spread Beyond pelvis or Recurrence → **RADIATION CHEMOTHERAPY** → 20%

A The cervix is the narrowed lower part of the uterus that opens into the vagina. It is made up of cells entirely different than those in the body of the uterus. Cancers of the cervix differ from those arising from the rest of the uterus. The cervix is the most common site of cancer in women.

B Cancers of the cervix often shed some cells into the vagina. By examining the secretions from the cervix under a microscope, the physician can often detect very early cancerous changes. This is the well known Papanicolaou (or "Pap") smear.

C When there is no visible tumor but the Pap smear is positive (indicates cancer), the physician usually removes a small cone or core of tissue from the cervix for more accurate diagnosis. This is called conization, and can be done under local or general anesthesia. If the cancer is so small it cannot be seen by the naked eye, conization itself may remove all the tiny tumor deposit. If the patient still has childbearing ahead of her and wants to keep her uterus, this procedure alone results in a 97% 5-year cure. If she is beyond the childbearing age, the uterus is removed, providing an almost 100% chance for cure.

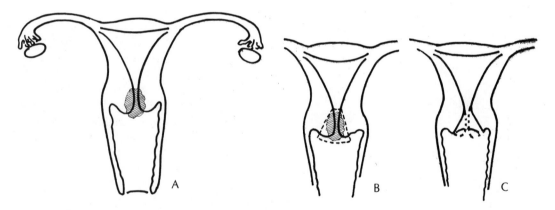

a) TUMOR OF THE CERVIX AT THE TOP OF THE VAGINA
b) PORTION OF THE CERVIX REMOVED WITH THE TUMOR
c) CERVIX FOLLOWING REMOVAL OF THE TUMOR

D If on microscopic study the specimen (cone) of the cervix shows any signs of spread (invasion), then the best chance of cure (about 98%), regardless of the age of the patient, is to remove the entire uterus (hysterectomy). Anything short of this carries too high a risk of tumor recurrence and spread.

E The chances of cure decrease as the cancer becomes larger and is found to have invaded the vagina or other organs near the cervis. A complicated system of staging (I through IV) is used as a handy way of describing how far a cervical tumor has spread. When limited to the cervix (Stage I), the cancer can be treated either by radiation alone or by removing the uterus and adjacent tissues. Both ways of treatment provide a 93% chance of cure. Some physicians prefer one treatment, some another.

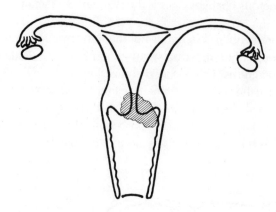

CANCER OF CERVIX SPREAD TO WALL OF VAGINA

F If the tumor has spread to the surrounding structures (Stage II or III), the chances of cure are 80% when the spread is only in that part of the vagina immediately adjacent to the cervix. The chances of cure are 50% if the tumor has extended to the more distant parts of the vagina.

G If the tumor has grown to the pelvic wall (Stage III) at the time radiation is started, the chances of cure are 30%.

H Advanced cervical cancer may invade the urinary bladder or rectum. This also may occur when radiation treatment fails. About half of these patients will have a chance for cure by operative removal of all the pelvic organs. This extensive operation (pelvic exenteration) requires removing both the rectum and the urinary bladder along with the tubes and ovaries. After operation, a colostomy (see "Colostomy," page 220) drains the stool into a bag on the left side of the abdomen. Urine is drained through a short length of intestine into a bag worn on the right side of the abdomen. This is a heavy price to pay, but many patients want the chance of cure despite the obvious drawbacks of this inconvenient way of disposing of urine and feces. Operative mortality for pelvic exenteration is 10%, and the chances of some type of complication in the early days following operation are about 66%. About half of the women undergoing this extensive salvage operation are alive five years thereafter.

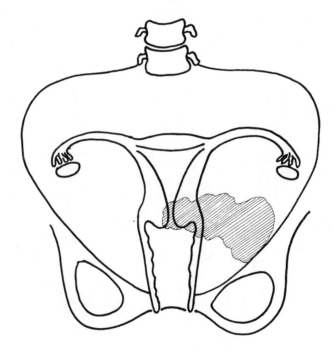

CANCER OF CERVIX SPREAD TO THE PELVIC WALL

4. *Endometrial Cancer*

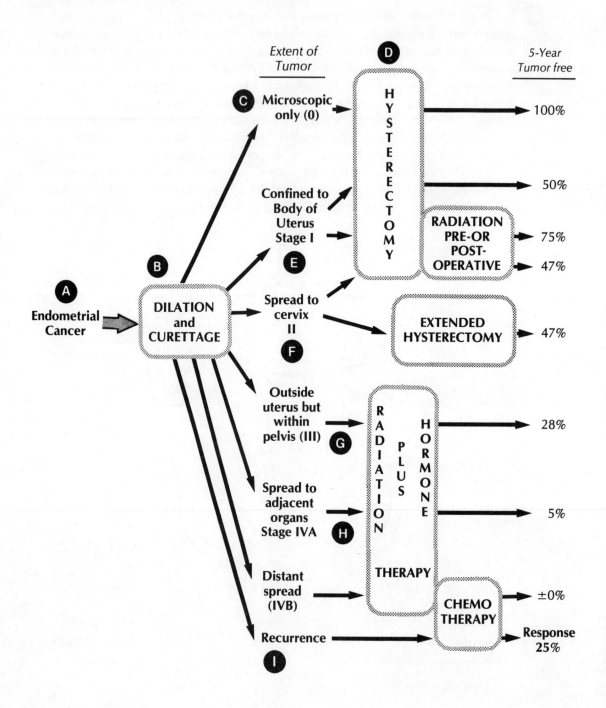

Extent of Tumor

5-Year Tumor free

A Endometrial Cancer

B DILATION and CURETTAGE

C Microscopic only (0)

D HYSTERECTOMY → 100%

E Confined to Body of Uterus Stage I → 50%

RADIATION PRE-OR POST-OPERATIVE → 75%
→ 47%

F Spread to cervix II

EXTENDED HYSTERECTOMY → 47%

G Outside uterus but within pelvis (III) → 28%

H Spread to adjacent organs Stage IVA

RADIATION PLUS HORMONE THERAPY → 5%

Distant spread (IVB) → ±0%

I Recurrence

CHEMO THERAPY → Response 25%

A There are two parts to the uterus; the narrow neck, or cervix, that opens into the vagina and the larger body, or fundus. Cancers arising in the two areas are very different. The tissue lining the body of the uterus is called the endometrium, and cancer from this area is called endometrial cancer.

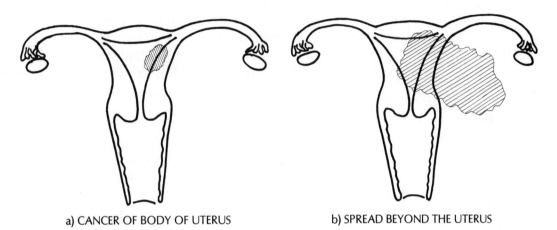

a) CANCER OF BODY OF UTERUS   b) SPREAD BEYOND THE UTERUS

B A common sign of endometrial cancer is abnormal vaginal bleeding. Dilation and curettage (see "Dilation and Curettage," page 314) provides a specimen of tumor for examination. Along with physical examination and other tests, it determines the extent or stage of the growth.

Chances for cure depend on three main factors:

- Age of the patient
- How widely the cancer has extended or spread (stage)
- How malignant the cells of the tumor appear under the microscope (tumor grade)

C Tumor cells that most closely resemble normal are Grade 1. Those that look most malignant are Grade 3. The chances of a patient being tumor-free after five years from all endometrial tumors is:

- All Grade 1: 80%
- All Grade 2: 75%
- All Grade 3: 40%

The overall chance for cure for a patient with endometrial cancer is over 70%.

Endometrial Cancer

D Occasionally, a small strictly localized cancer is found in the endometrial tissue obtained at the time of the D & C. Such a tumor is totally curable by removing the uterus (hysterectomy). Since 75% of endometrial cancers occur in women over fifty years of age, taking out the uterus is usually a reasonable form of treatment.

E When the tumor is still confined to the body of the uterus, treatment consists of removing the uterus plus radiation. Adding radiation to hysterectomy improves the likelihood of cure about 20%. Together, radiation and hysterectomy provide a 70% chance for cure. Some radiologists and gynecologists give radiation before hysterectomy and some after operation. The ovaries and surrounding structures are removed along with the uterus.

F When the cancer has extended from the body of the uterus into the cervix, it is necessary to take out the uterus along with the surrounding tissues. This is called an extended or radical hysterectomy. The chances of cure are about 45% after this operation.

G When endometrial cancer has spread into the tissues of the pelvis, it is beyond the limits where it can all be removed by operation. Radiation and hormone therapy is then used.

The normal uterine lining (endometrium) grows and decays monthly during a woman's menstrual cycle under the influence of sex hormones. A drug called progestin, similar to one of the sex hormones, limits growth of 45% of endometrial cancer. This drug is used in conjunction with radiation in treating Stage III tumors that have extended in the pelvis beyond the limits of operative removal. Twenty-five percent of patients so treated are tumor free in five years.

H When endometrial tumor has spread out of the pelvis, the chances of cure are less than 5%. In addition to radiation and hormone therapy, as described for Stage III tumors, these patients are given a course of anti-tumor drugs, such as cytoxan or adriamycin. These drugs are not curative, but they give symptomatic relief and decrease the size of the tumor in 20–30% of cases.

I About 5% of the time, endometrial cancer will reappear after treatment only in the vagina, where it can be locally excised with a 5–10% chance of cure. In most such cases, the cancer has spread widely, and the only treatment to provide relief of symptoms is radiation hormones and anti-cancer drugs. There is a 25% chance that endometrial cancer will decrease in size for several months after such treatment.

5. Ovarian Cancer

A Although each of the two ovaries is only about the size of a thumb nail, they are so active that they are the source of an inordinate number of tumors, some benign and some cancerous. Of all women who develop ovarian cancer, 80% can be cured.

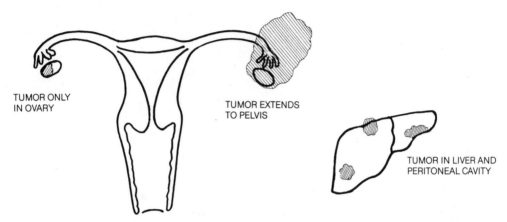

TUMOR ONLY
IN OVARY

TUMOR EXTENDS
TO PELVIS

TUMOR IN LIVER AND
PERITONEAL CAVITY

B There are many kinds of ovarian tumors, each with its unique chances for cure. Ninety percent are called epithelial tumors. More than half of these produce a thin, watery fluid and are therefore called serous tumors. Most of the remainder produce thick mucus and are called mucinous tumors.

C The basic treatment of ovarian cancer is by removal of both ovaries and the entire uterus and fallopian tubes. This operation is called total abdominal hysterectomy and bilateral salpingo-oophorectomy, a jawbreaker name that, for obvious reasons, is better known by its acronym, TAHBSO. (Details of this operation are described in "Abdominal Hysterectomy," page 320.)

D About 45% of ovarian cancers are still contained within the ovary when first discovered. Twenty-five percent of the time, a similar tumor appears in both ovaries simultaneously. When all of the tumor is confined to the ovaries, 50–70% of women can look forward to cure.

E A number of drugs shrink or slow the growth of ovarian cancer. About 70% of ovarian cancers are benefited by drug treatment for periods of one to five years. These drugs are given for five-day periods every month. At the end of a month, some gynecologists advise a "second-look operation" to see if any tumor remains in the pelvis and abdomen. If it does not, use of these powerful and potentially toxic drugs can be stopped.

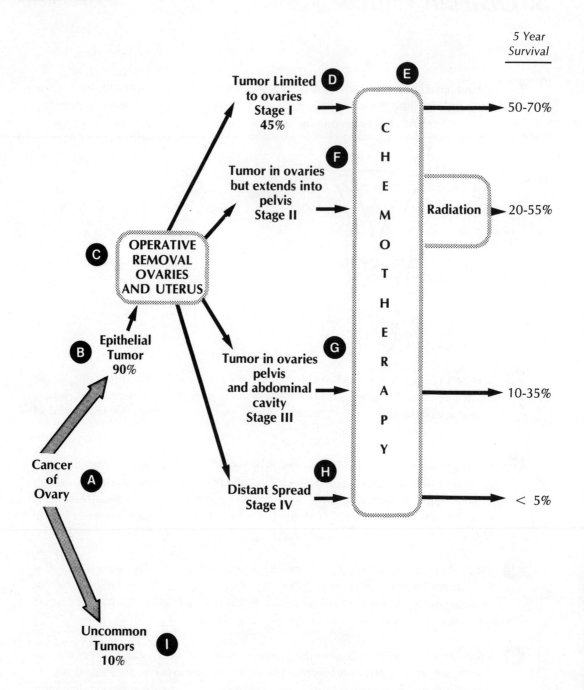

F When ovarian cancer has spread into the pelvis (Stage II), treatment consists of TAHBSO plus anti-tumor drugs given for twelve months. Many physicians also add a course of radiation to the pelvic area. The chances for cure vary from 20–55%, depending on the type of tumor cell. Mucus tumors have a better chance for cure than do the serous tumors.

G Ovarian tumors that extend outside the covering capsule of the ovary are likely to send tumor cells into the peritoneal cavity, where the cells grow and form new sites of tumor. When this happens, the chances of being able to remove all tumor are greatly decreased. With TAHBSO and chemotherapy, there is a 10–35% chance of five-year survival, even with such an advanced stage of the disease. Some physicians add X-ray treatment as well. With advanced ovarian cancer, all of the tumor cells cannot be removed by the surgeon. In contrast to most cancers, there is benefit to removing a part of ovarian cancer, even if a lot of tumor is still left behind. This is called "debulking" the tumor. The presumption is that taking out most of the tumor improves the body's ability, with the help of anti-cancer drugs, to cope with the smaller amount of tumor that remains. Without debulking, almost no patients with Stage III cancers of the ovary live two years. With debulking, this figure is increased to 50%.

H When ovarian cancer has spread throughout the body, it is incurable. Survival is measured in months. X-ray shrinks tumor size and provides relief of symptoms in about 70% of cases. Survival is usually no more than about six months, but some patients live one to two years.

I About 10% of ovarian cancers secrete some type of sex hormone. They are not epithelial tumors. Frequently, they cause change of menstrual habits. Treated with operative removal, radiation, and anti-cancer drugs, some (dysgerminoma, androblastoma, etc.) have a 90–100% chance of cure. Others are not so easily cured.

6. Ectopic Pregnancy

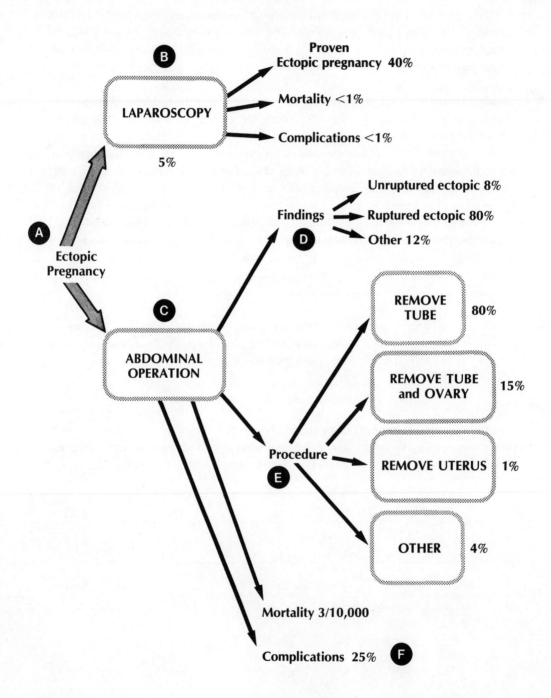

A The sperm normally has two trips through a fallopian tube. In the first, it travels upstream, like a salmon, from the body of the uterus to the egg near the ovary. The second trip takes it back down the tube, as a part of the fertilized egg, to the body of the uterus where it normally implants itself. There, like a young tree, it puts down roots and begins to grow for nine months. But occasionally, the fertilized egg gets delayed in its passage down the tube and begins to grow while still in the fallopian tube, short of its normal site of growth within the body of the uterus. This occurs once in every 200 (0.5%) pregnancies. In this abnormal location, it is known as an ectopic (abnormally placed) pregnancy.

The small diameter of the fallopian tube is not designed to support a growing embryo. Most such ectopic pregnancies simply lose their blood supply, die, and disappear. But others may bleed or break into the peritoneal cavity (ruptured ectopic pregnancy).

Factors that increase the likelihood of ectopic pregnancy include:

- Previous pelvic infection.
- Use of intrauterine contraceptive device (IUD). This is associated with a five-times-normal expectancy of ectopic pregnancy.
- Previous ectopic pregnancy, where there is a 10% likelihood of repeating the same condition.

B Many gynecologic conditions produce signs and symptoms similar to ectopic pregnancy. It is important to separate them, for they are treated differently. A unique technique is often utilized to differentiate such conditions. The gynecologist, places a lighted tube fitted with a lens system (laparascope) into the lower abdominal cavity and looks for blood coming from the ectopic site of pregnancy. Sometimes the tube is inserted through the back part of the vagina, where it is known as a culdoscope.

Laparoscopy is used to confirm the diagnosis in about 5% of ectopic pregnancies. The mortality rate and complication rate of this procedure is infinitesimal, and it can confirm an ectopic pregnancy about 40% of the time.

C Once the diagnosis of ruptured or bleeding ectopic pregnancy has been made, an abdominal operation is necessary to stop the bleeding. This requires general or spinal anesthesia and usually has to be performed as an emergency.

D A large number of variations of abnormally placed pregnancies may be found, some bleeding, some ruptured, some in the process of being absorbed. Each requires different management.

Ectopic Pregnancy

E Eighty percent of the time, the fallopian tube containing the abnormally placed pregnancy has to be removed (salpingectomy). In another 15%, the ovary on that side also has to be removed with the tube (salpingo-oophorectomy). In only about 1% of cases is it necessary to remove the entire uterus. In some cases, it is possible to remove the ruptured part of the tube and to sew the two ends back together (tuboplasty).

F Postoperative complications are usually mild but frequent:

- Wound infection: 6%
- Generalized infection: 15%
- Pelvic infection: 5%

Ectopic pregnancy, although rarely fatal (1 in 350), accounts for 10% of all maternal deaths caused by pregnancy.

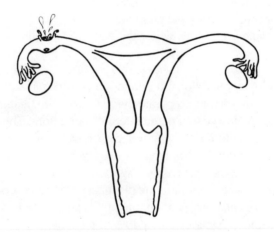

RAPTURED ECTOPIC PREGNANCY

7. Tubo-Ovarian Abscess

A Each ovary lies at the open end of an extended arm of the uterus called a fallopian tube, which serves as a pipe to carry the egg to the body of the uterus. The tube and ovary are a common site for infection and abscess formation. Four percent of all women in the United States have a tubo-ovarian infection at sometime during their life. This can result following pregnancy, from pelvic operations, as a result of abortion, or from gonorrhea. Use of an intrauterine device (IUD) for contraception increases the likelihood of a tubo-ovarian abscess.

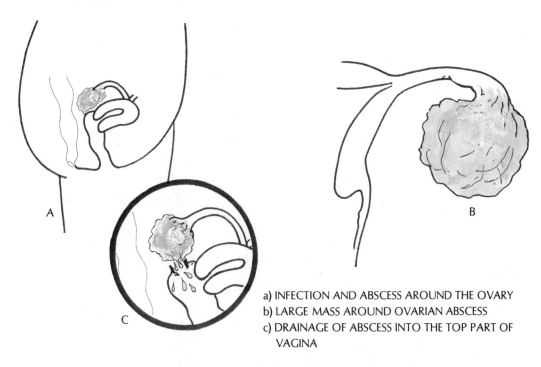

a) INFECTION AND ABSCESS AROUND THE OVARY
b) LARGE MASS AROUND OVARIAN ABSCESS
c) DRAINAGE OF ABSCESS INTO THE TOP PART OF VAGINA

B Antibiotics, if started early enough, cure about 80% of tubo-ovarian infections.

C Operative drainage is needed in the 20% that do not respond. If the infection is only on one side, such drainage can be done through the vagina (culpotomy) or through the abdomen. If the infection is on both sides, the drainage procedure is better performed through an abdominal incision. Drainage can be expected to cure about 70% of such patients.

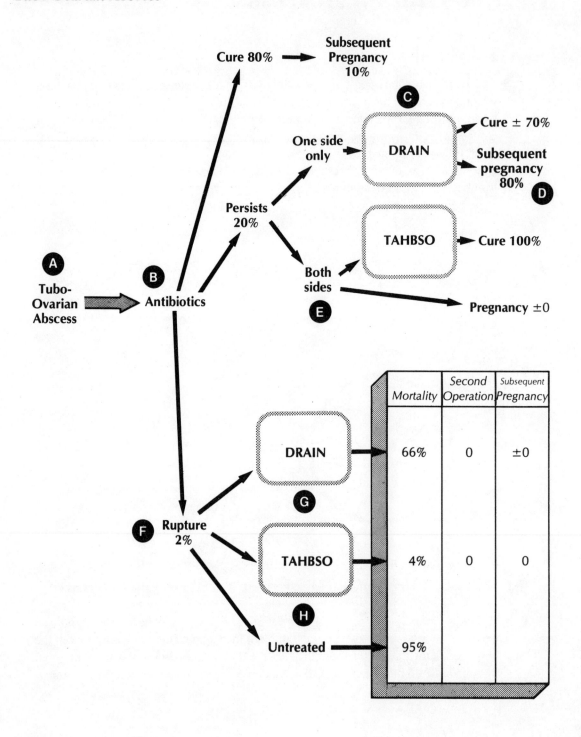

D But the abscess takes its toll by sealing the tubes so that they no longer can transport the ovum (egg) to the uterus.

If only one tube or ovary is involved in the abscess, the chances of later pregnancy is about 80%. But if both tubes are infected, the likelihood of a later pregnancy is almost nil. Much later, when all infection has been cured, it is possible to remove the sealed part of the tube and reattach the cut ends to provide a better passageway for the egg to the uterine body. The likelihood of a future successful pregnancy after such a procedure is about 20%.

E When the abscess and infection persist, patients usually develop a painful mass in the pelvis and have very painful menstrual periods. Ultimately, removal of their pelvic organs is required for cure. This operation is called total abdominal hysterectomy and bilateral salpingo-oophorectomy (TAHBSO). The tubes, ovaries, and the entire uterus are removed (see "Abdominal Hysterectomy," page 320).

F About 2% of patients with tubo-ovarian abscess will, despite treatment, break open (perforate) the abscess into the abdominal cavity, causing generalized peritonitis. This is a life-threatening emergency. Without operation, 95% will die.

G Emergency operation is obviously necessary. Simply draining the abscess would seem to be the most logical procedure, but it isn't, for these reasons:

- The chance of death is 66%.
- For those who survive, 30% will need a second operation because of complications of the infection.
- The chance of the uterus ever serving its function again is low. Only 10% ever can become pregnant, because the tubes have been sealed shut by the infection.

H Thus, in a ruptured tubo-ovarian abscess, most gynecologists remove the infected tubes, the ovaries and the uterus, which has the following ramifications:

- Operative mortality is about 4%, which is about two-thirds that of drainage alone.
- Since the infected tube and ovaries are gone, there is little threat of a second operation, whereas after simple drainage the likelihood is 30%.
- Removing the infection-destroyed uterus, tubes, and ovaries takes from the patient nothing that is of value to her. These organs no longer can function.
- Following removal of the ovaries, female sex hormones pills can be taken by mouth to substitute for the removed ovaries.

8. Sterilization

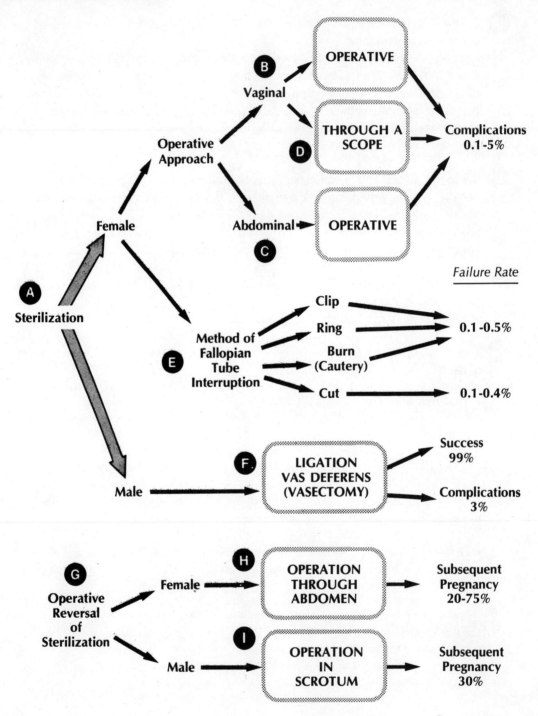

A Sterilization is the process of making either a woman or man incapable of reproduction or inducing pregnancy. There are obviously many ways this can be done. Operative sterilization of the female usually involves interrupting both fallopian tubes, thus preventing the sperm from reaching the ovary. Sterilization of a man usually involves preventing the sperm from leaving the male partner. Sterilization is 99% effective (far more so than contraception) in preventing pregnancy but, of course, is relatively irreversible.

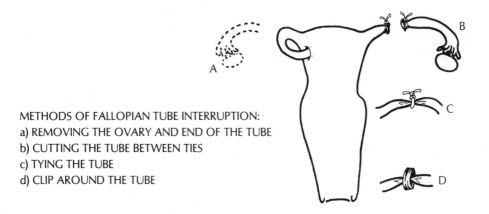

METHODS OF FALLOPIAN TUBE INTERRUPTION:
a) REMOVING THE OVARY AND END OF THE TUBE
b) CUTTING THE TUBE BETWEEN TIES
c) TYING THE TUBE
d) CLIP AROUND THE TUBE

B One approach to the fallopian tubes is through an incision in the back of the vagina (culpotomy). This usually requires one day of hospitalization. Mortality of the procedure approaches zero. The chances of complication are:

- Bowel perforation: 0.3%
- Infection requiring reoperation: 1%
- Bleeding: 2%

C The other approach to the tubes is through an abdominal incision (laparotomy). Because sterilization is often performed through a small incision, this is often called a mini-laparotomy. Hospitalization is one to two days. The possibilities of complication, though slight, include those of any laparotomy.

D Several of the simpler procedures for cutting the fallopian tubes can be performed through a small-caliber, lighted tube (endoscope), the diameter of the index finger. The tube can be inserted either through a small incision in the vagina (culdoscopy) or through a small abdominal incision (laparoscopy).

The likelihood of complications with endoscopic sterilization include bowel perforation in 1 out of 3,600 cases and heart irregularities in 5% of the cases.

Sterilization

E The fallopian tubes can be interrupted in a variety of ways, including various types of clips, bands, rings, or cutting and burning devices. Some can be applied through an endoscope, others require a larger incision. Each technique prevents pregnancy in well over 99% of patients.

F Sterilization of the male involves interrupting the tiny tube (vas deferens) that carries sperm from the testicles to the base of the penis. Vas ligation can be done under local anesthesia as an office or outpatient procedure, with minimal discomfort. Minor complications such as bleeding or infection occur in about 2% of cases. Success with this simple procedure is over 99%. Vas ligation in no way affects sex function, erotic drive, or "manliness."

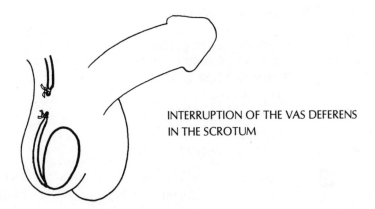

INTERRUPTION OF THE VAS DEFERENS
IN THE SCROTUM

G People should not seek sterilization if they anticipate wanting more children. Sometimes, however, a sterilized man or woman wishes to reverse the sterilization. Success is possible but not too probable.

H In women, reversal of sterilization depends on reattaching the tied, cut, burned, or buried ends of the fallopian tubes back together. This requires hospitalization for five to ten days, general anesthesia, and a long, meticulous operation. Success, judged by a subsequent pregnancy, varies between 20–75%, depending on the technique used for original sterilization and the possibility for revision and repair of the tubes.

I Reversing sterilization of the male requires finding the two ends of the cut vas deferens and joining them together so that this tiny tube will allow passage of the sperm. Chance of success is about 30%.

9. Abortion

A Abortion is the term used to describe the termination or interruption of pregnancy before the full, nine-month term is completed, resulting in a dead fetus.

B About 20% of all pregnancies spontaneously abort; that is, without any meaningful interference, the fetus never comes to term. Most occur within the first few weeks of fertilization of the egg, and the woman usually is not even aware that she was ever pregnant or thus lost her pregnancy (aborted). Other may occur at any time up to full term. The likelihood of miscarriage or abortion of all pregnancies is:

- First three months of pregnancy: 20%
- Second three months of pregnancy: 5%
- Third three months of pregnancy: premature delivery

C Induced abortions are those brought on voluntarily, by the physician's meaningful actions, to end an unwanted or dangerous pregnancy. Because the risks of induced abortion are so small during the first three months of pregnancy, all efforts are made to do it during this time. About 80% of induced abortions are performed during the first twelve weeks of pregnancy.

D Suction curettage (dilatation and evacuation) is the technique used for over 95% of abortions induced during the first twelve weeks of pregnancy. Under general or local anesthesia, a suction device is applied through the vagina to the opening of the uterus (cervix). The contents of the uterus, including the fertilized ovum, are sucked out with almost no damage to the uterus itself. Hospitalization is usually for only a few hours.

E After sixteen weeks of pregnancy, other techniques are used to induce abortion. Classic "sharp" curettage (as described in "Dilation and Curettage," page 314) is used to scrape out the contents of the uterus. Another technique involves instillation into the uterus of solutions that will cause the uterus to contract and empty itself.

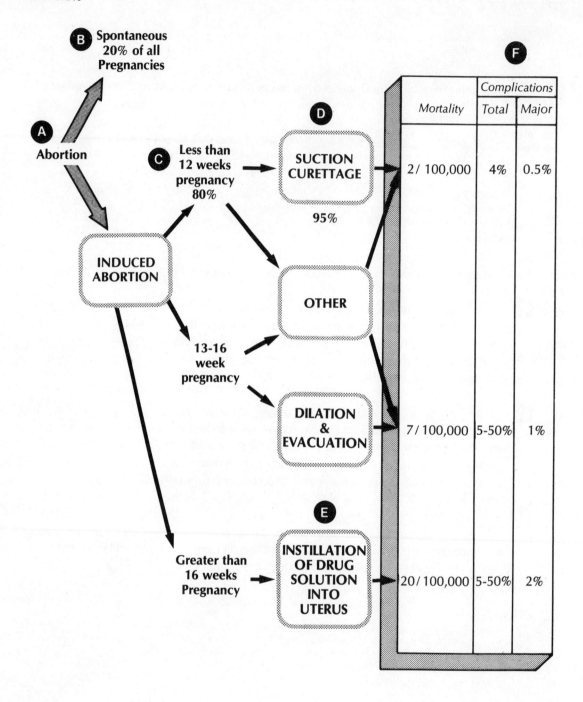

F The most common complications of dilatation and curettage for abortion are:

- Perforation: 0.5% (This may cause so little trouble that it goes unrecognized. The big advantage of dilation and evacuation (D&E) over curettage (D&C) is eliminating the threat of perforation.)
- Small tear (laceration) of the cervix: 0.5%
- Bleeding: 0.5%
- Infection: 1% (Occasionally requires a repeat operative curettage.)

After three months of pregnancy, dilation and curettage is the most common method of evacuating the uterus. It has a three-times-higher risk of complication than when performed before the third month of pregnancy, but the types of complications are about the same.

10. Dilation and Curettage (D&C)

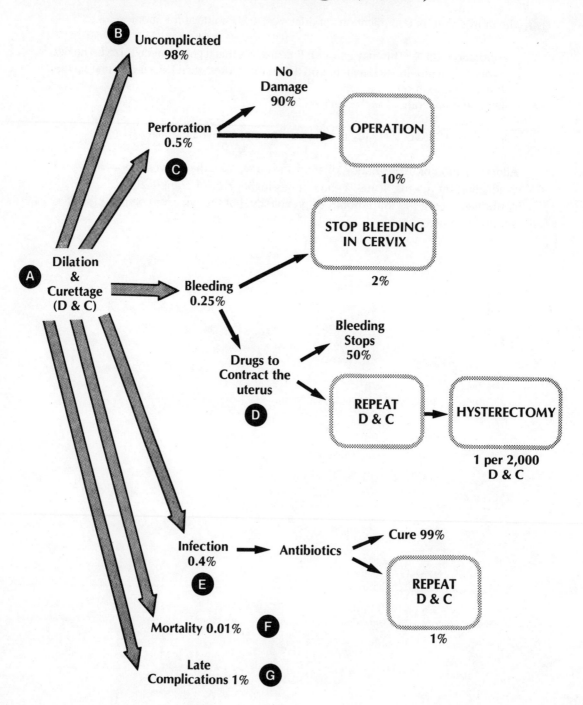

314

A Dilation and curettage of the uterus is the commonest operation performed on women. It consists of widening (dilating) the neck (cervix) of the uterus as it opens into the top part of the vagina and then removing the lining and contents of the uterine cavity. Because emptying the uterus is done with curettes, which scrape the side walls of the uterus, this part of the procedure is known as curettage. Hence, this procedure bears the well-known acronym D&C.

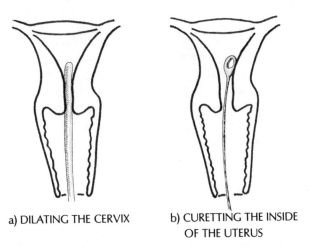

a) DILATING THE CERVIX

b) CURETTING THE INSIDE OF THE UTERUS

The procedure is performed for a variety of reasons, such as to detect cancer, to stop bleeding from the uterus, to empty the uterus, for infection, or to obtain a specimen (biopsy) of the endometrium for study under the microscope. The patient is usually hospitalized for only the day of the operation. Anesthesia is either spinal or general.

B D&C is a relatively benign procedure, 98–99% being uncomplicated. Occasionally, the sharp curettes make a small hole in the uterus wall. The overall likelihood of this is **C** about 0.5%. The exact incidence is unknown, because usually it does no damage, and both the gynecologic surgeon and the patient are unaware it happened. Expected perforation is:

- Overall: 0.5%
- Soon after delivery: 0.8%
- In the elderly woman with a small uterus: 2%
- In the presence of tumor or infection: 2%

Operation is necessary in less than 1% of women in whom there was uterine perforation from D&C.

In the rare instance where operation is necessary, the uterus must be removed in 15% of the cases. There is even a remote chance of death in neglected cases.

Dilation and Curettage (D&C)

D There is always some bleeding from the vagina following D&C. In over 99% of cases this will stop within twenty-four hours. In about 0.2% of patients, it is necessary to return the patient to the operating room and place a stitch in the cervix to stop the bleeding. In the rare instance where bleeding comes from the body of the uterus, drugs that contract the uterus and pinch off the bleeding vessels will stop bleeding in one-half of the cases. When this fails and a repeat D&C does not stop bleeding, it may be necessary (once in every 2,000 cases of D&C) to remove the uterus.

E In the hands of untrained illegal abortionists, infection used to be common. At the present time, however, with abortion made legal and usually performed in a hospital or in an office by trained gynecologic surgeons, the chances of serious infection following D&C is only about 0.3% for suction D&C and slightly higher for formal D&C performed with sharp curettes.

In about 1% of cases of infection following D&C, a repeat D&C will be necessary to be certain the uterus is entirely emptied of its contents and well drained. This usually stops the infection.

F Death following D&C is so uncommon that there are several reports of many thousands of cases without any mortality.

G Rarely are there any late complications following D&C, but occasionally painful menstrual periods or a tendency to miscarry have been blamed on a previous D&C. Most are, in fact, due to the disease for which the D&C was performed in the first place and not to the operation.

11. Vaginal Hysterectomy

A The uterus can be removed either through the abdominal cavity (abdominal hysterectomy) or through the vagina (vaginal hysterectomy). The choice of approach depends on many factors, including the reason for performing the procedure, the size of the uterus, etc.

B When the choice is made to perform vaginal hysterectomy, the woman can anticipate an 85% chance of a totally uncomplicated course following operation. Hospitalization is usually about four to six days.

Either general or spinal anesthesia is used, and the entire incision is made within the vagina so that there is no scar on the abdomen or external evidence of the operation, nor is the vagina disfigured.

Death due to operation is extremely rare, about 0.1%, but as with any operation, there are possible complications, such as wound infection, or bleeding from the operative area. These occur only 2% of the time.

C Both the bladder and the two ureters, which drain urine from the kidneys to the bladder, lie alongside the uterus and are in the operative field during vaginal hysterectomy. There is always a possibility that a small hole can be made in the bladder (about 2%) or that one of the ureters can be damaged during the operation (about 1%). Either of these possible complications will require reoperation.

In about one in every 200 patients, the operation that starts out as a vaginal hysterectomy must, for various technical reasons, be converted to an abdominal operation and a second incision made on the lower abdomen (see "Abdominal Hysterectomy," page 320).

D In about 4% of cases, some sort of second operation through the vagina is required either to control persistent bleeding or to drain a local infection. This may prolong hospital stay a few days, but does not usually interfere with an ultimately good result.

E Removing the uterus cuts some of the nerves to the nearby urinary bladder and removes some of its support, thus temporarily interfering with proper passage of urine. This, in turn, often causes a minor infection in the bladder. In about 10% of patients, there is some degree of urinary tract infection after vaginal hysterectomy, but in most cases, this is adequately managed by antibiotic and other drug therapy. After some weeks, the bladder regains its tone. Drugs can then be discontinued and the infection is cured.

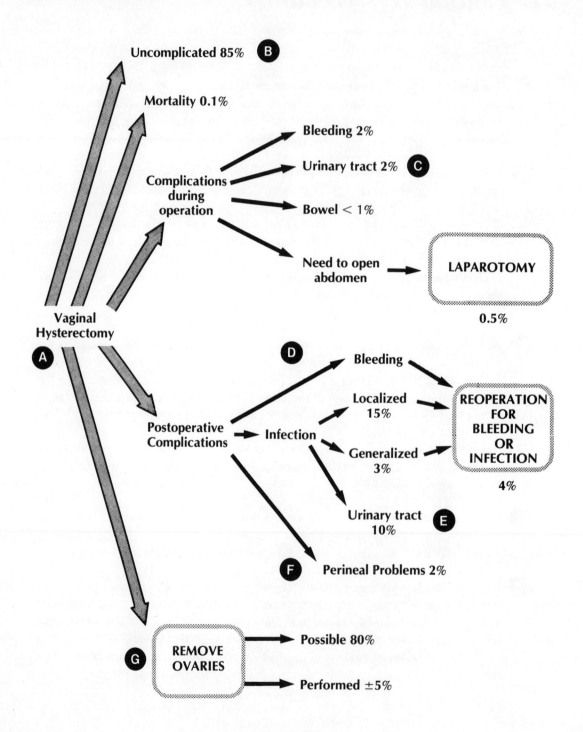

F In about 2% of cases after operation, there will be weakness in the area of the operation, allowing the bladder (cystocele) or rectum (rectocele) to slip down as a hernia under the skin. Occasionally, such perineal hernias have to be repaired by operation.

G It is technically possible to remove the ovaries along with the uterus at the time of vaginal hysterectomy. This is actually performed in about 5% of cases (see "Tubo-Ovarian Abscess," page 305).

12. Abdominal Hysterectomy

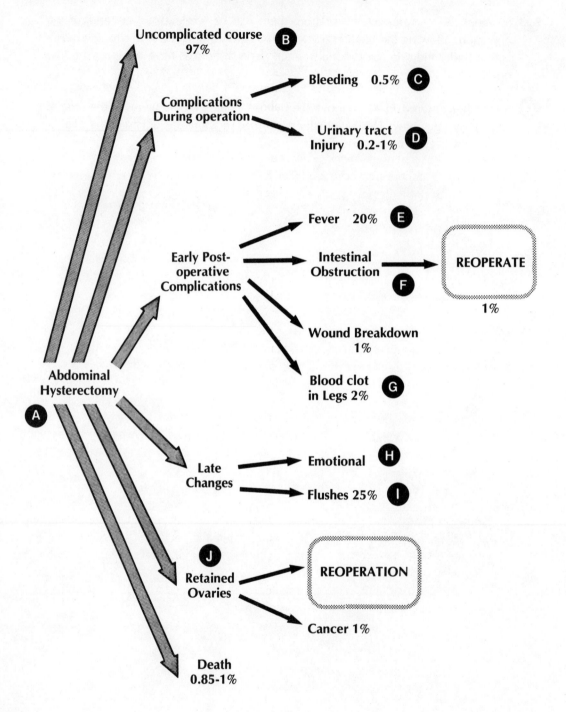

Uncomplicated course 97% **B**

Complications During operation

Bleeding 0.5% **C**

Urinary tract Injury 0.2-1% **D**

Early Post-operative Complications

Fever 20% **E**

Intestinal Obstruction **F**

REOPERATE 1%

Wound Breakdown 1%

Blood clot in Legs 2% **G**

Abdominal Hysterectomy **A**

Late Changes

Emotional **H**

Flushes 25% **I**

J Retained Ovaries

REOPERATION

Cancer 1%

Death 0.85-1%

A After childbearing is over, the uterus serves no useful purpose. If any significant disease thereafter involves the uterus, it might just as well be removed, if the small risk of hysterectomy outweighs the risk of the disease. Decision to perform hysterectomy, therefore, requires understanding the risks of the disease and the risk of the operation. Hysterectomy can be performed either through the vagina (vaginal hysterectomy) or through an incision that goes through the abdominal cavity (abdominal hysterectomy). Which technique is advisable in a given case depends on many factors.

B Normally, the patient is in the hospital for one to two days before and five to seven days following an uncomplicated abdominal hysterectomy. For one to three days after operation, the patient is given nothing to eat or drink by mouth and is fed intravenously until the intestines begin to function properly. About 97% of cases have an uncomplicated hospital course.

C After abdominal hysterectomy, about 1% of patients have significant postoperative bleeding, and in an occasional case, a second operation—usually made through the original incision — is needed to stop the bleeding.

D The ureters (the tubes carrying urine from the kidneys to the bladder) lie alongside the uterus, and in about 1% of cases, one or (rarely) both of the ureters are damaged during the hysterectomy. Many injuries to only one ureter go unrecognized, since a person gets along quite well with only one kidney.

E Postoperative fever is usually due to infection in the urinary tract or in the lungs after hysterectomy. A low-grade fever for one to four days is very common and usually of little significance; it gradually subsides. As with any operation, there is always a chance of infection in the wound or in the operative site.

F Following any major abdominal operation, the intestines are paralyzed for a few days. After abdominal hysterectomy, about 1–2% of patients will have intestinal obstruction, due to adhesive bands around the site where the uterus was removed. This is particularly likely to happen if there was infection, tumor, or bleeding around the uterus.

The need for treatment with a tube in the stomach or the chances for reoperation are as described in "Abdominal Operation," page 252.

G There is wide variation (0.6%–3%) in the reported probability of developing blood clots in the leg (thrombophlebitis) after hysterectomy. The discrepancy is due mainly to the criteria for making the diagnosis. Clots in the legs can be detected in almost every woman after a pelvic operation, but in only about 2% of patients is there any evidence to the patient that this exists. The significance of thrombophlebitis and the possibility of developing a pulmonary embolus is discussed in "Postoperative Thrombophlebitis," page 150.

H Even though the uterus is of no functional value to a woman after she has finished bearing children, it stands as a symbol of womanliness. It is no wonder that, following hysterectomy, many women experience some emotional tensions. To complicate the matter, many candidates for hysterectomy are in the midst of their menopause, with all the unpleasant adjustments that this inevitably entails. When functioning ovaries are removed at the same time as the uterus, surgical menopause is induced. Other factors that increase emotional problems following hysterectomy include previous emotional instability or misunderstanding of what the operation entails. Emotional complications following hysterectomy — or for that matter any operation — are just as real as is a wound infection!

I Sudden episodes of uncomfortable hot flashes are common in menopause and may also occur following hysterectomy, if the ovaries are removed.

J The ovaries lie close to the uterus and can be removed at the time of hysterectomy without additional operative risk. If the woman has completed her childbearing, the ovaries are of little benefit. Arguments in favor of routine oophorectomy at the time of hysterectomy in women who have completed childbearing are that there is a 0.2% chance of cancer developing in the remaining ovary and a 5% likelihood of requiring an operation on the ovaries for some other reason. Many gynecologists and surgeons conclude that the ovaries should be removed in post-menopausal women at the time of abdominal hysterectomy, because more is gained in avoiding future ovarian disease than is lost by removal. There is, however, controversy as to removing the ovaries in pre-menopausal women. Some women and gynecologists are not so cavalier about the loss of gonads (ovaries), even if their function can be adequately replaced with a pill.

XII
Children

1. Birth Defect

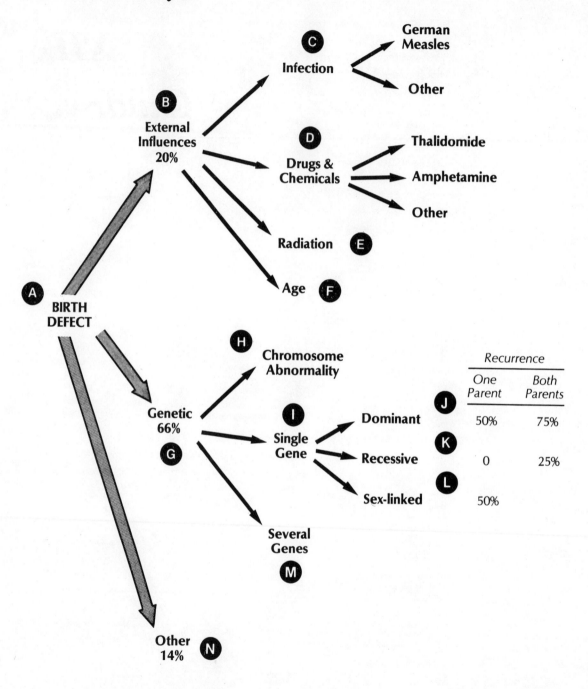

A Parents of a child born with a birth defect want to know what the chances are that a similar defect may occur if they have other children. Accurate prediction requires examination of the child, the parents, and review of similar defects among relatives and ancestors. Sometimes it is necessary to study the chromosomes in the white blood cells of the child and the parents. Genetic counselors specialize in defining these risks.

B Approximately 3% of all live newborn infants have some birth defect. About 20% are due to some infection or toxic influence on the mother, usually during the first three months of her pregnancy.

C If the mother has German measles (rubella) during the first month of pregnancy, there is a 50% chance that the child will have a birth defect; if during the second month, 22%; and during the third month, 7%. About one-third of these children will have cataracts of the eye, and an equal number, hearing loss. Other infections of the mother known to cause defects include syphilis (if untreated), toxoplasmosis, cytomegalovirus, and herpes. Mumps in the mother is suspected, but not proven, to increase the likelihood of a defect.

D Certain drugs taken during pregnancy increase the likelihood of birth defects. The most notorious is thalidomide, primary cause of limb deformities in about 1% of cases. The evidence is questionable concerning the effect of amphetamine ("speed"). Mothers who drink over 50 grams of alcohol (three to four mixed drinks or whiskey) per day have about a 50% chance of having a child with brain damage. There is a possible increased incidence of birth defects in women taking drugs for control of epilepsy or convulsions. There is no evidence, despite all that has been written, that LSD, marijuana, heroin, or cigarettes increase the likelihood of birth defects in an unborn child. Cigarette smoking by the mother decreases the child's birth weight but does not increase the chance of a birth defect.

E X-radiation of a pregnant fruit fly certainly produces some very odd baby fruit flies, but there is no hard evidence that it increases the likelihood of birth defects in humans. It increases the remote chance of infant mortality by about seven times, as well as the risk of leukemia, but there is no proof it increases the risk of human birth defects.

F The older the mother, the more apt she is to bear a child with a birth defect. For example, the likelihood of Down's Syndrome (a serious defect involving mental retardation) is 0.1% in children of mothers of all ages. However, if the mother is thirty-seven years of age, the probability is 1%, an increase of tenfold. If the mother is forty-five years of age, the chance is about 6%. A woman releases her best eggs from the ovary when she is young.

G Genes are the unit of genetic function that determine our inherited characteristics. They are strung along the length of twenty-three different sets of chromosomes in each cell, which under the microscope look like oddly bent pairs of matchsticks.

In about 66% of newborns with birth defects, there is an identifiable abnormality with one or more of the genes. When a genetic abnormality is identified, it increases the accuracy of predicting whether the defect will be repeated in another child. But even then, it may be difficult to predict categorically the probability of recurrence. Each child and his parents must be considered individually. Likelihood of repetition of cleft lip and palate, for example, averages about 4%, but depending upon the specific genetic abnormality involved, the chance of repetition may vary from less than 1% to 50%.

H In about 0.4% of live births and in 13% of children with birth defects, an abnormality can be seen by examining one or more of the chromosomes within the white blood cells. Some of the conditions produced by this abnormality are known by the man's name who first described the condition, such as Down's syndrome or Turner's syndrome. Others go under more confusing titles such as Triple-X or 47XXY. Such strange names describe, in the shorthand of the geneticist, which chromosome is abnormal and in what way. More than half of newborns with chromosome abnormalities have some degree of mental retardation. Precise definition of the chromosome defect is necessary for accurate prediction of the likelihood of repetition in another child.

I In about 1.9% of live births and 36% of children born with a birth defect, a single gene is at fault.

J There are several hundred types of birth defects known to be transmitted by a dominant single gene defect in one of the parents. There is a 50% chance that the child will have the disorder if one parent only has the defective gene and a 75% chance if both do. An example is certain types of dwarfism.

K Recessive single gene defects are only transmitted to the child if *both* parents are carriers. If both parents have the trait, there is a 25% probability the child will have the disorder. There are about 800 such recognized disorders, such as sickle cell anemia and phenylketonuria (PKU).

L About 150 disorders, such as hemophilia and certain types of muscular dystrophy, are carried on the X or sex chromosome. If the mother has this trait, she has a 50% chance of passing it on to a son but not a daughter.

M Several genes are at fault (polygenetic) in about 17% of infants with birth defects. Environmental factors may influence the likelihood that polygenetic disorders actually produce a defect in a child at risk. Some polygenetic disorders include cleft lip and palate (a 0.1% chance when polygenetic), club foot (a 0.02% chance), diabetes, hydrocephalus, and urinary tract malformations.

N Over a thousand types of birth defects are now recognized. In about 14%, the cause is still unclear. The overall likelihood of repetition in a representative group of conditions is as follows:

LIKELIHOOD OF A SUBSEQUENT CHILD HAVING A SIMILAR BIRTH DEFECT IF PARENTS ARE UNAFFECTED

Atrial Septal Defect		3.2%
Biliary Atresia		??—very rare repetition
Cleft Lip and Palate (overall average)		2.24%
Coarctation of Aorta		1.8–2.4%
Cystic Fibrosis		25%
Cystinuria		25%
Down's Syndrome	1% repetition for	96% of cases
	5–20% repetition for	4% of cases
Hirschsprung's Disease		6%
Hypospadius and Extrophy Bladder		±12%
Imperforate Anus, when autosomal recessive		25%
Patent Ductus Arteriosus		3.4%
Pectus Excavatum, if parent affected and autosomal dominant		50%
Port Wine Stain, if parent affected		50%
if parent unaffected		not increased from random
Phenylketonuria		25%
Polydactyly (extra finger or toe) dominant		50%
Tetralogy of Fallot		2.7–3.2%
Thalassemia		25%
Tracheo-Esophageal Fistula		not increased from random
Ventricular Septal Defect		4.4–5.0%

---

2. *Tracheo-Esophageal Fistula*

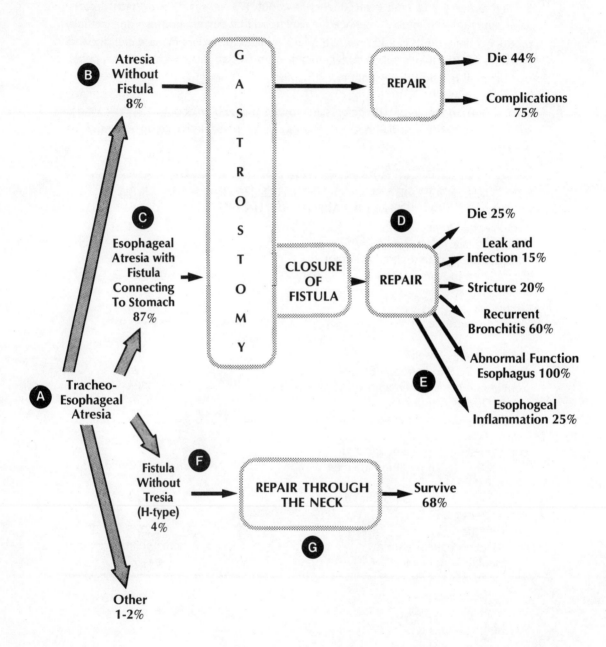

A Tracheo-Esophageal Atresia

B Atresia Without Fistula 8%

C Esophageal Atresia with Fistula Connecting To Stomach 87%

F Fistula Without Tresia (H-type) 4%

Other 1-2%

G A S T R O S T O M Y

CLOSURE OF FISTULA

REPAIR → Die 44%
→ Complications 75%

D REPAIR
→ Die 25%
→ Leak and Infection 15%
→ Stricture 20%
→ Recurrent Bronchitis 60%
→ Abnormal Function Esophagus 100%
→ Esophogeal Inflammation 25%

E

F REPAIR THROUGH THE NECK → Survive 68%

G

A The tube that carries food from the mouth to the stomach (esophagus) is totally separated in the chest from the trachea, which carries air to and from the lungs. Occasionally, a child is born with a connection (fistula) between these two tubes. The results on the infant can be appreciated by anyone who by mistake has inhaled (aspirated) water or irritating stomach contents after vomiting. There is a great deal of coughing and irritation of the lungs. This is what happens in these newborn infants, most of whom, to make matters worse, are premature, underweight, and have other inherited abnormalities. There are several anatomic variations of how the esophagus is abnormal.

ONE TYPE OF DEFECT: A BLIND END OF ESOPHAGUS WITHOUT CONNECTION TO THE LUNGS.

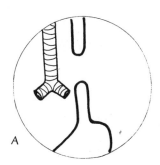

B In 8% of cases, the upper esophagus ends in a blind pouch in the upper part of the chest. There is no connection of the airway to the stomach. Treatment of these infants begins by placing a tube in the stomach in an operation (gastrostomy) performed on the abdomen. The infant is fed by this means for one to twelve months until he gains weight. In the second operation, the two blind ends of the esophagus are connected together, allowing the infant to swallow food into the stomach. There is a 65% chance that the neonates will survive these two operations. Full term, nine-month infants have a much better chance than those premature—some of whom only weigh 1–2 kilograms when born.

C By far the most common type of defect (87%) involves a similar blind end of esophagus high in the chest but a connection (fistula) between the lower end of the esophagus and the trachea and airway. Stomach juice can back up through this fistula to the lungs. Treatment of this type of defect first involves placing, for feeding, a gastrostomy tube through the abdominal wall into the stomach. The fistula tract carrying stomach contents to the lungs is then closed, thus protecting the lungs from further insult. Later, the two ends of the esophagus are connected within the chest, and the child can swallow normally.

Tracheo-Esophageal Fistula

D The exact type and timing of surgical repair depends on the size and general condition of the baby and the presence of other associated inherited problems. Only in relatively healthy, full-term infants can all the defects be repaired within a week after birth.

E Complications are many following *any* repair of a tracheo-esophageal fistula. If there is a leak at the site where the two ends of the esophagus are joined together, a dangerous infection in the chest cavity occurs. It is fatal in about 35% of cases in these infants. In about 20% of these children, narrowing (stricture) occurs at the point where the ends of the esophagus are sewn together. This can, in 75% of cases, be successfully managed by passing a dilator through the mouth to and then beyond the narrowed point. In the other 25% of patients with a stricture, another operation is required to open the narrowed point in the esophagus when the child is older.

F Although many of these children do well, none ever has a totally normal swallowing mechanism in the esophagus, even though the operations were well performed. About 5% of such children will have so much discomfort from the esophagitis that they will require an operation to prevent stomach contents from going into the esophagus just as do adults with reflux esophagitis (see "Esophagitis," page 84).

G Rarely (9% of the time), a small fistula tract connects an intact esophagus to an intact airway. The fistula forms the cross bar of an H, connecting the two parallel tubes within the chest. This odd fistula can be closed with almost uniform success by an operation performed through an incision in the neck.

THE COMMON TYPE
OF DEFECT WITH A BLIND
END OF UPPER ESOPHAGUS
AND A FISTULA CONNECTING
THE TRACHEA AND LUNGS
TO THE LOWER ESOPHAGUS
AND STOMACH.

TRACHEA

ESOPHAGUS

3. *Upper-Intestinal Obstruction*

A There are many reasons why newborn infants vomit. But if vomiting persists and the more common causes such as infection or brain injury are excluded, then a mechanical obstruction to the outlet of the stomach or duodenum must be suspected.

B Very rarely, the end of the stomach or adjacent duodenum is blocked by a thin diaphragm. Another rare cause is a curious saclike opening, resembling a double stomach, which blocks food passage. These very rare lesions can be removed or repaired with an expected risk of about 5%, depending mainly on the condition of the infant before operation.

C Of far greater frequency is a thickening of the muscle at the outlet of the stomach (pylorus), which after one to four weeks of life, blocks exit of food and water. This is called hypertrophic pyloric stenosis. Associated other serious congenital anomalies are relatively rare (2%). After operation, the babies are perfectly normal. Fortunately, this is the commonest cause of obstruction.

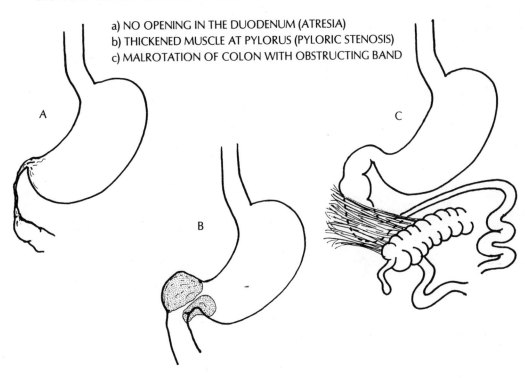

a) NO OPENING IN THE DUODENUM (ATRESIA)
b) THICKENED MUSCLE AT PYLORUS (PYLORIC STENOSIS)
c) MALROTATION OF COLON WITH OBSTRUCTING BAND

A

C

B

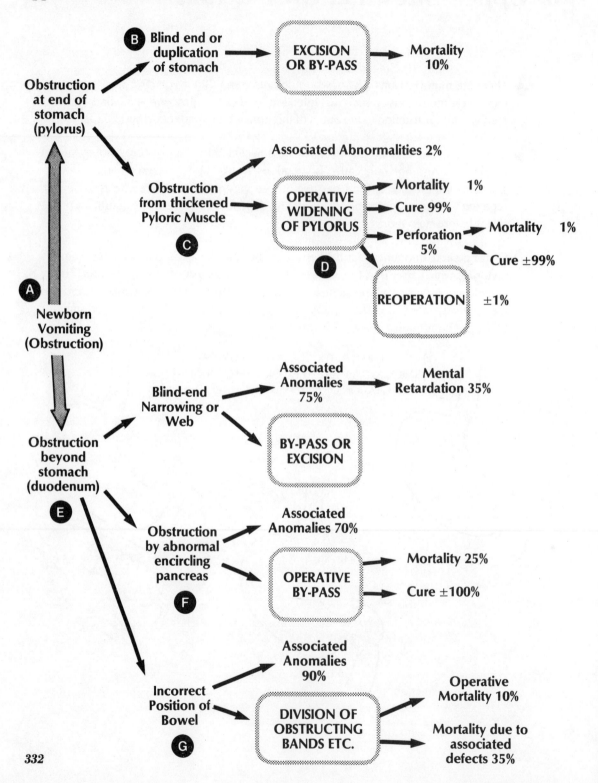

D Operative repair of hypertrophic pyloric obstruction involves splitting the thickened muscle that surrounds and obstructs the pylorus, thus permitting food to pass out of the stomach in a normal manner. This relatively simple and safe operation will almost immediately restore the infants to normal. Operative mortality approaches zero. In less than 1% of the cases, reoperation is necessary to cut the muscle a little more widely. In another 5%, the operation leaves a small hole in the lining of the stomach that underlies the muscle. If such a perforation is recognized at the time of operation, no subsequent trouble results, except that hospitalization may be prolonged one to two days.

E The duodenum is that part of the intestinal tract that lies immediately beyond the stomach. Congenital abnormalities of the duodenum can produce a narrowing (stenosis), a thin obstructing diaphragm or web, or even a totally blind segment of this part of the gut (duodenal atresia). Each of these abnormalities obstructs the passage of food out of the stomach and causes vomiting immediately after birth. In each, there is a very high (45–75%) likelihood of a serious coexisting deformity of some kind. Thirty-five percent of these infants are mongoloids, a serious mental and general handicap, which limits the capacity of such a child to live a full or socially productive life.

F Occasionally, a misshaped pancreas is wrapped all the way around the duodenum and, like a tightened fist, blocks passage of food. Infants with such an annular pancreas have a 70% probability of associated serious congenital anomalies. Seventy percent of the time, the annular pancreas produces only partial duodenal obstruction, which may not become evident in the immediate newborn period.

The safest operation for both annular pancreas and duodenal atresia is to connect the stomach to the small intestine, thus bypassing or short-circuiting food around the block of the duodenum. This permits the infant to eat normally. Even this bypassing operation for annular pancreas has an operative mortality of 25%, because of coexisting, crippling, inherited defects.

G The normal colon lies firmly attached to the back part of the abdominal cavity, well clear of the stomach and duodenum. In about one infant in 500, the bowel lies in an abnormal site because its normal attachments are lacking. Usually, this causes no difficulty, but occasionally a band from the misplaced colon falls across the duodenum and obstructs passage of food. About half (55%)of such infants start vomiting within the first week of life. The other 45% have trouble later on.

Although operative cure of duodenal obstruction due to such malrotation of the colon is relatively simple. The overall hospital mortality is about 35%, because of other associated inherited abnormalities frequently encountered.

Upper-Intestinal Obstruction

The frequency of coexisting congenital abnormalities in newborn infants with duodenal obstruction raises a difficult clinical, moral, and economic problem for the parents and the physician. Decision must be made whether to take extraordinary measures to operate and keep such neonates alive for what at best may be a miserably dependent and very expensive future existence. The dilemma is not unique among infants with duodenal obstruction, but is particularly poignant where coexisting inherited abnormalities of many other parts of the body are so great. Because some of the defects have a predictably high likelihood of occurring in future pregnancies, the parents of these children should consult a genetic counselor. If the genetic counselor quotes a very high likelihood of another child being similarly afflicted, the parents may want to consider sterilization and adoption rather than running the known high risk of producing another child with similar handicaps.

4. Imperforate Anus

A An occasional child is born without an opening at the anus, where the rectum normally opens to the skin between the buttocks. The lower end of the colon may either end in a blind pouch or connect, by a small abnormal tunnel or sinus tract, to the vagina or into the urinary tract.

ANATOMY OF THE DEFECTS:

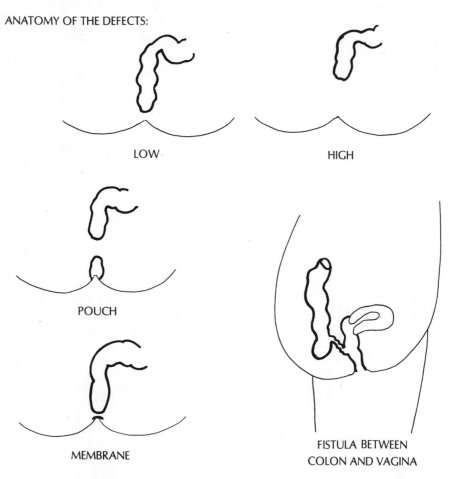

LOW

HIGH

POUCH

MEMBRANE

FISTULA BETWEEN
COLON AND VAGINA

There are several types of imperforate anus, each treated by slightly different means and each with its own probability of yielding a good result. As with most inherited defects, newborns with imperforate anus are apt to have other anatomic abnormalities. One in three such infants has an abnormality in the urinary tract; 25%, a defect in the spine; and 10%, a heart defect.

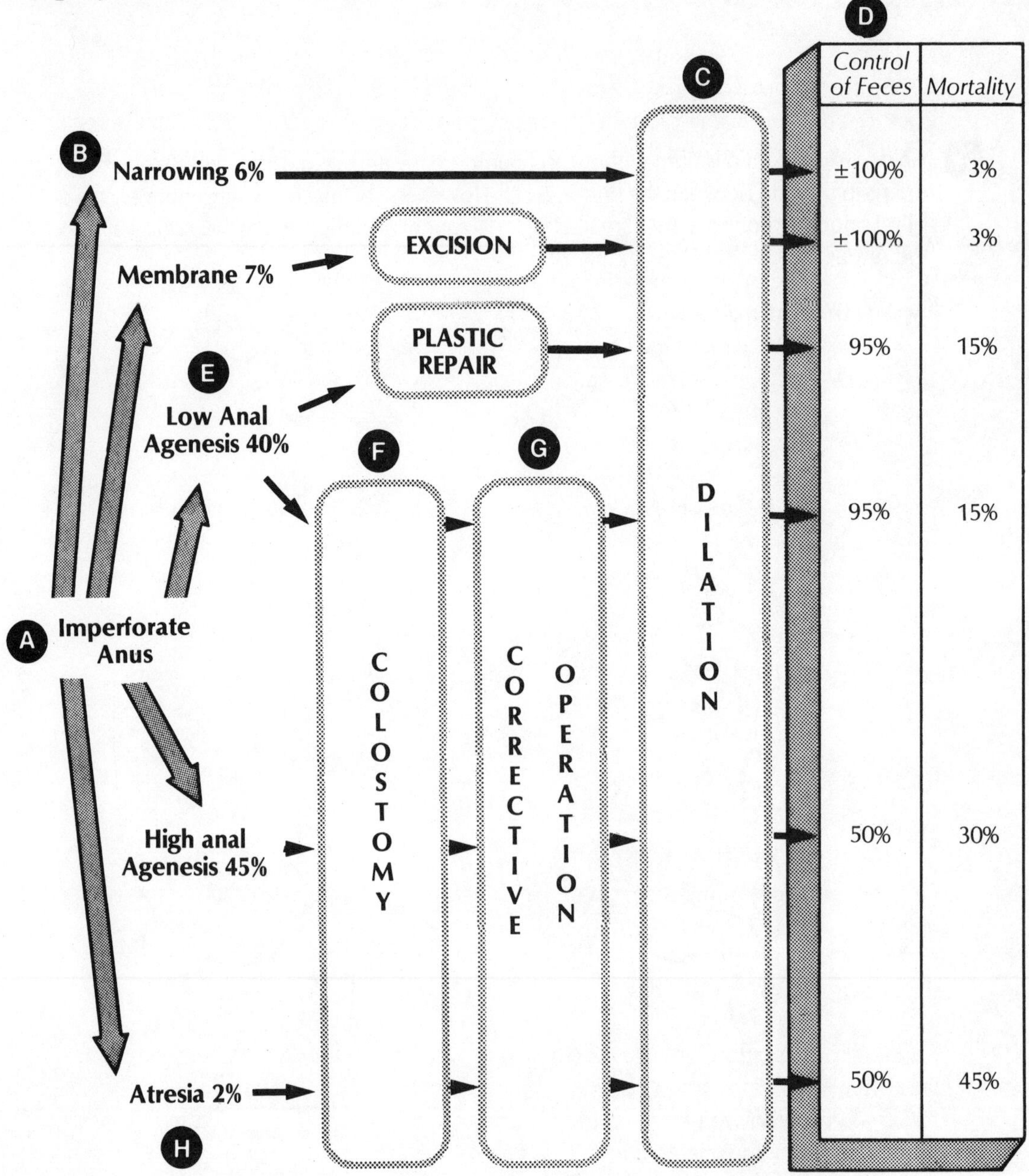

D | Control of Feces | Mortality

B Narrowing 6%

Membrane 7%

EXCISION

PLASTIC REPAIR

E Low Anal Agenesis 40%

F COLOSTOMY

G CORRECTIVE OPERATION

C DILATION

A Imperforate Anus

High anal Agenesis 45%

Atresia 2%

H

	Control of Feces	Mortality
	±100%	3%
	±100%	3%
	95%	15%
	95%	15%
	50%	30%
	50%	45%

B Where the rectum is separated from its normal anal opening by a thin sheet of tissue, this membrane need only be cut open to release the stool. If the operation is performed promptly after birth, the mortality should be very low, but many such defects are overlooked, and if so 3% of the infants may die. Once the opening is assured, ultimate control of bowel movements should be normal.

C Even with simple imperforate anus defects there is a tendency for a scarlike narrowing (stenosis) to develop at the anal opening. With all complicated defects, there is at least a 35% likelihood of this occurring, even after good operative care. The infant's mother must be instructed to dilate the opening daily for at least six months after the operation.

D Fecal continence means the ability to control the bowel movements. Following repair of imperforate anus, control may not be normal until the child is in his teens.

E In the commonest type of defect, a blind pouch of rectum ends above the skin of the buttocks. In half of male infants having this defect, a small tract will connect the pouch of bowel with the urinary tract. In females, 80% will connect the pouch by a similar narrow tunnel into the vagina. Although gas and small amounts of stool may pass out through these tracts, neither is usually wide enough to function as a vent for stool, and a colostomy is required soon after birth to permit normal emptying of the bowel.

The pouch may end at any distance from the buttocks. In 40% of cases, it is near the skin (low anal agenesis), and in another 45%, high up within the abdominal cavity. The level of the end of the pouch affects the chance for an ultimately good result.

F A blind rectal pouch, even if it connects by a thin fistulous opening to the vagina or urinary tract, causes obstruction and must be relieved soon after birth with a decompressing colostomy (see "Colostomy," page 220). Complications of colostomy in infants are 25% more frequent than in adults. Five percent of infants with a colostomy will need a second operation to revise or change the colostomy before it is finally closed.

G A number of operations are used to bring the rectum out to the skin of the buttocks at the normal site of the anus. With a previously constructed colostomy, this can be performed on a bowel pouch empty of feces. These operations are usually delayed until the child is about eight months old. After the rectum is brought down to its normal position and the wound well healed, the colostomy can later be closed, and the child can pass his stool in the normal manner.

Infants with a low-lying rectal pouch (low anal agenesis) have a 95% chance of ultimately having good fecal continence. Those with pouches high above the normal position have about a 50% chance of ultimately having a good result. Repair of defects that are far from the anus are difficult, with a 30% complication and mortality rate, twice that of low-lying pouches.

H Other rare variations of imperforate anus exist that do not have as good a chance of successful results as do the more common defects in this area.

5. Jaundice in the Newborn

A The liver produces a golden-colored fluid called bile, which drains through a tube (the bile duct) to the intestine. Anything that blocks the disposal of bile, whether in the liver or in the drainage duct, causes its retention, producing a yellow color to the skin and to the normally white part of the eyeballs. This is called jaundice.

B Ten percent of children who become jaundiced within the first twenty-four hours after birth have a so-called Rh blood group incompatibility. The jaundice is due to abnormal breakdown of the child's red blood cells, releasing a pigment that causes a yellor color. The first-born child of a mother is not under risk for jaundice due to Rh problems.

 If tests show that the mother might have Rh problems with subsequent children, an injection of a material called RhoGAM after delivery of the first child will diminish this risk to about 1%. If the sensitized mother is not treated, she has a 20% chance of having her next child jaundiced from Rh incompatibility.

C If the jaundiced infant is not treated, 50% will survive, and there will be significant brain damage in 35% of those who live.

D Treatment of Rh disease depends on the degree of jaundice. If the degree is mild, the infant may require no treatment or can be cured by exposure to ultraviolet light. If the jaundice is severe, the infant's blood is removed and exchanged for new blood through a catheter placed in the umbilical vein. About 65% of infants so treated will survive. The others will die because of previous damage to organs while the infant was within the womb. There is a 10% likelihood of complication following exchange transfusion, including the possibility of a clot forming in the vein that leads from the belly button (umbilicus) to the liver.

E Infections of the fetus while within the womb with diseases such as german measles (rubella) and other blood group incompatibilities may also cause jaundice immediately after birth.

F Jaundice that appears between the second and fourth day after birth is due, in about 90% of cases, to so-called "physiologic jaundice." The liver in these newborns has not developed sufficiently to process the material from red blood cells which is deposited in the infant's skin, giving it the yellow color. Virtually all such infants (about 98%) will

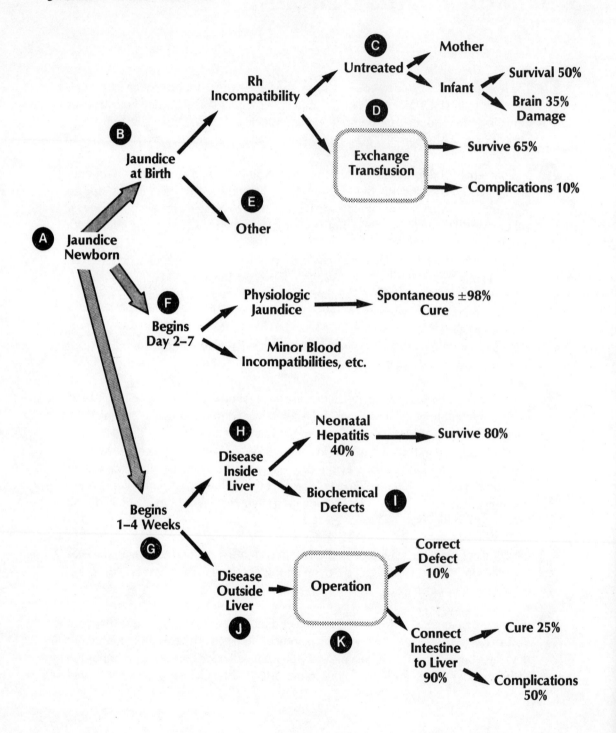

get rid of their jaundice within one week and be normal thereafter. Premature infants born before their full nine-month developmental period inside the mother's uterus are particularly apt to be jaundiced for this reason.

G Jaundice that does not become noticeable until one to four weeks after birth can be caused either by disease within the liver or by obstruction of the ducts that carry bile from the liver to the intestine.

H About 40% of jaundiced infants with disease within the liver suffer from neonatal hepatitis, a disease of unknown cause. They have an 80% chance of survival.

I An occasional infant will be born without certain biochemical mechanisms within the liver to dispose of bile. Bile accumulates and the infant becomes jaundiced. The most common disease has the difficult name alpha-one-antitrypsin deficiency. Such infants live an average of about two years. There is no known treatment.

J If all tests indicate that the jaundice is due to a block of the bile passage *outside* the liver, an operation is performed. In 10%, the defect in the bile duct can be corrected and the child has a 50% chance of cure.

K Much more frequently, (90%) the biliary atresia is uncorrectable by common operations. In these infants, the surgeon brings a piece of intestine up to the edge of the liver, and bile works its way out of the liver into the intestine.
   The chances of success depend on the age at which the operation is performed.

Age	Chance for Success
Less than 2 months	90%
2–3 months	40%
3–4 months	10%
Over 4 months	±0%

When these operations are unsuccessful, the only hope for benefit is by liver transplantation.

XIII

Orthopedics

1. Shoulder Problems

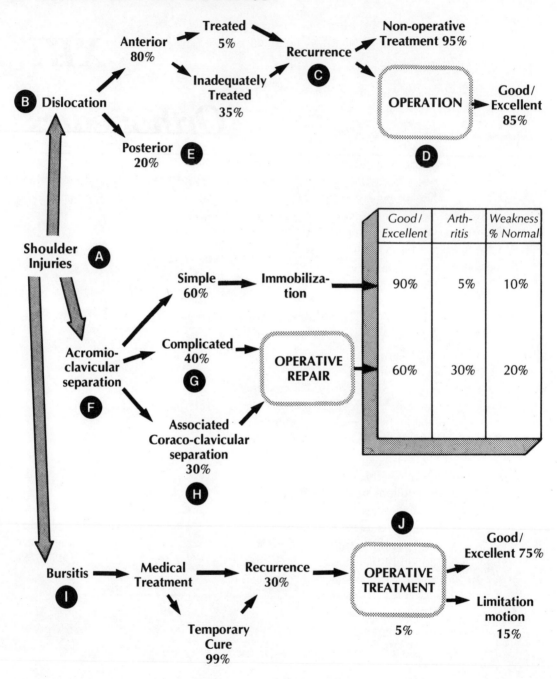

A People need good, pain-free motion in their shoulders in order to take care of themselves and earn a living. Try combing your hair or even dressing yourself with a painful shoulder joint!

B During some sports activity or after a fall, the upper arm will pop out of its ball-and-socket joint in the shoulder girdle. This is a dislocated shoulder. Some individuals are particularly prone to dislocating their shoulder. In over 90% of cases, the arm dislocates onto the front of the chest wall (anterior dislocation). This is painful and frightening, but usually not dangerous. In 10% of cases, there may be an accompanying break (fracture) in the bone. Putting the shoulder back in place can be performed by an experienced physician, without the use of general anesthesia and even without hospitalization in over 90% of cases. The earlier the attempt is made to reduce the dislocation, the easier it is to be successful, for the big muscles around the shoulder go into spasm and make reduction difficult. There is often some soreness in the arm for several days after reduction, when the pain has gone. Damage to accompanying nerves and blood vessels to the arm occurs in less than 1% of cases.

C If the shoulder is reduced then immobilized for six weeks after the initial anterior dislocation, there is only a 5% probability of a recurrence. If, however, the patient starts using his arm again as soon as the pain is gone, the chances of a recurrent dislocation is about 35%. Once there is a recurrence, the shoulder dislocates with progressively less exercise or injury, much to the discomfort and disgust of the patient.

Ninety percent or more of patients will simply give up the sport or activity (such as overhand serves in tennis or getting basketball rebounds off the backboard) that provokes dislocation. The tendency to dislocate gradually diminishes.

D In about 5% of patients with chronic dislocation, operation is performed because of constant discomfort and distress caused by the dislocation. The many available operations are designed to strengthen the joint capsule and use various muscles around the shoulder to contain the bone in the upper arm (humerus) in its proper location in the joint. They prevent recurrence in 90% and give good to excellent results in 85%. Motion of the shoulder can be expected to be about 75% of normal, and complications of the operation, such as infection, occur in about one percent of cases.

E In less than 5% of shoulder dislocations, the arm bone (humerus) slides out behind the shoulder joint. In about 25% of such posterior dislocations, there is a broken bone with this injury.

Shoulder Problems

F The bones around the shoulder are held in position both by muscles and by tough ligaments that run like anchoring cables between the bones. When the ligaments are torn, the shoulder joint is apt to weaken, and the bones separate. One of the main ligaments runs from the acromion process of one bone to the clavicle (collar bone) is called, quite logically, the acromio-clavicular ligament. The popular term for a torn acromio-clavicular ligament is shoulder separation. About two of three such patients have only slight to moderate separation of the bones and can be treated with a sling to immobilize the arm for a few days because of pain. Good to excellent results can be expected in 90% of patients, and subsequent pain from arthritis resulting from the injury can be expected in 5%.

G In perhaps 40% of patients, the separation is so wide and the shoulder so weakened that operative repair of the ligament may be required. Expectancy after such repair is good to excellent strength in 90% of patients, recurrence of ligamentous tear in 10%, some residual arm weakness in 5%, and, ultimately, some painful arthritis in the joint in 20%. The patients must refrain from full, violent exercise for three months.

H In about 30% of patients with an acromio-clavicular injury, there is simultaneous tear of another nearby ligament that runs from the clavicle (collar bone) to the so-called coracoid process of the shoulder. A tear of this coraco-clavicular ligament usually is repaired along with the nearby acromio-clavicular band, to give stability to the shoulder.

I All the muscles and soft tissues around the joints slide back and forth over each other every time there is motion. Between such neighboring tissues, there is often a thin, slitlike envelope that facilitates such a sliding motion. Usually these smooth, shiny, bursal envelopes are filled with just a few drops of lubricating fluid, but when they become inflamed (bursitis), as from over-use of the shoulder in an unaccustomed activity, they can become painful. The early days of the tennis season is a favorite time for this complaint.

Putting the joint at rest allows the inflammation to subside and temporarily, at least, cures many such patients. Recurrence can be expected in about 30% of cases, depending on repetition of the activity. Injecting anti-inflammatory drugs directly into the painful joint gives relief in about 90% of patients.

J Only in about 5% of all persons with bursitis will operation ever be necessary. It consists of removing the entire swollen inflamed sac. The chances of a good to excellent result with relief of pain, full motion, and no recurrence are about 75%.

2. *Fractures Around the Shoulder*

(A) There are three different bones that may be broken following injury to the shoulder: 1) the collar bone or clavicle; 2) the big bone on the back of the chest—the scapula; and 3) the long bone of the upper arm that fits into the socket of the shoulder joint—the humerus. The human race has graduated from using the forelegs for weight-bearing and locomotion, but the trade-off is heavy reliance on these upper limbs for earning and enjoying a living for which a full range of pain-free shoulder motion is needed.

(B) The treatment and anticipated results of fractures of the humerus near the shoulder depend primarily on the number of bone fragments that result from the injury, whether or not the fragments are displaced, what part of the bone is involved, whether the fracture extends into the shoulder joint, and what the age of the patient is.

Luckily, 80% of the fractures of the humerus have only two fragments, and usually, the strong muscles hold the bones in reasonably normal position with each other. Therefore, in only 2% of cases is it necessary after this type of fracture to do more than immobilize the shoulder for three to six weeks to obtain good healing and good to excellent motion and use of the arm thereafter.

(C) Classic treatment for fractures of the upper end of the humerus may vary from a simple sling for a few weeks of relative immobilization to manipulation of the arm and bone fragments under anesthesia, immobilization in a cast, and prolonged physical therapy. In the elderly, strict immobilization may produce beautifully aligned bone fragments on X-ray study after six weeks, but a frozen and useless shoulder. As so often happens in clinical decisions, a compromise is necessary. In this case, one trades some slight bony deformity for a movable, functioning shoulder by encouraging early motion exercises two to three weeks after injury.

(D) Non-union or delayed union in this area is usually due to major separation of bone fragments.

(E) Complications of fracture or its treatment usually follow three- and four-part fractures where open, operative correction is necessary. This may involve infection (5% of the time); adhesions that will restrict motion and be painful; imperfect union of the bone ends, somewhat restricting full motion; and rarely, about 1% of the time, loss of the blood supply (avascular necrosis) of the head of the humerus.

Fractures Around the Shoulder

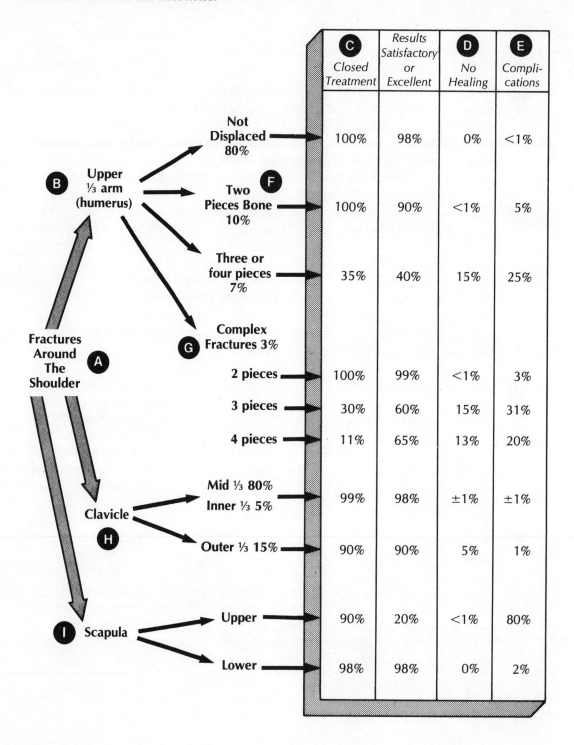

	C Closed Treatment	*Results Satisfactory or Excellent*	**D** No Healing	**E** Complications
Not Displaced 80%	100%	98%	0%	<1%
Two Pieces Bone 10%	100%	90%	<1%	5%
Three or four pieces 7%	35%	40%	15%	25%
Complex Fractures 3%				
2 pieces	100%	99%	<1%	3%
3 pieces	30%	60%	15%	31%
4 pieces	11%	65%	13%	20%
Mid ⅓ 80% / Inner ⅓ 5%	99%	98%	±1%	±1%
Outer ⅓ 15%	90%	90%	5%	1%
Upper	90%	20%	<1%	80%
Lower	98%	98%	0%	2%

Upper ⅓ arm (humerus) — **B**

Fractures Around The Shoulder — **A**

Complex Fractures 3% — **G**, **F**

Clavicle — **H**

Scapula — **I**

F The more the number of pieces of bone fragments after a fracture, the less effective the ultimate expected function and the greater the likelihood of poor healing. In four-piece fractures, the probability of delayed union is 15%. Open reduction involves placing the bone fragments in good position, then fixing them there with wires, pins, screws, or plates.

G Complex fractures of the shoulder include those fracture-dislocations that destroy the smooth surface of the head of the humerus, which normally fits like a ball into the socket of the shoulder joint. A smooth surface is necessary for the shoulder to move in full range and without pain. Total shoulder replacement with a prosthesis is occasionally indicated for a destroyed shoulder joint. The likelihood of a successful result is 50% following this operation. Range of motion and strength are both about 30% of normal.

H Fractures of the collar bone (clavicle) almost always heal with nothing more than simple immobilization of the shoulders by any one of several available methods. Even the thickened callus or heaped-up bone around the fracture site, which seems unsightly some weeks after injury, will usually spontaneously mold itself into a normal contour after a few months. Very rarely is it necessary to operate on these fractures to reduce the bone ends and fix them in position with a wire. This is done most frequently for fractures of the outer 10 centimeters of the bone.

I The upper part of the scapula includes all the structures that go into forming the socket of the shoulder joint. Fractures involving the socket result in less-than-perfect, pain-free motion in eight of ten cases, even if they almost always heal. The lower half of the scapula is not involved in motion of the shoulder and usually heals without disability.

3. *Wrist Fracture*

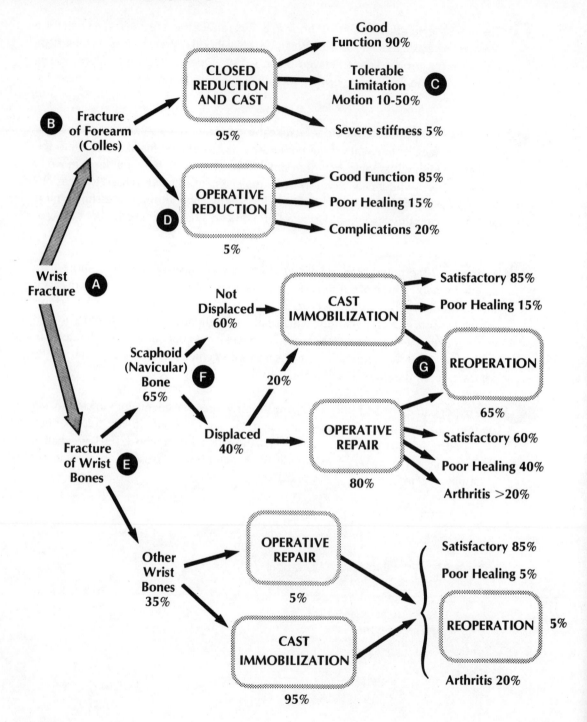

A A broken wrist usually results from a fall on the outstretched hand. There are two bones in the forearm (the radius and ulna) that connect with a set of wrist bones (the carpal bones).

B The commonest wrist fracture is of both forearm bones just above the wrist joint. Ninety-five percent of such so-called Colles' fractures are treated by putting the bones back in proper position (reduction), using local or general anesthesia, and immobilizing the arm and wrist in a cast for four to six weeks. Vigorous use of the hand should begin immediately to avoid the complications listed below.

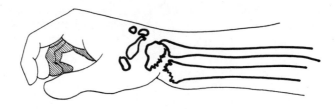

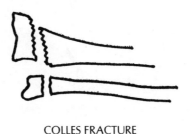

COLLES FRACTURE

Complications of a Colles' fracture include:

- Some visible deformity (crookedness): 75%
- Measurable but not functionally limiting decrease in wrist and forearm motion: 95%
- Minor decrease in motion of the fingers: 45%
- Decreased grip strength: 30%
- Slow healing of bone ends: 30%
- Severe disabling stiffness of wrist, hand, and fingers: 1–5%

C These limitations are more frequent in the elderly.

D Operative repair of a Colles' fracture is used in only an occasional young vigorous person with such a fracture.

E The eight wrist bones are arranged in two rows and fit between the bones of the forearm on one side and the bones of the hand on the other.

F The boat-shaped navicular (or scaphoid) bone is the wrist bone most commonly broken (70% of the time) with a fall on the outstretched hand. Although there is tenderness to pressure at the base of the wrist, there may be no sign of fracture on X-ray examination of the bone for several weeks after injury. If not immobilized promptly, wrist function can be very unsatisfactory. For this reason, a sprained wrist is often put in a cast for a few weeks, even if there is no demonstrable fracture line visible on the X-ray study.

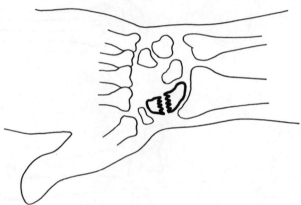

FRACTURE AT NAVICULAR BONE

In 65% of patients with a scaphoid fracture, the bone fragments are in good position and require only prolonged (three months or more) cast immobilization. When the bones are out of position, 80% require operative repair and some sort of operative fixation of the fragments.

G When the fragments of the scaphoid do not heal properly, operative repair may be required weeks or months after injury. A variety of methods of fusing the bones together or replacing them are available, and about 50% of the time a good wrist will result.

4. Cut Tendons

(A) When a muscle shortens, the force is transmitted to the bone through an extension of the muscle called a tendon. These tough, white tendons act like a steel cable to move the bone. The big muscles of the forearm largely stop at the wrist, where they fan out in an array of tendons that lead to various parts of the bones in the fingers. Tendons are covered by a delicate sheath, which keeps them from sticking to adjacent soft tissue as they move back and forth. Although intact tendons are tough, they contain few blood vessels. When they are cut, they do not heal either quickly or kindly, unless treated with great surgical care. Infection is disastrous.

(B) If the cut goes only partway through the tendon, it should be repaired to provide full strength in the future. Results are usually excellent, if there is no subsequent infection.

(C) Tendons that extend the fingers on the back of the hand are less critical than those on the palm and are not subject to the powerful muscle forces that apply to the flexors on the palm side. Repair of extensor tendons can be expected to give good straightening of the finger in 95% of cases.

(D) The complex anatomy of the tendons on the palm side of the hand make their repair and the expected result different at each zone of the hand.

Zone 1 extends from the middle crease in the finger to its tip. Cut tendons in this area can either be reattached to the small bone at the end of the finger or the cut ends sewn together. The chance of a good result is about 85%.

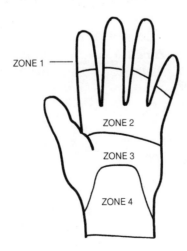

ZONE 1

ZONE 2

ZONE 3

ZONE 4

Cut Tendons

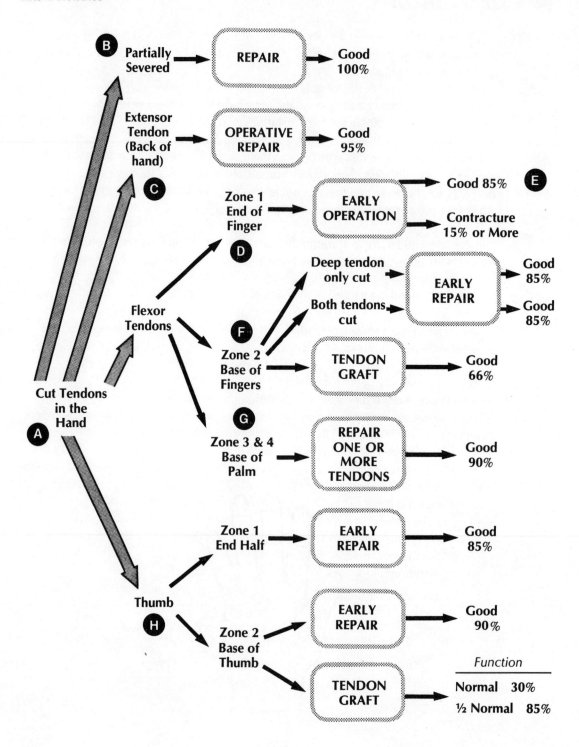

B Partially Severed → **REPAIR** → Good 100%

Extensor Tendon (Back of hand) → **OPERATIVE REPAIR** → Good 95%

C

A Cut Tendons in the Hand

D Flexor Tendons

Zone 1 End of Finger → **EARLY OPERATION** → Good 85% **E**
→ Contracture 15% or More

F Zone 2 Base of Fingers

Deep tendon only cut → **EARLY REPAIR** → Good 85%
Both tendons cut → Good 85%

Zone 2 Base of Fingers → **TENDON GRAFT** → Good 66%

G Zone 3 & 4 Base of Palm → **REPAIR ONE OR MORE TENDONS** → Good 90%

H Thumb

Zone 1 End Half → **EARLY REPAIR** → Good 85%

Zone 2 Base of Thumb → **EARLY REPAIR** → Good 90%

→ **TENDON GRAFT** →

Function

Function	
Normal	30%
½ Normal	85%

E Good result with a severed flexor tendon is measured by the ability to flex (bend) the fingertip to within 1.4 centimeters of the palm. There is no significant disability if this amount of motion is possible.

F The outlook for good function is worst when the tendons are cut in Zone 2, which lies between the middle of the palm and the middle crease in the fingers (as illustrated on page 353).

There are two sets of flexor tendons in this area, one lying on top of the other (the superficial and the deep). If only the superficial tendon is cut, then there is little disability, for the deep tendon can assume all functions. If both sets of tendons are cut, eight out of ten patients will have good function after repairing the critical deep tendon only.

When, after injury, a gap separates the cut ends of the tendon, a tendon unimportant for function can be taken from the foot or forearm and spliced into the gap as a free graft to connect the ends. Sixty-six percent of such patients can anticipate having good flexion of the fingers after about three months.

G When a tendon is cut at the base of the palm or wrist (Zones 3 and 4), nerves and blood vessels are usually damaged at the same time. Tendon repairs in this area have a better expectancy for a good result (90%) than do injuries in the mid-palmar area.

H Monkeys hang very nicely from trees with hands whose thumb cannot be rotated around to oppose the little finger. Only man has this ability, and here lies all the difference. When thumb tendons are cut and not adequately repaired, the injured hand begins to resemble that of a clever monkey. If the severance is near the top of the thumb (Zone 1), repair has an 85% chance of expected good result. But when the tendon is cut at the base of the thumb, only half can be expected to have good function after the ends are sewn together. Subsequent operations to shorten or lengthen the tendons so that they apply the best tension on the thumb will improve this expectancy to 80% good result. When the injury has produced a gap in the tendon and a graft is needed in the thumb, only one in five will have normal range of motion, and 80% will have only half normal motion.

5. Hip Fracture

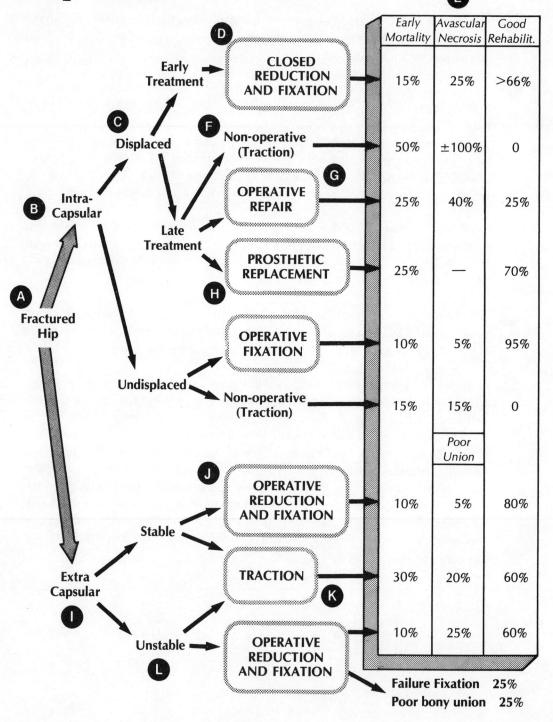

	Early Mortality	Avascular Necrosis	Good Rehabilit.
D CLOSED REDUCTION AND FIXATION	15%	25%	>66%
F Non-operative (Traction)	50%	±100%	0
G OPERATIVE REPAIR	25%	40%	25%
H PROSTHETIC REPLACEMENT	25%	—	70%
OPERATIVE FIXATION	10%	5%	95%
Non-operative (Traction)	15%	15%	0
		Poor Union	
J OPERATIVE REDUCTION AND FIXATION	10%	5%	80%
TRACTION	30%	20%	60%
L OPERATIVE REDUCTION AND FIXATION	10%	25%	60%

Failure Fixation 25%
Poor bony union 25%

E

A Fractured Hip

B Intra-Capsular

C Displaced

Early Treatment

Late Treatment

Undisplaced

I Extra Capsular

Stable

Unstable

K

A Old people are particularly apt to slip, fall, and break their hips. Injuries that might only bruise their grandchildren may frequently fracture the thigh bone near where it fits into the hip joint. Old people's bones are both brittle and weak. In the past, a broken hip in an old person almost always led to pneumonia and early death.

B The femur around the hip is divided into two sections, one within the hip joint capsule (intracapsular portion) and the other outside the capsule (extracapsular). That portion within the joint (intracapsular portion) has a poor blood supply and, therefore, heals slowly after being broken. That outside portion (extracapsular) gets plenty of blood from the muscles that attach to the bone, and fractures in this part of the bone usually heal well.

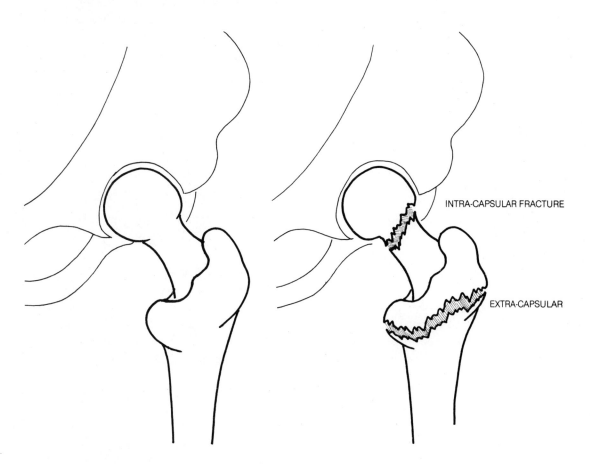

INTRA-CAPSULAR FRACTURE

EXTRA-CAPSULAR

NORMAL ANATOMY

C. As with any broken bone whose pieces are displaced (i.e., in abnormal position), manipulation of the leg or operation is needed to line up the bone fragments. The hip being a most important weight-bearing area, where muscles pull with forces exceeding body weight, it is important to know whether the broken pieces of bone tend to remain in position (are stable) with weight-bearing, or whether putting weight on the leg tends to deform the fragments (unstable fracture). All of these categorizations of hip fractures are important in determining how the fractures are treated and the chances of proper healing.

D. Intracapsular fractures heal poorly, are usually displaced, and often are unstable. All three of these factors are reasons to operate and to manipulate and fix the fragments into good position with wires, nails, or screws passed into the bone. The early mortality of this operation (15%) is primarily from associated heart disease in these elderly patients. If all goes well, as can be anticipated in 80% of these patients, they can walk on crutches in one week and without crutches in three months.

Important major complications and their chances of occurrence following operation include:

- Urinary tract infections: 15%
- Pneumonia: 5%
- Heart attack: 5%
- Blood clot in leg (thrombophlebitis) clinically evident: 25%
- Wound infection: 1–5%

E. In about one fourth of all displaced intracapsular fractures, everything will seem to be going well for several months after injury and operation when a suspicious change begins to take place on the X-ray and pain may begin to develop in the hip. This is evidence of so-called avascular necrosis of the head of the femur, where it fits into the socket of the pelvis. Ultimately, the head of the femur collapses and no longer fits the socket. If the fracture is not treated by operation and the bone fragments fixed to each other, avascular necrosis is almost inevitable. The likelihood of this occurring in an undisplaced intracapsular fracture is about 5%. Avascular necrosis is now usually treated by total hip replacement (see "Hip Replacement," page 360).

F. Occasionally, a patient has such a poor life expectancy from other causes, such as heart disease, that the risk of operation is thought too great. Treatment then consists of traction, which consists of pulling the leg away from the hip in order to line up the bone ends. This gives relief from pain by immobilizing the leg during the six or more weeks of healing. During this period, about half of the patients can be expected to die, and those who survive have a less than 20% chance of ever walking without crutches. Almost all of these intracapsular fractures treated by traction will have subsequent avascular necrosis of the femoral head.

G One method of repair (endoprosthesis) is to remove the fractured head of the femur and to replace it with a metal ball attached to the shaft of the femur. The ball fits into the normal socket of the hip. In essence, it is half of a total hip replacement. There is a 10% chance of hospital mortality, but 75% of patients will have good rehabilitation and ultimately walk without crutches.

H If there are complications in healing, such as avascular necrosis or delayed union, the head of the femur and the hip socket can be replaced (as described in "Hip Replacement," page 360). Total hip replacement in these elderly people following fracture is much riskier than when performed on younger patients who have arthritis.

I Fractures outside the capsule (extracapsular) have a better chance of good healing than those within the capsule, largely because the blood supply to the fragments from the surrounding tissues is better. There is essentially no chance of avascular necrosis in this type of fracture. One type of extracapsular break is referred to as an intertrochanteric fracture, because of its location.

J The operation to reduce and fix an extracapsular fracture is performed through an incision on the outside of the thigh. The fragments are realigned and then held in position with screws, wires, plates, or nails. The expected hospital mortality is 10%, and the chance of infection is 5%. Eight out of ten of these old people can be anticipated to walk. The other 20% will have various problems with bone healing.

K Traction, rather than operation, is reserved for those patients too sick to undergo operation. Patients so treated have a poor outlook. The chance of dying in the hospital is 30%. Only about one-half of those who survive will ultimately walk independently.

L An unstable fracture, in which bone fragments tend to slip apart with weight-bearing, understandably has a lesser chance of good healing than in a fracture where the bone fragments are stable. Failure of fixation can be expected in 25% of patients, and poor union in an equal number. Only 60% have a chance of walking without crutches, even after operation and fixation of the broken bone fragments.

6. Hip Replacement

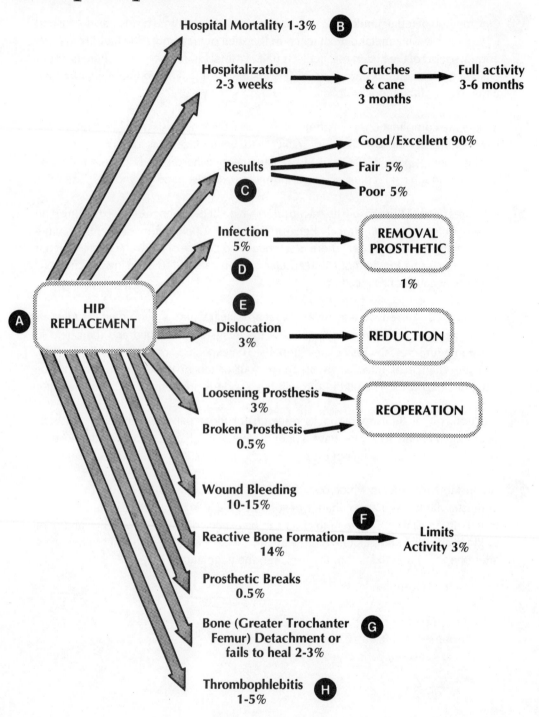

Hospital Mortality 1-3% **B**

Hospitalization 2-3 weeks → Crutches & cane 3 months → Full activity 3-6 months

Results **C** → Good/Excellent 90%
→ Fair 5%
→ Poor 5%

Infection 5% **D** → REMOVAL PROSTHETIC 1%

E
Dislocation 3% → REDUCTION

Loosening Prosthesis 3% → REOPERATION
Broken Prosthesis 0.5%

Wound Bleeding 10-15%

Reactive Bone Formation 14% → **F** Limits Activity 3%

Prosthetic Breaks 0.5%

Bone (Greater Trochanter Femur) Detachment or fails to heal 2-3% **G**

Thrombophlebitis 1-5% **H**

HIP REPLACEMENT **A**

A The hip joint can become so painful and activity so limited by arthritis that it is best to remove the whole joint and replace it with a plastic and metal ball-and-socket device. This procedure has been performed since approximately 1960 and is now an extremely common operation.

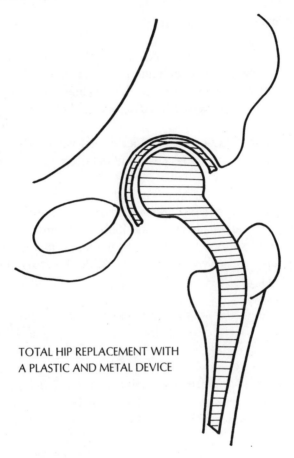

TOTAL HIP REPLACEMENT WITH
A PLASTIC AND METAL DEVICE

B Operative and hospital mortality of 1–3% is primarily due to associated heart disease or blood clots from the leg to the lung.

C A painless hip and normal gait without the need for crutches or cane can be expected in 90% of patients after total hip replacement. Even mild exercise is possible after six months. In nearly all patients, there will still be some minimal residual pain in the hip, but this will rarely require pain medicines. In 5%, the hip joint will be worse than before operation, due to some serious complication.

D Whenever a foreign substance is placed within the body, there is an increased chance of bacterial infection. If the hip has not been operated upon before, the chances of infection are less than 5%. If previous surgery has been done on the hip, the likelihood of infection is much greater. Two-thirds of the infections will occur within the first year. If the hip does become infected, 80% of the prostheses must be removed, in which case, patients are committed to using crutches thereafter. In 5–20% of the instances, after six to twelve months, when the infection has cleared, another try at hip replacement can be made with a 70% chance of success.

E Dislocation of the plastic ball-and-socket joint occurs in 1–3% of patients, but can usually be reduced under anesthesia without need for an open operation.

The metal and plastic-bearing surfaces of current artificial joints are bound tightly to the bone with a special type of bone glue or cement. Just like the caulking around a bathtub, this may gradually crack and loosen with time. In about 30% of cases, the device becomes so loosely attached to the femur that it requires reoperation and replacement within ten years. This is particularly likely to occur in patients who weigh over 180 pounds.

F In 14% of patients, the plastic device inserted into the bone will stimulate an over-growth of bone, but in only 3% does this require operative intervention to increase motion.

G The bony prominence (greater trochanter) along the upper-outer margin of the femur is often temporarily removed during the operation, and in 2–3% of cases, it fails to heal. In rare instances, reoperation is necessary to reattach the trochanter to the main part of the femur.

H Following any operation around the hip, there is always a chance that a clot will form in one of the leg veins, producing what is known as thrombophlebitis (see "Thrombophlebitis," page 150). The danger lies in the possibility that a clot will be thrown off from the leg vein and lodge in the lung, producing a pulmonary embolus. The exact chance of developing thrombophlebitis after a hip replacement is difficult to determine, because there are so many ways of deciding whether such a clot exists. About 20% of patients with a hip replacement will have clinical evidence (pain, swelling, and tenderness) of such clotting, and about 10% of these will develop clinical evidence of a pulmonary embolus.

7. Knee Injury

A Knee injuries usually occur during sports activities. This discussion includes only four of the more common types of injury and does not deal with the many kinds of fractures that can occur around the knee.

B Two thin crescent-shaped plates of cartilage lie in the knee joint between the thigh bone (femur) and the two bones in the lower leg, below the knee. Each cartilage (meniscus) acts like a gasket or shim, bearing much of the body weight and moving each time the knee moves. It is no surprise that the menisci occasionally tear under this constant stress. When they do, the knee may temporarily lock and be painful. Once such a tear occurs and the knee locks, there is a 90% chance it will recur and an 85% likelihood that the knee will have to be operated upon and the cartilage removed. The operation requires three to five days of hospitalization, followed by a four to eight week period of protected activity before full activity is resumed.

C Although about 80% of patients will have good to excellent results immediately after removal of the cartilage, there is a 25% chance of arthritic changes in the knee ten to twenty years later, because the protection of the meniscus has been removed.

D A pair of tough bandlike ligaments run within the knee joint holding the thigh bone (femur) to the leg bone (tibia). Because they cross, they are called the cruciate ligaments. When either is torn, the knee loses a good deal of its fore-and-aft stability.

TORN CRUCIATE LIGAMENT

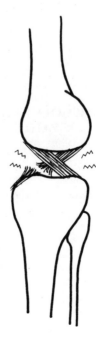

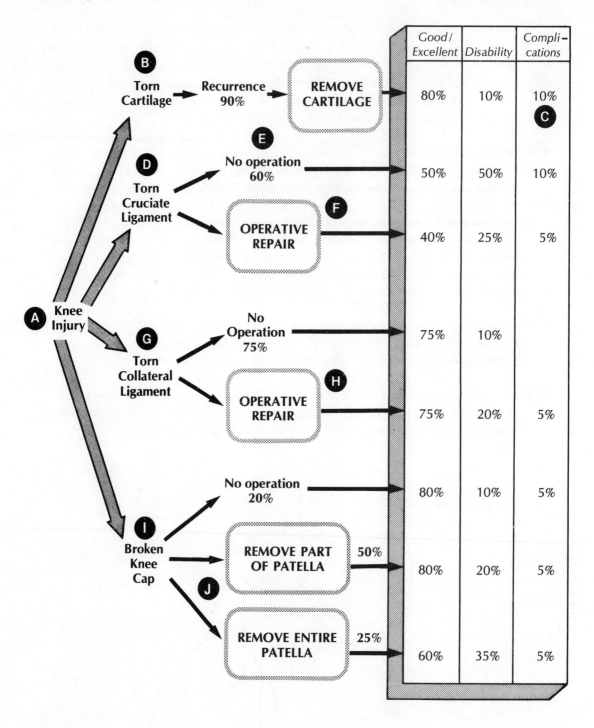

	Good/ Excellent	Disability	Compli- cations
B Torn Cartilage → Recurrence 90% → REMOVE CARTILAGE	80%	10%	10% **C**
D Torn Cruciate Ligament → **E** No operation 60%	50%	50%	10%
→ OPERATIVE REPAIR **F**	40%	25%	5%
G Torn Collateral Ligament → No Operation 75%	75%	10%	
→ OPERATIVE REPAIR **H**	75%	20%	5%
I Broken Knee Cap → No operation 20%	80%	10%	5%
→ REMOVE PART OF PATELLA 50%	80%	20%	5%
→ **J** REMOVE ENTIRE PATELLA 25%	60%	35%	5%

A Knee Injury

E Without operation, a person with a torn cruciate ligament has an unstable but usable knee, if he does not engage in strenuous athletics. Building up the strength of the knee muscles can partially compensate for damaged cruciates. About 60% of patients do not choose to have cruciate ligament repair. Of these, about one-half will have troublesome instability of the knee.

F Operative repair of the cruciate ligaments requires three to seven days of hospitalization, and six to twelve weeks in a cast, and another twelve weeks of rehabilitation. These ligaments often do not heal very firmly. Only 50% of patients can expect good to excellent results, with a powerful, stable, pain-free knee after operation. There is significant knee instability in about 35%. In all of these operations inside the knee joint, there is always about a 5% risk of infection of the skin wound or deeper inside the joint itself. Infection within the joint can cause serious arthritis and limitation of motion.

G The knee joint is also stabilized by two broad, flat, and very tough ligamentous bands (the collateral ligaments), which run like a harness on either side of the knee joint from top to bottom. The one on the middle side of the leg is called the medial collateral ligament, and the one on the outside, the lateral collateral ligament. They are often torn by twisting injuries.

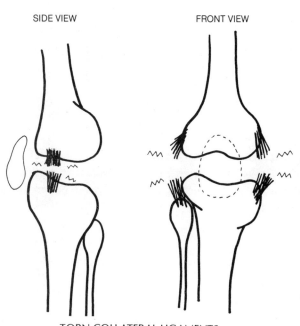

SIDE VIEW   FRONT VIEW

TORN COLLATERAL LIGAMENTS

H In only about 25% of cases is it necessary to repair tears of collateral ligaments. The operation requires three to seven days hospitalization and a cylinder cast to immobilize the knee for six to eight weeks. Full activity can be resumed after twelve to sixteen weeks. Good to excellent results after repair occur in about 75% of cases and weakness or discomfort in about 15%.

I The knee cap (patella) can be broken by a direct blow to the knee. This bone is enclosed in a tendon and helps give strength and efficiency to the muscles that straighten the lower leg.

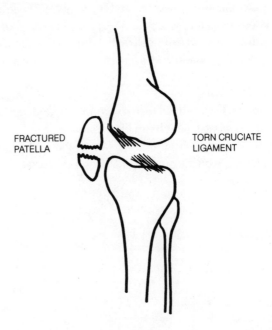

FRACTURED
PATELLA

TORN CRUCIATE
LIGAMENT

J Depending on the type of fracture, the patella can be left in place and immobilized for four to six weeks until healed, or part or all of it can be removed. Each type of fracture is treated differently. If the entire bone is removed, power to straighten the leg is reduced about 25–40%.

8. Ankle Injury

A A person's entire weight is precariously balanced on his two thin and highly flexible ankles, where a complex array of muscles, tendons, ligaments, nerves, and blood vessels converge. Precise alignment of the ankle bones is necessary for perfect ankle motion. It is no wonder that ankle injury often produces later disability.

B A ligament is a tough, white band that binds but allows motion between two adjacent bones. A series of ligaments holds the bones around the ankle in the precise alignment necessary for a good gait. When the ligaments are over-stretched, some of the fibers are torn. This is referred to as a sprain. In severe sprains, the ligaments may be completely severed, creating a loose ankle joint.

C Most sprains can be treated by immobilizing the ankle, allowing the ligaments to heal while the ankle is completely at rest. This can be accomplished by using crutches, by applying a bandage that will stop motion in the ankle, or by putting the ankle in a plaster cast. By the end of three weeks, 95% of such patients with an ankle sprain will have complete healing of the ligament and can ultimately anticipate normal ankle function. After severe sprains, there may be some permanent stiffness and limitation of motion.

D Rarely, when the ankle ligaments are totally torn, it is advisable to repair them surgically. This requires six weeks of immobilization in a cast, but provides a 90% probability of a normal pain-free ankle.

E The only vulnerable spot on the Greek warrior Achilles was behind his heel. This precise spot was where he was shot by the Trojan hero Paris. Ordinary mortals suffer injury in many other places, but they too can tear the Achilles tendon behind the heel, which is named in the Greek warrior's honor. The Achilles tendon pulls the foot down when one stands on tiptoe. After years of wear and tear, it may snap, requiring treatment by either of two methods.

F Fixing the foot with the ankle and toes pointing down relaxes the Achilles tendon and permits the torn tendon ends to come together and heal. Casting the foot in this awkward position for at least six weeks provides 75% of patients with good healing. In the other 25%, the tendon may not be as tight as it should be and the ankle is weakened. The tendon may re-rupture in 1–5% of cases treated by immobilization, requiring an operation in which the ends of the tendon are sewn together.

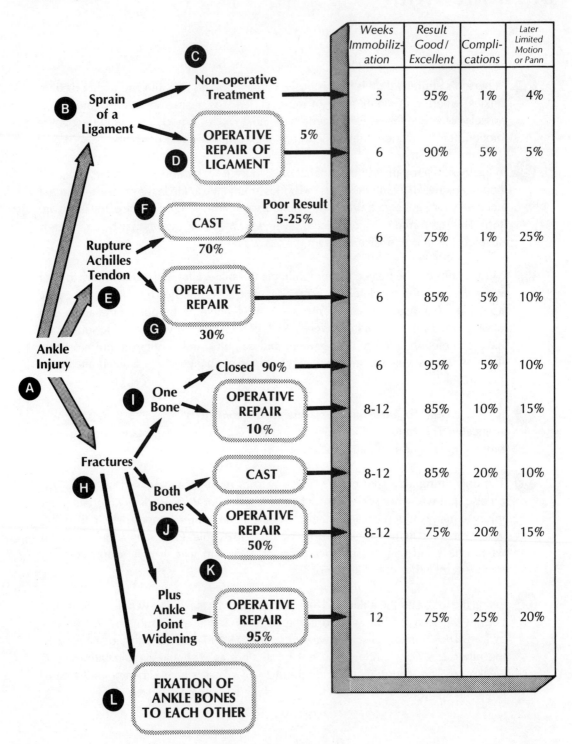

	Weeks Immobiliz-ation	Result Good / Excellent	Compli-cations	Later Limited Motion or Pann
Non-operative Treatment	3	95%	1%	4%
OPERATIVE REPAIR OF LIGAMENT	6	90%	5%	5%
CAST	6	75%	1%	25%
OPERATIVE REPAIR	6	85%	5%	10%
Closed 90%	6	95%	5%	10%
OPERATIVE REPAIR 10%	8-12	85%	10%	15%
CAST	8-12	85%	20%	10%
OPERATIVE REPAIR 50%	8-12	75%	20%	15%
OPERATIVE REPAIR 95%	12	75%	25%	20%

Sprain of a Ligament — B

C — Non-operative Treatment

D — OPERATIVE REPAIR OF LIGAMENT — 5%

Rupture Achilles Tendon — E

F — CAST — 70% — Poor Result 5-25%

G — OPERATIVE REPAIR — 30%

Ankle Injury — A

Fractures — H

One Bone — I

Both Bones — J

K

Plus Ankle Joint Widening

L — FIXATION OF ANKLE BONES TO EACH OTHER

G The more common method of treatment of a ruptured Achilles tendon is to sew the two ends of tendon together soon after injury. This is followed by six weeks of immobilization in a cast. A strong ankle can be expected in about 85% of cases treated by such operation. Once an Achilles tendon has ruptured, there is about a 10% chance that the tendon on the other ankle will rupture sometime in the future. Rupture of this tendon is a sign of tendon degeneration—unpleasant though this fact may be to a middle-aged athlete!

H Each of the two bones of the lower leg (tibia and fibula) end in a bulbous swelling called the malleolus, which can be felt on either side of the ankle. Together, they form a bony groove or mortice that fits snugly over the bones of the foot. This provides both a free-gliding motion of the bones and a stable ankle joint. Fractures of the ankle may involve one or both of these malleoli. If the malleoli are pulled apart by the fracture, the mortice, or groove for the ankle, is widened and the joint made unstable.

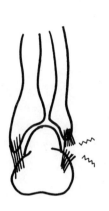
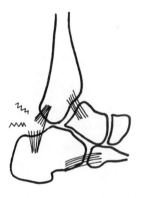

TORN LIGAMENTS AROUND
THE ANKLE

FRACTURES OF THE LEG BONES
AROUND THE ANKLE

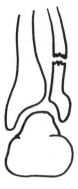
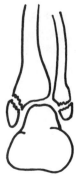

Ankle Injury

I When only one malleolus is broken, the orthopedist can usually press the bones of the ankle into their correct position and then immobilize the ankle in a cast during the six weeks' healing period. In about 95% of cases, this will result in an essentially normal ankle. In about 10% of cases, there will be residual pain, arthritis, or some limitation of motion. Operative repair of a fracture of only one malleolus is needed in only about 5% of cases, where the bone fragments cannot be brought into good position or the ankle mortice remains widened.

J When both malleoli are broken (bimalleolar fractures) there is less chance of being able to put the bony fragments in good position and keep them there without operation. In about one-half of the cases, operation is required, fixing the bones in position with some type of nail, screw, or plate. After eight to twelve weeks of immobilization in plaster, a good result can be anticipated in about 75% of cases. There is some limitation of motion or pain in about one in seven patients. The 20% chance of complication includes an occasional delay in healing of the bone ends or the need for a second operation to achieve better realignment or better bone healing.

K Sometimes, the leg bones around the ankle are broken in three places (trimalleolar fracture). The ankle mortice is invariably widened with this type of injury. Although 5% of the time such severe injuries can be treated without operation, most (about 95%) require fixation of the bone fragments in position using screws, nails, or plates put into the bone. After twelve weeks of immobilization in a plaster cast, 75% of patients will have a good functioning ankle. In the other 25%, complications may vary from pain, limitation of motion, delay in healing, need for reoperation, or even rarely (1–2%) infection.

L When all other measures fail and ankle pain is seriously disabling, decision may be made to join (fuse) the bones around the ankle to each other. This prevents all motion in this joint. Such an operation is called ankle arthrodesis, or fusion of the joint.

The operation is successful in achieving bony union across the joint in about 85% of cases. Reoperation is needed in the remainder. After about sixteen weeks of immobilization in a cast, while the bones heal together across the joint, 90% of patients will have a pain-free ankle. A limp-free walking gait can be anticipated in 75% within three months. Because the ankle cannot move freely in a forward and backward plane after fusion, there is limitation in ability to run. But the other joints in the foot compensate for many of the other motions that normally occur in the ankle.

Replacement of the ankle joint with an artificial joint (prosthetic) may be the procedure to use in the future, but this operation has not been performed long enough to permit certainty of its long-term results.

XIV
Urology

1. Kidney Cancer

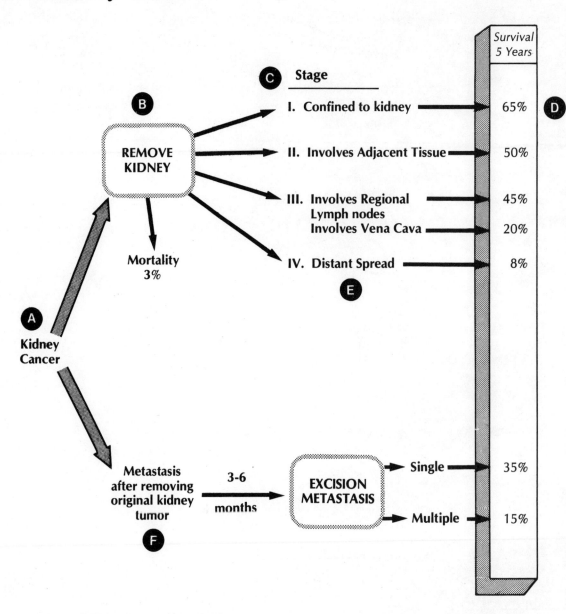

Survival
5 Years

C Stage

B

**REMOVE
KIDNEY**

I. Confined to kidney — 65% **D**

II. Involves Adjacent Tissue — 50%

III. Involves Regional
Lymph nodes — 45%
Involves Vena Cava — 20%

IV. Distant Spread — 8%
E

Mortality
3%

A

Kidney
Cancer

Metastasis
after removing
original kidney
tumor
F

3-6

months

**EXCISION
METASTASIS**

Single — 35%

Multiple — 15%

A The two kidneys lie beneath the rib cage in the flank on each side of the backbone. Their purpose is to secrete urine. Each kidney functions so well that removal of one in no way effects the health of the person.

B Treatment of kidney cancer involves removing the kidney and all the surrounding tissue that might be invaded by the tumor. This is called a radical nephrectomy (see "Nephrectomy," page 378).

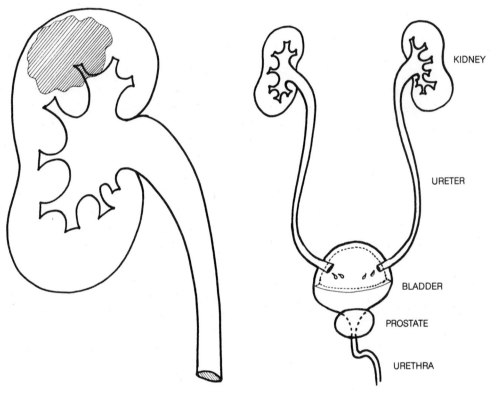

TUMOR AT THE UPPER PART OF THE RIGHT KIDNEY

NORMAL ANATOMY OF KIDNEY, URETER, BLADDER, PROSTATE AND URETHRA

C The chance for cure of a kidney tumor is determined by how far the tumor has spread when treatment is started (stage of the tumor), and by the appearance of the tumor cells when examined under the microscope (grade of the tumor). The two methods of measuring tumor growth and chance of survival usually correspond.

Microscopic Appearance	Extent of Spread
Grade I	12% spread to lymph nodes
Grade II	28% spread to lymph nodes
Grade III	34% spread to lymph nodes

D When the tumor is still within the kidney (Stage I), 65% are cured by nephrectomy. When it has broken through the kidney capsule but is still in the soft tissue around the kidney, half of the patients are cured by removing the kidney and that tissue containing tumor.

Lymph nodes draining the kidney run along the backbone and can be removed by an incision through the chest and abdomen. If these regional nodes are involved with tumor, but removed, there is a 45% chance of cure. The kidneys lie next to the big vein (vena cava) that drains the lower part of the body. If the tumor involves the wall of the vena cava, but can be removed, there is still a 20% chance of cure.

E When kidney cancers have spread to distant parts of the body, such as the lung, liver, or bones, all the tumor cannot be removed. However, this type of cancer sometimes grows very slowly, and about 8% of patients, even with such widespread disease, will be alive in five years.

Radiation will decrease pain and slow the growth of almost all localized tumor deposits (metastasis). Anti-cancer drugs are relatively ineffective.

F Occasionally, the original tumor will have been removed and only a single metastatic deposit of cancer will remain in the lung. If after about three to six months there is no other evidence of tumor, it is worth removing the solitary tumor nodule (metastasis) in the lung. About 35% of such patients will be alive five years later.

2. Kidney Transplant

A End-stage kidney disease exists when a patient can no longer excrete urine well enough to support life. Under these circumstances, there are two choices of treatment available. The first is reliance on a kidney machine two to three times a week for the rest of one's life. The second is a kidney transplant. Most patients undergoing transplant require some period of support on the artificial kidney (hemodialysis) before operation.

B The patient's diseased kidneys must be removed in about 20% of cases before transplant, because they are a source of infection or will otherwise interfere with function of the kidney transplant. Removing both kidneys (nephrectomy) is usually done some weeks before the transplant.

C Life can be maintained in a person whose kidneys have been removed using a device (artificial kidney) that pumps the patient's blood over a plastic membrane that filters out toxins, just as kidneys excrete these wastes into the urine. This is called dialysis. Blood is taken from an artery, then pumped through the machine and back into a vein.

Several techniques are used to provide efficient access to a big artery and vein every three days, as is needed for dialysis. One involves placing a plastic tube in an artery and nearby vein in the forearm, forming a small shunt outside the skin, which can be readily opened during dialysis. Another method involves connecting a small artery to a vein beneath the skin. A needle is put into the high flow connection between the artery and vein through the skin for each dialysis. Creating and revising these shunts are tedious, but not dangerous to the patient. They require operative revision at least once a year and, often, even more frequently.

Two to three dialysis sessions each, requiring five hours attachment to the machine, are needed each week. Drawbacks to dialysis, in addition to the time required, include anemia (abnormally low amounts of red blood cells) in 95% of cases, weakness in 50%, and bone problems in 25%. Dialysis in a center costs about $25,000 per year. Dialysis performed at home costs about $15,000 a year. About 10% of patients on dialysis hold a paying job.

D Frequently, a relative will donate one of his kidneys to a sick recipient. This requires a major operation on the donor, but the operative risk is small, and a normal person can safely lose one kidney. Kidneys from close relations have a better chance of good function as a transplant than those from unrelated persons. The risk of the kidney recipient dying during the hospitalization for receiving the kidney transplant is less

Kidney Transplant

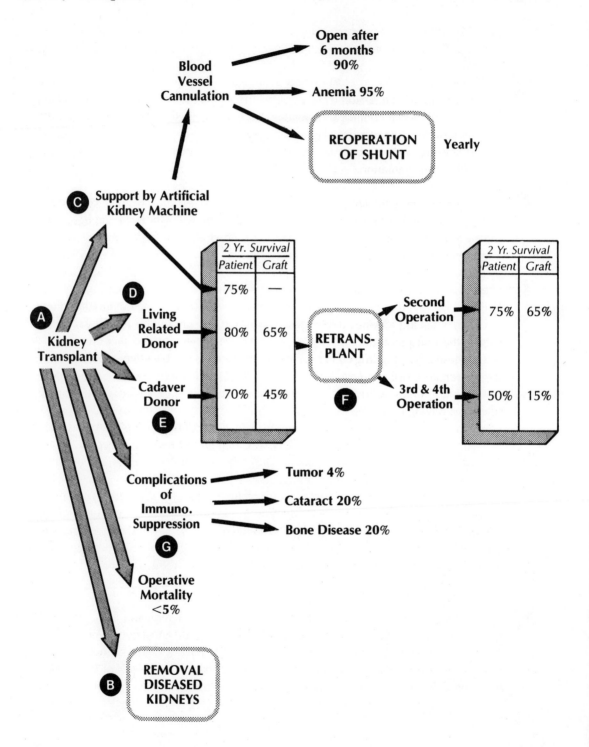

Blood Vessel Cannulation

Open after 6 months 90%

Anemia 95%

REOPERATION OF SHUNT — Yearly

C Support by Artificial Kidney Machine

A Kidney Transplant

2 Yr. Survival
Patient	Graft
75%	—
80%	65%
70%	45%

D Living Related Donor

E Cadaver Donor

RETRANSPLANT **F**

Second Operation

3rd & 4th Operation

2 Yr. Survival
Patient	Graft
75%	65%
50%	15%

G Complications of Immuno. Suppression

Tumor 4%

Cataract 20%

Bone Disease 20%

Operative Mortality <5%

B REMOVAL DISEASED KIDNEYS

than 5%. When kidneys from living, related donors are used, the probability of the patient surviving two years is 80%, and the chance of that kidney functioning after two years is about 65%.

E A kidney taken from a person soon after death (cadaver donor) can be kept alive for a few hours by special cooling and washing techniques. The chances of such cadaver kidneys working are not quite as good as when the kidney is taken fresh from a living donor. Seventy percent of patients receiving cadaver donors are, however, alive two years after transplantation.

F The main reason a transplant kidney fails is the reaction of the body against the transplanted (foreign) organ. Special drugs are given to suppress this rejection of the kidney transplant but still to allow immune defense against infection.

Sometimes a second kidney must be used to replace an original transplant. Such a second transplant has almost as good a chance of success as the original replacement, if the patient for retransplantation is carefully selected.

G A person receiving a kidney transplant must stay on immunosuppressive drugs for as long as the transplant functions in order to allow the foreign organ to survive in his body. These powerful drugs involve severe but not crippling problems. Among them are an increased risk of developing infection, an eighty-fold increase in the chance of developing a tumor, a 20% chance of developing cataracts in the eyes, and a 20% chance of having problems with bone fractures.

3. *Nephrectomy*

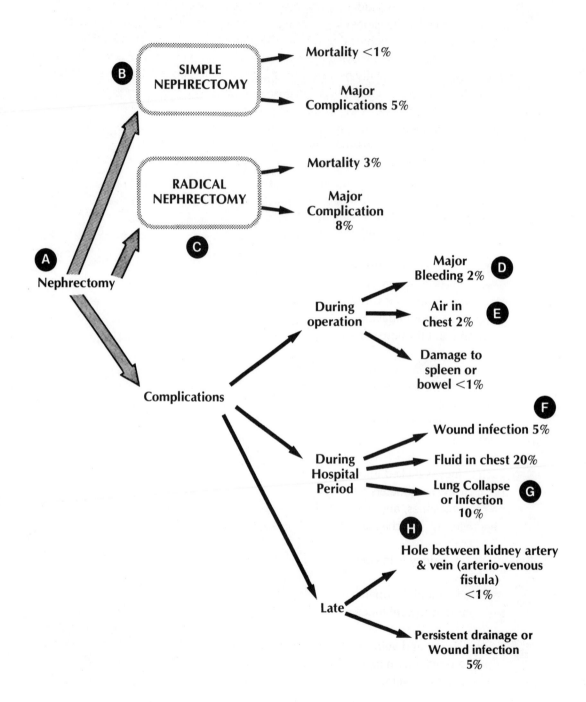

B SIMPLE NEPHRECTOMY → Mortality <1%

Major Complications 5%

RADICAL NEPHRECTOMY → Mortality 3%

Major Complication 8%

C

A Nephrectomy

Complications

During operation → Major Bleeding 2% D

→ Air in chest 2% E

→ Damage to spleen or bowel <1%

F

During Hospital Period → Wound infection 5%

→ Fluid in chest 20%

→ Lung Collapse or Infection 10% G

H

Late → Hole between kidney artery & vein (arterio-venous fistula) <1%

→ Persistent drainage or Wound infection 5%

A There are normally two kidneys, one on each side of the backbone in the flank. They can be removed by incisions either through the back, through the chest, or through the abdomen. There are technical advantages and indications for each approach.

Common causes for removing the kidney include tumor, infection, certain types of kidney stone, injury totally destroying the kidney, or the desire to donate a healthy kidney to someone as a transplant. Because of the enormous reserve capacity of each kidney, the loss of one is of no danger to a patient. In fact, two out of every one thousand people are born with only one kidney, and most such people never even know that one kidney is missing, unless for some reason they undergo special studies.

Hospitalization for nephrectomy is, characteristically, five to fourteen days.

B Simple nephrectomy means removing only the kidney itself, not all the tissue around it. This is the procedure usually performed for injury, infection, and stone. The anticipated mortality is about 1%.

C Radical nephrectomy implies taking out the kidney and all the tissue that surrounds it. It is usually done to remove a kidney tumor and any cancer that might have spread into the surrounding tissues. The operation can be performed either through the chest or through the abdominal cavity. The chances of mortality (3%) and complication (8%) are higher in this more extensive operation than with a simple nephrectomy.

D One-quarter of all the blood put out by the heart goes through the big arteries and veins that supply the two kidneys. These are big vessels, and there sometimes is bleeding during nephrectomy. In about 1% of simple nephrectomies and 5% of radical nephrectomies, it is necessary to give blood transfusions due to blood loss during operation.

E Each kidney is tucked into a conveniently protected anatomic nook in the flank, but within a few centimeters from it lie the chest cavity, the abdominal cavity, the spleen, and the intestines, any one of which occasionally may be injured or entered during nephrectomy. The chances of this occurring are about 1%.

F When the kidney is infected, there is a 5% probability of wound infection.

G Reaction around the operative site may produce fluid in the chest after operation or a slow return of bowel function.

H The big artery and vein serving each kidney lie side by side. Rarely, a hole appears between them after nephrectomy, allowing high-pressure arterial blood to pour into the low-pressure vein. Such an arteriovenous fistula requires surgical repair.

4. Kidney Stones

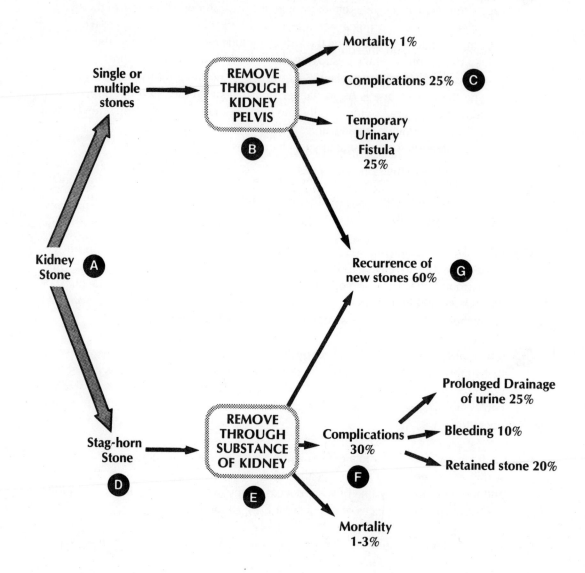

Single or multiple stones → **REMOVE THROUGH KIDNEY PELVIS** (B)

Kidney Stone (A)

Stag-horn Stone (D)

REMOVE THROUGH SUBSTANCE OF KIDNEY (E)

Mortality 1%

Complications 25% (C)

Temporary Urinary Fistula 25%

Recurrence of new stones 60% (G)

Complications 30% (F)

Prolonged Drainage of urine 25%

Bleeding 10%

Retained stone 20%

Mortality 1-3%

A The urine is almost saturated with minerals and chemicals filtered out of the blood by the kidney. When the urine becomes oversaturated, stones begin to form in the kidney. If small, they may pass into the bladder. If they get too large, they stay suspended in the kidney causing pain, bleeding, and infection.

B Urine made in the kidney drains into a funnel-shaped kidney pelvis, which narrows down to a small caliber tube — the ureter, which extends from the kidney to the bladder. Stones made in the kidney may either remain in the kidney pelvis or fall down into the ureter. When stones are loose in the funnel-shaped kidney pelvis, they usually can be removed rather easily by an operation performed in the flank. The surgeon simply cuts onto the stone and removes it from the kidney pelvis, not even disturbing the working part of the kidney. Hospitalization is usually about seven to ten days.

There is only a 5% probability of leaving any stones behind after such an operation. Expected mortality is about 1%, but complications after operation, such as wound infection or temporary drainage of urine out the wound, occur in about 25% of cases.

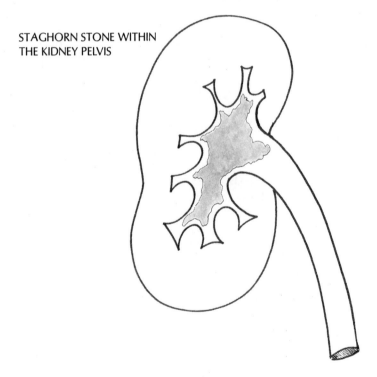

STAGHORN STONE WITHIN
THE KIDNEY PELVIS

C Leakage of urine from the wound after operation normally stops by the fourteenth day. If drainage persists, as it does in about 25% of cases, a small catheter may have to be passed up to the kidney from below, through the bladder, to assure good urine drainage. This almost always stops drainage of urine through the wound within a few days.

D Sometimes, a stone forms deep within the kidney and will not pass into the broad funnel-shaped kidney pelvis. Such stones assume the branching shape of the central part of the kidney drainage system and are, therefore, called stag-horn stones (calculi).

E Stag-horn stones fit snugly, like a cast, within the kidney and are difficult to remove. In contrast to stones rattling around loose within the kidney pelvis, the stag-horn stones are caught in the fleshy part of the kidney substance, like a fish hook. To remove them, the kidney has to be cut wide open and the stones picked out of the kidney substance. This is a tedious technical procedure.

F There is a 30% chance of complication following operation for a stag-horn stone. This includes a 25% chance for prolonged leak of urine through the wound. In about 20% of cases, tips of the stag-horn stone lodged deep in the substance of the kidney may have to be left there. Expected mortality is about 1% in this difficult operation.

G Once a patient forms a kidney stone, he has a 60% chance of forming others. Some people are just stone-formers. In others, where a specific cause for forming stones can be found and corrected, there may be no further trouble.

Overactivity of the parathyroid gland and gout are two diseases that cause recurrent kidney stones. Treatment of the underlying disease decreases the chance of forming future stones. But everyone who has had one urinary tract stone must realize he is at high risk to form other new ones in the future.

5. Ureteral Stones

A Small stones formed in the kidney may drop down the funnel-shaped part of the drainage system (kidney pelvis) into the small-caliber tube (ureter) that leads from the kidney to the bladder. Such urinary tract stones may be a symptom of an underlying disease. Therefore, even if the offending stone is removed, there is a 60% probability that such a person will have another stone at a future date.

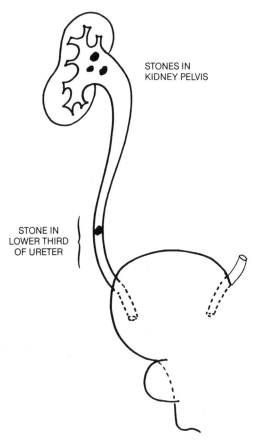

STONES IN
KIDNEY PELVIS

STONE IN
LOWER THIRD
OF URETER

B Stones passing down the ureter cause colicky pain in the flank and side. But if they are small enough, they will go through the ureter to the bladder in a day or so, and the pain will disappear. Eighty percent of all stones small enough to get into the ureter will pass spontaneously into the bladder. If less than 0.5 centimeters in diameter, there is a 95% chance that the stone will pass. Larger stones may move part way down the ureter and then become stuck and have to be removed by the urologist.

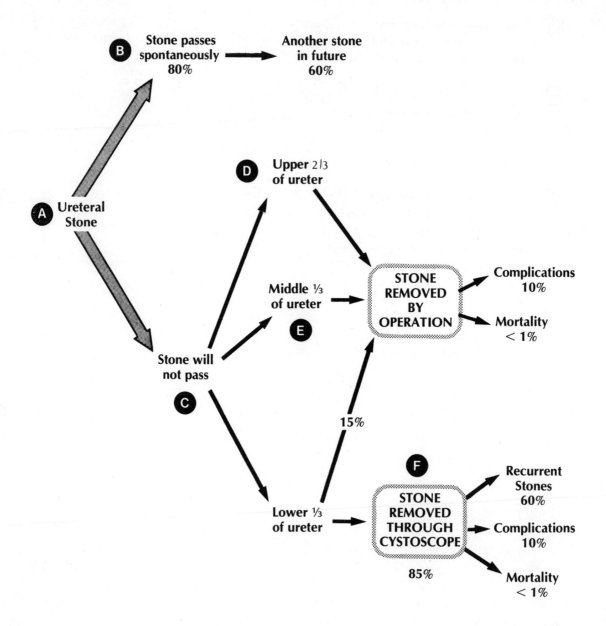

C Stones in the ureter may be removed either by operation or by pulling the stones down the ureter, using a lighted tube (cystoscope) and special instruments passed up the ureter from below, through the bladder.

D Stones in the upper two-thirds of the ureter that will not move have to be removed by operation. Trying to pull them down using a cystoscope is too apt to rupture the ureter. Expected operative mortality is less than 1%, and hospitalization about one week. There is a 10% chance of prolonged drainage of urine from the operative incision where the stone was removed, but this ultimately stops.

E Stones in the lower one-third of the ureter often will pass into the bladder within a day or two. If they will not and the stone is less than 0.8 centimeters in diameter, there is an 85% chance that the stone can be released and removed through a cystoscope and other small instruments passed from the bladder into the ureter.

There is about a 3% chance of making a small hole in the ureter while prying loose such a stone. If this occurs, the site of the perforation must be closed by an operation.

F Fifteen percent of stones in the lower one-third of the ureter cannot be dislodged with instruments passed through the bladder and must be removed by an operation, just as are stones in the upper and middle one-third of the ureter.

6. Bladder Cancer

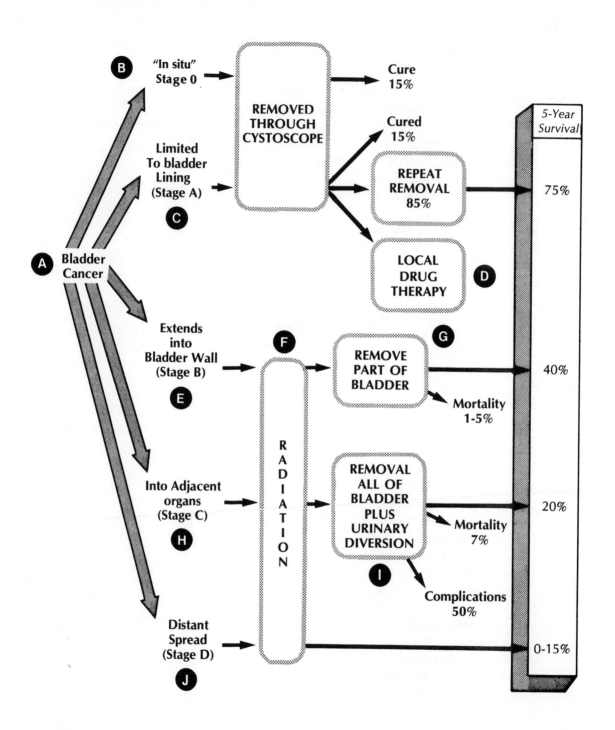

B "In situ" Stage 0

A Bladder Cancer

C Limited To bladder Lining (Stage A)

E Extends into Bladder Wall (Stage B)

H Into Adjacent organs (Stage C)

J Distant Spread (Stage D)

REMOVED THROUGH CYSTOSCOPE

Cure 15%

Cured 15%

D REPEAT REMOVAL 85%

LOCAL DRUG THERAPY

F RADIATION

G REMOVE PART OF BLADDER

Mortality 1-5%

I REMOVAL ALL OF BLADDER PLUS URINARY DIVERSION

Mortality 7%

Complications 50%

5-Year Survival

75%

40%

20%

0-15%

A Bathed for years in urine filled with all the toxic substances that come out of the kidneys, it is no surprise that the lining of the bladder is frequently the site of cancer. Its environment is miserable.

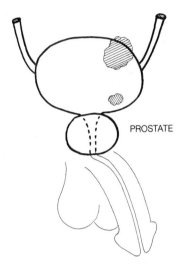

PROSTATE

TWO BLADDER CANCERS: *Above,* TUMOR GROWING THROUGH BLADDER WALL ; *Below,* SMALL TUMOR STILL WITHIN BLADDER

A common sign of bladder cancer is blood in the urine. The diagnosis is confirmed by looking into the bladder with a lighted tube (cystoscope) that is passed into the bladder from below. A piece of the tumor is removed and examined under the microscope to confirm the diagnosis.

B The extent of tumor spread (stage) when first treated is important in determining the probability of cure. The most localized form is called "cancer in situ," and by the name, would suggest it is easy to cure. But it is a bad actor, largely because many islands of in-situ tumor are usually dotted around the bladder. Only 15% of patients with in-situ cancers can be cured by removal of these islands of cancer through the cystoscope.

C Stage A tumor, localized in the bladder lining, usually grows slowly. Fifteen percent can be cured by burning or cutting the tumor out through the cystoscope. But in the other 85% of patients, new tumors develop or the tumor reoccurs. Repeated local excision through the cystoscope provides a five-year cure for 75% of such patients. This requires cystoscopic examination every three months thereafter.

D When these locally recurrent tumors turn up in several sites throughout the bladder, an anti-cancer drug, such as thio-tepa, can be placed in solution in the bladder to bathe the tumor sites with the drug. This helps control growth.

E When the tumor extends into the bladder wall (Stage B), it is best treated with X-ray before any part or even the entire bladder is removed surgically. Combining radiation and surgery is better than either alone.

	Radiation alone	Removal of bladder (cystectomy) alone	Combined radiation and cystectomy
5-Year Survival	20%	20%	40%

F Radiation for bladder cancer is given over the lower abdomen and requires about one to six weeks of treatment. This causes a good deal of discomfort in the weeks following treatment, but in only about 15% of patients will this pain persist.

G When tumor occurs in only one part of the bladder but burrows into the bladder wall, that part of the bladder involved with tumor can often be removed following radiation. Removing part of the bladder (a partial cystectomy) cures about 40% of patients. The bladder stretches easily, and even large parts of it can be removed without affecting its ability to store and expel urine. Operative mortality of partial cystectomy is 1–5%, and the chances of complications after operation are 12%.

H When bladder cancer has spread to the nearby pelvic organs (Stage C), the only chance for cure is to remove the entire bladder (total cystectomy), along with the involved organs. Such a tumor is best treated with X-ray before operative removal. The first step is to divert urine from the bladder into a short, isolated segment of bowel that, like a drainage pipe, carries the urine to a bag worn outside of the body. The patient empties the bag of urine whenever it fills. The next stage in treatment is X-ray therapy to the empty urinary bladder, and the final stage is total removal of the bladder by operation (total cystectomy).

I The expected mortality from total cystectomy and the procedure called ileal loop urinary diversion is 7%. About 50% of patients will have some sort of complication from the extensive operation. This may include temporary leakage of urine from the wound.

J When bladder cancer has spread beyond the limits of operative removal, it is incurable, but X-ray treatment will provide a 10% chance of relief from pain.

7. Prostatism

A The prostate gland in men surrounds the tube that drains urine from the bladder (urethra) to the penis. The size of the gland is affected by male sex hormones and often gradually enlarges during adult life. By age seventy, 75% of men will have non-cancerous enlargement of the prostate, causing difficulty in expelling urine from the bladder. This is called prostatism.

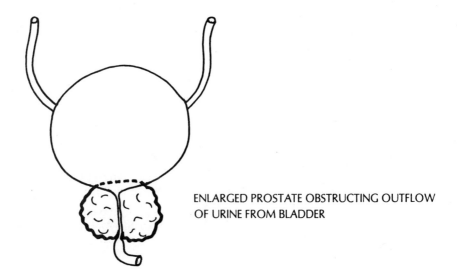

ENLARGED PROSTATE OBSTRUCTING OUTFLOW
OF URINE FROM BLADDER

B Simple enlargement—called benign hypertrophy—accounts for 75% of prostatism. However, 10% of patients thought to have benign prostatic hypertrophy will be found at operation to have cancer in the gland. The physician often suspects this cancerous change before operation by the hard consistency of the gland when felt during a rectal examination (see "Cancer of the Prostate," page 392).

C In 15% of patients with prostatism, a localized narrowing of the urinary bladder neck causes the obstruction rather than generalized enlargement of the prostate gland. Bladder-neck contraction is treated by removing the enlarged part of the gland through a lighted tube (cystoscope) inserted in the urinary passage of the penis. This is called transurethral resection (see "Transurethral Resection," page 400).

Prostatism

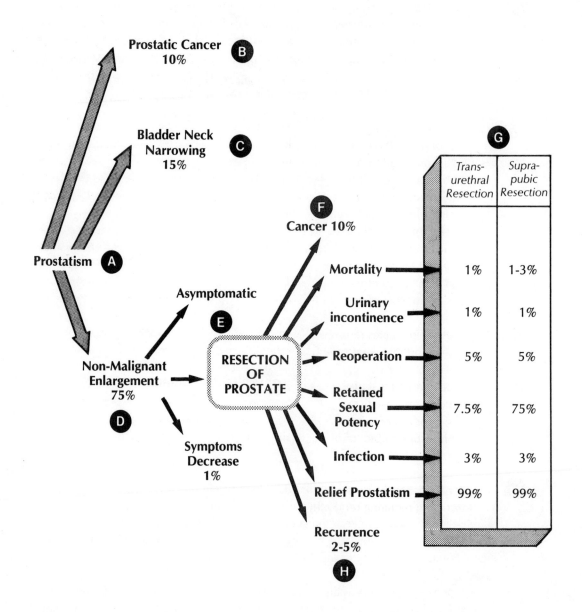

Prostatic Cancer
10% **B**

Bladder Neck
Narrowing **C**
15%

Prostatism **A**

Asymptomatic

E

RESECTION
OF
PROSTATE

Cancer 10% **F**

Non-Malignant
Enlargement
75%

D

Symptoms
Decrease
1%

Recurrence
2-5%

H

| | **G** | |
	Trans-urethral Resection	Supra-pubic Resection
Mortality	1%	1-3%
Urinary incontinence	1%	1%
Reoperation	5%	5%
Retained Sexual Potency	7.5%	75%
Infection	3%	3%
Relief Prostatism	99%	99%

D The early stages of benign prostatic hypertrophy are usually detected by rectal examination ten to twenty years before the enlargement begins to produce symptoms of prostatism. When symptoms become noticeable, they generally are progressive, although they may wax and wane in severity. As the condition progresses, the patient is made miserable by the constant need to pass small amounts of urine and the inability to totally control it. In the end, he also suffers kidney damage.

E There are several ways of removing the prostate gland: Transurethral resection (TUR) is the most common. It is performed under general or spinal anesthesia, requires three to ten days hospitalization, and is done through a lighted tube (cystoscope) passed up the penis to the prostate gland, which lies at the bottom of the bladder. The prostate is burned away under direct vision, giving a wide passage for urine. Ninety-nine percent of the time, it immediately relieves the symptoms of urinary obstruction.

Another common technique for resecting the prostate is through an incision in the lower part of the abdominal wall. The urinary bladder is opened and the prostate gland, lying at the bottom end of the bladder, is removed. This is a more formidable operation than transurethral resection because of the need to open the abdomen, but is used for certain types of very large glands. This is called a suprapubic prostatectomy.

F About 10% of prostates removed operatively will turn out to contain areas of cancer within the gland that were unsuspected or unproved by all tests before operation.

G Both techniques almost guarantee relief (99% of the time) of urinary obstruction and the symptoms of prostatism. The incidence of infection (3%), retained sexual potency (75%), and control of urine are almost the same for both operations. The mortality of 1–3% with suprapubic prostatectomy is slightly higher than with transurethral resection.

H In 2–5% of patients, the prostate gland will regrow after prostatectomy, causing return of prostatism and requiring reoperation.

8. Cancer of the Prostate

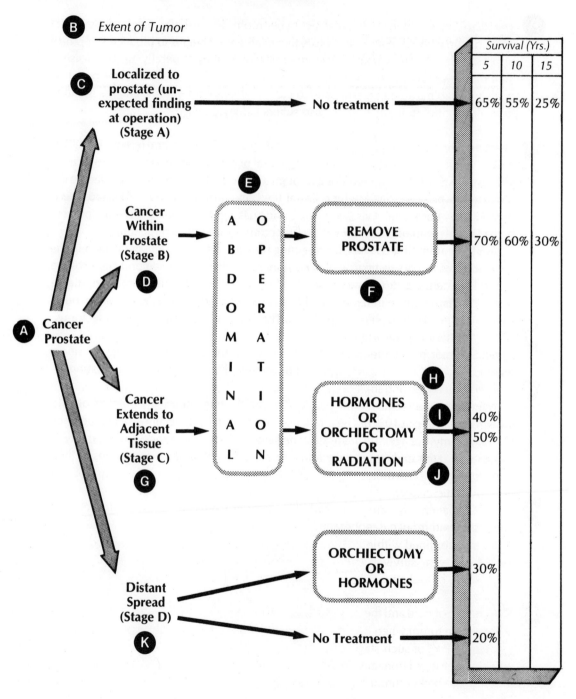

Survival (Yrs.)		
5	10	15

C Localized to prostate (un-expected finding at operation) (Stage A) → No treatment → 65% | 55% | 25%

A Cancer Prostate

D Cancer Within Prostate (Stage B) → E ABDOMINAL OPERATION → F REMOVE PROSTATE → 70% | 60% | 30%

G Cancer Extends to Adjacent Tissue (Stage C) → ABDOMINAL OPERATION → H I J HORMONES OR ORCHIECTOMY OR RADIATION → 40% 50%

K Distant Spread (Stage D) → ORCHIECTOMY OR HORMONES → 30%

→ No Treatment → 20%

392

A Cancer of the prostate is so common in older men that it can almost be considered a part of the aging process. Even when present, it does not necessarily kill the patient. The likelihood of a man having prostatic cancer as he grows older is:

Age (years)	Chance of having cancer in the prostate gland
40–49	4%
50–59	7%
60–69	12%
70–79	18%

The usual symptoms of prostatic cancer are an enlargement of the prostate, causing difficulty in urinating. When the physician feels a hard area in the prostate on rectal examination, he usually takes a specimen (biopsy) of the gland to determine whether it is cancer. There is a 25% chance that the biopsy may not show the tumor, even if tumor exists somewhere else in the gland. This type of biopsy is obviously not perfect.

B When the tumor is still within the gland, the chances for cure are better than if it has spread. Tumor boundaries are defined by Stages A through D.

C The most localized and smallest tumor (Stage A) is where unexpected tumor is found in the prostatic tissue removed for what was thought to be benign prostatic obstruction. This occurs in about 10% of transurethral resections of the prostate (see "Transurethral Prostatectomy," page 400) for what was thought to be benign disease. When discovered at this early stage, only 2% of men will die of the disease and only 10% will ever even develop symptoms of the tumor. Many old men get along reasonably well with prostatic cancer.

D In about one third of cases, cancer of the prostate is suspected by rectal examination, but is still confined within the prostate when first discovered. The likelihood of cure (five to ten year survival) is 60–70%, whether treated by hormones, removing the prostate, or by radiation.

E The chance of cure and the decision as to the best method of treatment depends on the extent of the tumor when it is first discovered. This is determined by a series of tests for "staging." Part of such staging involves an abdominal operation, where samples of tissue are removed from around the prostate and elsewhere in the abdominal cavity to determine whether tumor has spread.

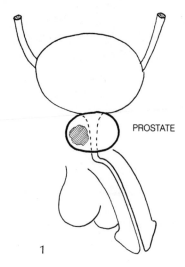

PROSTATE

1

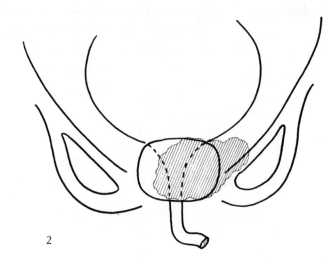

2

CANCER OF PROSTATE
1 NODULE STILL WITHIN THE PROSTRATE GLAND
2 EXTENDING INTO BONES OF PELVIS
3 CAUSING DIFFUSE ENLARGEMENT OF PROSTATE
  GLAND

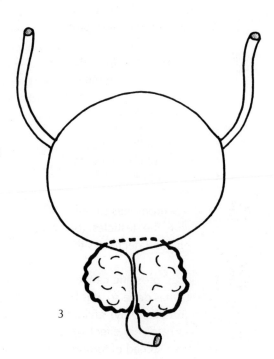

3

F When no tumor is found outside the prostate gland, wide excision of the prostate gland and surrounding tissue (radical prostatectomy) is often performed. In these elderly men, the mortality and expected rate of complications from radical prostatectomy is:

- Mortality: 25%
- Urinary incontinence (unable totally to control passage of urine): 10%
- Wound infection: 5%
- Sexual impotence: 100%
- Hospitalization: 10–21 days

There is a 60% chance of ten-year survival from this operation.

G When prostatic cancer has spread beyond the capsule that surrounds the prostate and extends into the surrounding tissue (Stage C), there is a 40–50% chance of five-year cure, whether treated by hormones, removing the testicles (orchiectomy), or radiation.

H Female sex hormones stop the growth of the prostate and slow the growth of most prostatic tumors. They, therefore, are used in the treatment of early cancers of the prostate and to control pain in advanced prostatic cancers.

I Radiation can be administered either by radioactive pellets injected into the prostate or by X-rays directed at the tumor. Expected complications of radiation include:

- Irritation of the bladder (cystitis): 20%
- Irritation of the rectum: 20%
- Swelling of the leg: 5%
- Swelling of the penis: 5%
- Sexual impotency: 40%

J Male sex hormones stimulate the growth of prostatic tissue and prostatic cancers. By removing the testicles (orchiectomy), the surgeon removes one source of such hormone and decreases the rate of growth of some such tumors.

K Advanced prostatic cancer often spreads (metastasizes) to the backbone (vertebrae). When it has done so, it is beyond cure, but often is very slow growing. Removing the testes (orchiectomy), giving female sex hormones, and radiation do little to prolong life but often are very effective in controlling bone pain from metastases. Even with such advanced spread of tumors, five-year survival is 20–30%.

9. Testicular Tumor

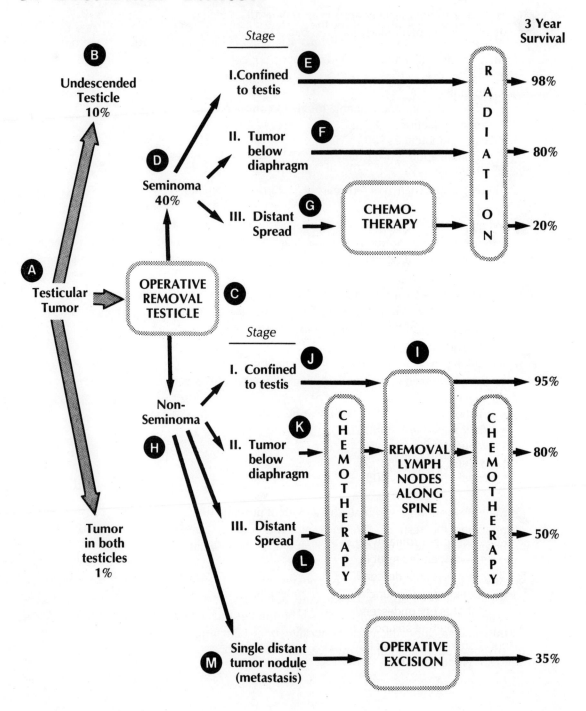

Stage   3 Year Survival

B Undescended Testicle 10%

A Testicular Tumor

C OPERATIVE REMOVAL TESTICLE

D Seminoma 40%

E I. Confined to testis → RADIATION → 98%

F II. Tumor below diaphragm → RADIATION → 80%

G III. Distant Spread → CHEMO-THERAPY → RADIATION → 20%

Tumor in both testicles 1%

H Non-Seminoma

Stage

J I. Confined to testis → **I** REMOVAL LYMPH NODES ALONG SPINE → 95%

K II. Tumor below diaphragm → CHEMOTHERAPY → REMOVAL LYMPH NODES ALONG SPINE → CHEMOTHERAPY → 80%

L III. Distant Spread → CHEMOTHERAPY → REMOVAL LYMPH NODES ALONG SPINE → CHEMOTHERAPY → 50%

M Single distant tumor nodule (metastasis) → OPERATIVE EXCISION → 35%

A Testicular tumors usually appear as non-tender swellings in the scrotum in young men. They are particularly likely to occur in undescended testicles.

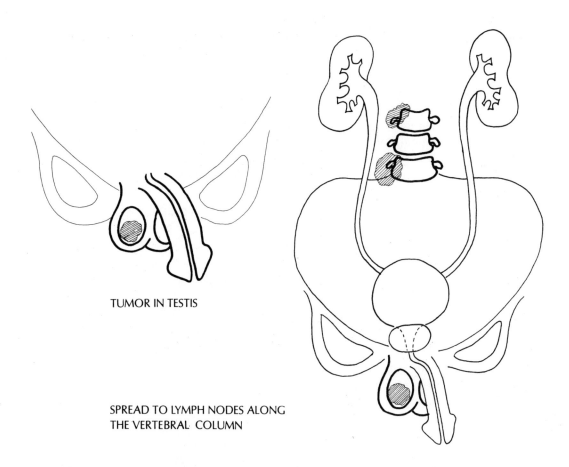

TUMOR IN TESTIS

SPREAD TO LYMPH NODES ALONG
THE VERTEBRAL COLUMN

B Men's testicles ordinarily lie in the scrotum. When one lies in the groin, it is referred to as an undescended testicle, since in fetal life, both testicles arise inside the abdomen and later normally descend to the scrotum. For some reason, a testicle that does not descend into the scrotum in adult life has a tendency to form a cancer. But this does not mean that every undescended testicle is or will be a cancer; only that it is suspect.

Merely putting an undescended testicle down into the scrotum by an operation will not change its chance of forming a tumor. It is abnormal, with a high risk for forming a tumor wherever it lies.

Testicular Tumor

C When the surgeon suspects that a mass in the scrotum is a testicular tumor, he removes the entire testicle by an operative incision in the groin, so as to get well around any tumor tissue. The scar is like that of a hernia repair.

D About 40% of all testicular tumors are of a type called seminoma. They are extraordinarily sensitive to X-ray therapy.

E The boundaries of the tumor determine the treatment. In Stage I seminoma, the tumor is confined to the testicle. After removing the testicle (orchiectomy), radiation therapy is given to the pelvic region and along the backbone. Ninety-eight percent of these young men can be expected to be cured.

F Even if the seminoma has spread up the groin and into the lymph nodes along the backbone (retroperitoneal nodes), 80% of patients still can be cured, by removing the tumor in the testicle (orchiectomy) and given x-radiation treatment along the vertebral column where the tumor has spread.

G When seminoma has spread to distant organs, such as the lungs or liver (Stage III), all tumor cannot be removed by operation. After removing the tumor in the testicle (orchiectomy), anti-cancer drugs can be first given followed by x-radiation to the metastasis. Survival at three years is 20%

H About 60% of testicular tumors are other than seminomas. Each type of tumor has a slightly different chance of cure. None is as sensitive to radiation as are seminomas. The untreated, five-year survival of the various types of tumors is:

- Embryonal cell cancer: 20%
- Teratoma: 9%
- Teratocarcinoma: 10–45%
- Choriocarcinoma: 1%

I These tumors, like seminomas, spread from the testicle to the lymph nodes behind the peritoneal cavity along the backbone. After removing the testicle containing the tumor, the lymph nodes that are apt to contain metastasis from the tumors are also removed by an operation that goes into both the chest and the abdominal cavity. Operative mortality is about 1% and hospitalization about seven to ten days.

J When these tumors are still confined to the testes (Stage I), cure after orchiectomy and removal of the lymph nodes is 90–98%, depending, in part, on the type of tumor involved.

K When all tests indicate that the tumor has spread beyond the testicle, but still has not gone above the diaphragm into or behind the chest cavity, treatment is first by chemotherapy (anti-cancer drugs), and then by operation, removing the lymph nodes behind the abdomen and chest. The chances of cure then are 80–85%.

L When tumor has spread to distant organs, such as the lung or bones, there still is a 50% chance of three-year survival after excising the tumor in the testicle and the lymph nodes along the vertebral column and giving anti-cancer drugs.

M Occasionally, when the tumor in the scrotum has been totally removed, only a single metastasis can be found in the lung, even several months after operation. Removing the single tumor in the lung under these unusual circumstances gives about a 50% chance of cure.

10. Transurethral Prostatectomy

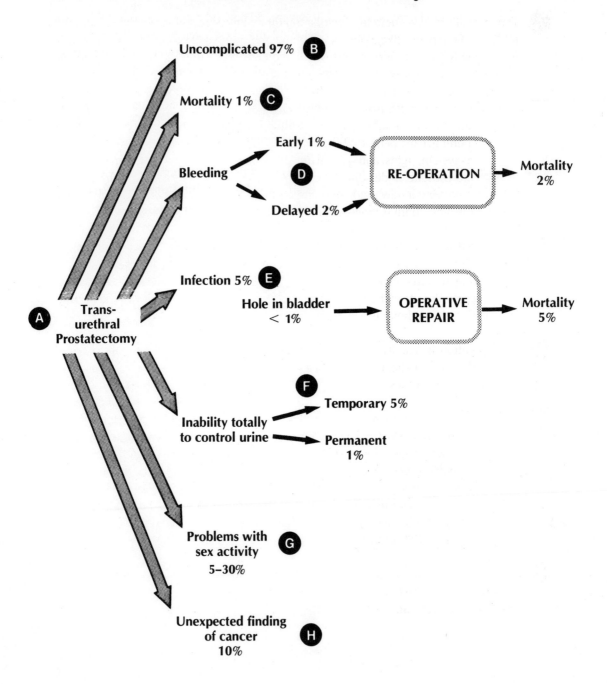

Uncomplicated 97% **B**

Mortality 1% **C**

Bleeding

Early 1% → RE-OPERATION → Mortality 2%

D

Delayed 2% →

Infection 5% **E**

Hole in bladder < 1% → OPERATIVE REPAIR → Mortality 5%

A Trans-urethral Prostatectomy

Inability totally to control urine

F

Temporary 5%

Permanent 1%

Problems with sex activity 5–30% **G**

Unexpected finding of cancer 10% **H**

A The normal prostate encircles the tube (urethra) that carries urine from the bladder to the base of the penis, like a pipe held lightly in the palm of the hand. As man ages, the fist gradually tightens and squeezes shut the urethra in the prostatic grip, producing obstruction to free flow of urine (see "Prostatism," page 389). This may occur either by a benign process (benign prostatic hypertrophy) or as a result of prostatic cancer. A common way of reestablishing a wide passage for urine flow is by burning out most of the prostate through a lighted tube—an endoscope or resectoscopy—passed up the urinary opening in the penis to the area where the prostate surrounds the urethra. Fitted with a lens system, lights, and special devices for resecting the gland, the urologist can remove the prostate under direct vision. A stream of water washes out the burned fragments, leaving a new, wide opening for the bladder. Like cleaning out a clogged drain in the sink, there is then free unobstructed flow.

B The patient usually must be in the hospital for three to ten days after the operation, which is performed under general or spinal anesthesia. A catheter passed up the penis drains urine from the bladder for three to five days after operation. A certain amount of bleeding from the site of the resected prostate colors the urine for a few days. When the urine clears, the catheter is usually removed.

C This operation is usually performed on old men, and death following operation is usually due to coexisting heart disease. Pre-existing kidney failure increases the mortality rate five times.

D Normally, bleeding from the bed of the resected prostate slows down and stops within a few days. In about 1% of cases, however, bleeding continues and requires operation through the cystoscope. This will stop the bleeding in 95% of such cases, but in the other 5%, it will be necessary to open the bladder through an abdominal incision to get control of the bleeding vessel. Mortality from this complication is about 2%.

Two to three weeks after operation, when the patient has left the hospital, the scab comes off from the burned prostatic bed, and a little blood may appear in the urine. This occasionally (2% of the time) requires reoperation for control.

E Infection in the urine is rare after prostatectomy, but when it occurs, there are easy pathways for bacteria to enter the blood stream from the operative site, and the patient often becomes very ill.

Transurethral Prostatectomy

F The nerves and muscles that control the release of urine from the bladder are located near the prostate and can be disturbed by the operation. For a few days after transurethral prostatectomy, the patient may not be able completely to stop leaking a little urine after he empties his bladder. Urinary continence usually returns within a few weeks, but in about 1% of cases, there is some permanent loss of control of urine flow. Usually, control of urine flow is improved by the operation performed on men with prostatism.

G Most of the older men who undergo transurethral prostatectomy will not notice any difference for better or worse in their sexual activities after the operation. A few temporary changes may occur in 40%, but after a few weeks, sex activity is resumed at about the same pace and fashion as before operation.

H Cancer of the prostate is common in old men. In about 10% of persons having a transurethral prostatectomy, there is a chance of finding cancer in the removed tissue, even though it was not suspected before operation. For the implications of such finding see "Cancer of the Prostate," page 392.